AYURVEDIC REMEDIES

for the Whole Family

By Dr. Light Miller

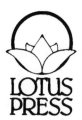

LOTUS
PRESS

Published by:
Lotus Press
P.O. Box 325, Twin Lakes, Wisconsin 53181 USA

DISCLAIMER

This book is not intended to treat, diagnose or prescribe. The information contained herein is in no way to be considered as a substitute for a duly licenced health care professional.

For inquiries contact Lotus Press:
P.O. Box 325, Twin Lakes, Wisconsin 53181 USA
e-mail: lotuspress@lotuspress.com
web: www.lotuspress.com
800-824-6396

Cover & Page Design/Production: Paul Bond, Art & Soul Design
Illustrations: Sage Sanson

First Edition, 1999
Printed in the United States of America

Library of Congress Cataloging-in-Publication-Data
Ayurvedic Remedies for the Whole Family
includes bibliographical references.
ISBN 0-914955-80-2   99-73001
                                                   CIP

TABLE OF CONTENTS

Chapter 13: 75 Health Conditions and Their Treatments 243

DEDICATION

With sincere and deep gratitude, this book is dedicated to all the families of this earth, and to all great teachers who have crossed my path, giving their knowledge and assisting in my growth.

Heartfelt appreciation for my Guru, Swami Shyam, and all my clients who allowed me to share in their life journey, as well as to my devoted secretary, Elizabeth Catenacci, for her support and encouragement and the ever so long hours of computer projects.

To my husband, Bryan, with his edits, as well as to my sons, Bodhi and Cedar, and to my daughter-in-law, Blair, who has blessed me with one of life's greatest gifts, my grandson, Noah. To my mother for giving me life.

Grateful acknowledgement also to my devoted apprentices, Sage Sanson, Katya Kudrov, Jenny Granell, Fanny Rose, and Jan Newton who have all assisted with the research of this book. The lovely artwork was created by the very talented, Sage.

To Dianna Daffner, Mary Murphy, Linda Johnson, Mary Katherine Wainwright, James Minckler, who have all so lovingly contributed to this book.

Deep gratitude to all those who constantly reflect the beauty of spirit in order for me to continue to awaken and expand and to Sandy Levey Lunden, Charisma, Duane O'Kane, Michael and Mary Jo Rice, and Martin Dahlborg.

FOREWORD

AYURVEDA PRESENTS AN ELABORATE and many-sided approach to the treatment of disease. It begins with a firm assessment of individual constitutional types that considers the entire range of bodily frame and weight, digestive and elimination patterns, immune function, disease history, psychological characteristics and spiritual inclinations. Then it determines the signs, symptoms and development of the particular disease afflicting the person - how it affects bodily organs and systems, activity and mental state, how it is related to environmental stresses, seasonal changes, and emotional imbalances. It determines the signature of the disease in terms of its interaction with individual constitutional energies - not simply what pathogen may be involved but the unique patterns that the disease manifestation creates within the person's own life, feeling and metabolism.

Once these factors are clearly determined Ayurvedic doctors prescribe a diet that addresses both the individual constitutional needs and the changing particularities of the disease condition. After all, the body is composed of food, so that all treatment must begin with the appropriate dietary regimen to address the body as a whole. Without appropriate changes in foods eaten and in eating habits real healing on a physical level becomes very difficult to sustain. Ayurvedic diets are primarily vegetarian in nature and emphasize natural foods and home cooking. They show us how to use oils and spices to make vegetarian eating both tasty and as strengthening as any meat diet. Through Ayurveda we can learn to use food as a medicine and cooking as a therapeutic method. On the foundation of right diet Ayurveda prescribes specific herbal measures to treat the disease and to maintain balance for the person's constitution in the process. Ayurvedic doctors may prescribe single herbs or elaborate herbal formulas. They may make up their own herbal mixtures or may prescribe ready-made herbal pills or powders from the vast Ayurvedic pharmaceutical industry. Ayurvedic herbal products may contain whole herbs, extracts, resins, herbal wines and various other herbal preparations. In India Ayurvedic products contain specially purified and potentized minerals (rasas and bhasmas) whose influences extend deep into the brain and nervous system.

Herbs are prescribed not only for internal usage but also for external usage in the form of massage oils, nasal washes, compresses, poultices, or enemas. As the skin is the largest organ in the body, applying oils directly to it reaches the body as a whole and helps balance all bodily systems.

The nasal passages are the gateway to the mind and govern all the senses. They are the first point of entry for the prana, or life-force, so treating the nose through oils, herbs and washes has an immediate and powerful effect on many conditions. Most disease begins with a breakdown of the immune system that, like the common head cold, usually begins with an obstruction in the nasal passages.

The colon is important not only for elimination but also for the absorption of prana from the food. Ayurveda affords much importance to colon therapies through enemas and purgatives, which also have significant cleansing powers, particularly for reducing vata dosha, the main culprit in most long term health imbalances.

On top of these usual physical treatment modalities Ayurveda possesses an entire range of subtle and sensory therapies. Perhaps the most important of these is aromatherapy, the use of essential oils to open the mind and senses, to clear the channels particularly of the lungs and chest, or to stimulate specific sensitive marma points. Color therapy is also used both through using special colored lights and through visualization of special colors.

On a deeper level Ayurveda prescribes the practices of Yoga, particularly pranayama, mantra and meditation for removing the psychological component of disease and helping us better to manage stress and pain. Through pranayama, Ayurveda shows us how to direct our prana or life-force to improve our energy, increase circulation, stimulate weak organs or areas in the body, and to strengthen the lungs and sinuses. Mantra helps focus our mental energy so that our mind is calm and one-pointed, attentive to disease and directed to wellness. Meditation helps clear the mind of negative thoughts and emotions that underlie and sustain the disease process. It helps us detach from our bodily compulsions and gain a new outlook on life so that we can change our life in the appropriate manner to eliminate life-style indiscretions that eventually result in disease.

Along with these treatment methods Ayurveda prescribes a certain life-style regimen to support them. This covers such diverse factors as what type of clothing to wear, what kind of exercise to do, patterns of sleep, type of work or occupation to follow. It involves adjustments to daily and seasonal changes and to changes of life and the aging process. Ayurveda engages our total being in the pursuit of harmony and happiness. Once we are engaged in right living on all these levels there is little from the external world that can harm us and many new internal sources of creativity and insight that open up for us, improving the quality of our entire lives.

Yet along with all of its unique healing methods Ayurveda remains eclectic. It can also use and recommend homeopathy, Western herbs, Chinese medicine and acupuncture, at times even surgery - whatever is best, necessary or easiest available for the individual and able to counter the disease. Ayurveda helps us use and mobilize all possible resources for health and wellness. It provides a comprehensive energetic model of health and disease that has a place for all forms of healing. In the course of a normal human life we all come down with a variety of common diseases. Most of these are not so severe that they require medical intervention or a visit to a doctor. Many of them, like the common cold, though common, have no real cure or treatment from modern medicine anyway. Here Ayurveda has a special importance. Its basis in diet and life-style therapies and its use of safe and mild herbal measures makes it ideal for treating diseases whose main origin is in our everyday activity and in seasonal adjustments.

In addition are chronic and long-term diseases from allergies and arthritis to cancer for which modern medicine has little to offer by way of a cure. Here also Ayurveda and its array of life-style therapies can offer much relief without the corresponding side effects of chemical medicines.

Ayurvedic Remedies for the Whole Family by Light Miller addresses this broad range of common diseases, everyday health concerns, and chronic conditions with the whole gamut of Ayurvedic approaches. In terms of diseases there is little that it does not consider. It covers everything from the common cold to cancer and heart attacks. But this wonderful book is not simply a collection of recipes for different diseases. It also addresses the general health concerns of the stages of life starting with childbirth and ending with old age, methodically going over conditions and problems involved including life-style and external disease factors. It notes such modern issues as the health effects of everything from computers to immunization. It addresses the issue of sexuality and of women's health in a deep way. Not merely prescriptive in nature the book explores the causes of disease and shows us how to prevent disease from arising in the first place.

The book is not simply limited to traditional Ayurvedic formulas, which are often hard to get in the West. It recommends a whole array of Western herbs, and addresses modern concerns of vitamins and minerals and their usage from an Ayurvedic standpoint.

The book is broad in its scope, well thought out in its details, and innovative in its approach. It is an important reference guide not only for every Ayurvedic home but also for all individuals and families concerned with health and right living. It is one of the most comprehensive books of its type and an important addition to the growing literature on Ayurveda.

Light Miller is to be commended for her painstaking research and thorough analysis that such an extensive volume indicates. No doubt it has taken her years of study, compilation and verification to produce such an important text. The book contains many important herbal formulas for treating diseases, using both Western and Ayurvedic herbs that will be of great interest to all types of herbalists and help in further research and development in this area.

As an expert in aromatherapy and co-author of Ayurveda and Aromatherapy, she provides a special place for the use of essential oils, not only for external usage but also as part of herbal formulas for internal usage. This occurs by putting a couple of drops of essential oil formulas in a cup of warm water. Such aroma based formulas have a special effect upon the prana and are able to preserve subtle herbal constituents that are often lost in storage or in cooking.

Ayurvedic Remedies for the Whole Family will bring the everyday wisdom of Ayurveda into the grasp of everyone. For those tired of dependency on chemical and drug based medicine it provides a clear way out to the natural light of healing. For those already engaged in such natural healing methods the book offers an Ayurvedic perspective that is both integrative and complementary and will take their healing knowledge and modalities to a higher level.

The new movement towards natural healing in the West is also creating an Ayurvedic renaissance, with new books on the subject coming out every year. The present volume takes that Ayurvedic renaissance to a larger audience where it can become part of the mainstream of healing in America. Certainly most of us are in need of this ancient wisdom and the wellsprings of life that flow through it. May we all embrace it not only for our own benefit but also for how it can heal our families, our communities, our environment and our planet.

Dr. David Frawley
Author of Yoga and Ayurveda, Ayurveda and the Mind, *and co-author of* Yoga of Herbs
Santa Fe, NM
August 1999

AYURVEDIC REMEDIES FOR THE WHOLE FAMILY

INTRODUCTION

RAISING A FAMILY IN TODAY'S challenging world can be a combination of many different experiences. It can be an opportunity to enhance our family legacies, to heal our relationships from the past by choosing differently than our parents, or a thrilling adventure of unlimited possibilities. A great philosopher of our times said our first job is to heal ourself, then the family, then the community, nation, and finally, the world (Rudolf Steiner founder of Anthroposophy). Ayurveda teaches us that we come to this earth to heal, to serve, and to remember who we are. In the process, the job of the family is to provide the most intimate environment in which to accomplish our life's mission.

As each of us commits to break the patterns of our own family system, the patterns that we know do not work for us, we release the old and allow for the new. An opening of ourselves for a new way of possibility to create a healthy and holy life - for us and for our families. It is of utmost importance that we remember our purpose, to know what we came here for, and to tap into the source of strength while holding a vision of peace. As this unified vision begins to permeate each family's life, a domino effect takes place for creating a better world for everyone.

The Divine Mother (the feminine principal of universal God) has given us many gifts from nature to heal ourselves, such as herbs and foods. The American Indians believe that every plant has a "give-away"; a gift that we can use to nurture ourselves. There has been a reawakening once again to the wholistic and spiritual practice of life called Ayurveda. This Ayurvedic health care system is over 5,000 years old and is the oldest recorded medicine practiced in India. While growing up I personally experienced this medicine which unlocked many secrets of alternative ways. Consequently, I offer my experience of thirty-one years experience in health care, family diagnoses, and recipes which have been tested with 1,000 clients. I can personally attest to the validity of the Ayurvedic health care system, as my children and myself have never needed allopathic medicine, not even aspirin nor immunization shots.

My years of experience I offer to you as my gift for the wellbeing of the family unit and for each individual therein. You will discover as you move through the pages of this book that it was the creation of the "Universal Family" as many loving individuals contributed to its unfoldment.

May your journey be blessed.

Dr. Light Miller

TESTIMONIAL

May I extend to you, the reader, an invitation to experience these time-tested remedies and to embrace an alternative approach to a healthier lifestyle. Taking responsibility for your family's wellbeing can bring new possibilities to the lives of everyone. The totality of healing which this book integrates is important for each family and each individual to understand and to choose. To make a real choice, one must be at a "knowingness" level, and this book provides invaluable information upon which an educated choice can be made. Read the book. Choose. Experience.

Sandy Levy Lunden
"On Purpose"
California & Sweden

CHAPTER 1

WHAT IS AYURVEDA AND WHY SHOULD I USE IT?

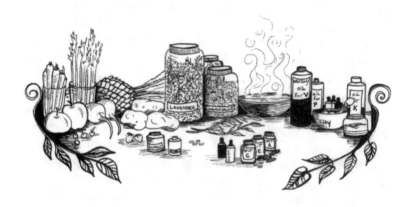

TODAY IN THE WEST, we are experiencing a health crisis. There are many diseases for which there are no cures. Modern medicine can only temporarily relieve the disease symptoms and have not yet been able to discover their cause. More and more people are searching for answers away from modern medicine. Statistics show that people in mainstream America spend between $1,000 - $2,000 a year on holistic health care, on top of their medical insurance. This holistic care includes such treatments as massage, acupuncture, chiropractic, naturopathic, Chinese Medicine, Therapeutic Touch, herbal and diet regimens.

Ayurveda is the 5,000 year old medical system that has been used in India on over a billion people. Ayurveda is a common sense medicine which can assist the individual with simple home routines which are preventative in nature and promote good health. Individuals learn to care for themselves. Dr. Mom is the home health practitioner for the whole family using at-home therapies including thoughtful application of foods, spices, herbs, massage, vitamins and minerals to correct problems and maintain health. Also available at a higher level for more severe conditions, are Ayurvedic doctors, practitioners, and clinics with advanced diagnostics and therapies.

Ayurveda is the only medical system that recognizes individual metabolic types. "One man's food is another man's poison" is a western phrase which explains this. This difference in metabolism is the reason why some people can eat anything and everything and not gain weight, while others have only to look at food to put on pounds. This knowledge of differences in individuals can be used to make food, herb and vitamin therapies rational and effective. Finding out what agrees with you, and what doesn't, is the difference between increasing health or losing it.

Modern medicine is less than 100 years old. One-third of doctor visits involve iatrogenic disease (disease caused by medicines and doctors). Modern medicine is still working out its bugs. We have placed our trust in medicine to find "magic bullets" for all diseases. It hasn't happened, and it won't. Ayurveda, on the other hand, is time tested and places its trust in basics; good food, appropriate herbs, clean water, peaceful thoughts, and appropriate lifestyle. When we embrace Ayurveda, we take back control of our own health. We rebuild it. We maintain it. Ayurveda teaches us that when we create balance, we can attain perfect health. As we understand our body-mind-spirit connection we are able to extend the span of life and create longevity. The main purpose of this science is to create self-knowledge and mastery. When we awaken to our true potential, we create freedom in our bodies. With practice and mastery of ourselves we can become free of suffering.

Ayurveda recognizes that we came here to this earth to accomplish specific purposes. Our true nature is Divine and everything that we need to know is already available within us. When we support our body with these principles, we are open to the unlimited possibilities and potential to live our life in health and awareness.

THE THREE DOSHAS

In Ayurvedic philosophy, Doshas are the primary life forces or biological humors created when the pairing of two of the five elements create three dynamic forces or interactions. The word Dosha means "that which changes," a term which refers to the way the elements are constantly in motion while retaining a dynamic balance. The word Dosha also means "that which darkens" or "spoils," a reference to the way an imbalance among the elements can cause dis-ease.

ETHER	AIR	FIRE	WATER	EARTH
VATA		PITTA	KAPHA	

VATA (va-ta) is created by a combination of the elements Ether (space) and Air. The driving force behind the other two Doshas, Vata ("that which moves things") is responsible for balance, energy, breath, movement, sense perception, thought, and will. As movement, Vata manifests itself in life in the movement of air, blood, food, nerve impulses, thoughts, and waste. The seven Vata characteristics which affect the body are cold, light, dry, irregular, mobile, rarefied, and rough. Excessive Vata force causes confusion, gas, high blood pressure, and nerve irritation. Insufficient Vata force can create congestion, constipation, nerve loss, and thoughtlessness.

AIR, UNRESTRICTED BY SPACE (AS IN THE OPEN OCEAN), CAN GAIN ENOUGH MOMENTUM TO BECOME A HURRICANE.

AIR CONFINED TO A BOX CANNOT MOVE AND BECOMES STAGNANT

The PITTA (pit-ta) Dosha or life force is created by the dynamic movement between the two elements which symbolize transformation, water and fire. The transforming nature of Pitta ("that which digests") is evident in our bodies by the digestive enzymes and hormones governing metabolism. Pitta works in our minds by transforming chemical and electrical impulses into thoughts. Pitta characteristics affecting the body include hot, light, fluid, subtle, sharp, malodorous, and clear. Excessive Pitta causes acne, anger, hormonal imbalance, and ulcers. Insufficient Pitta results in indigestion, sluggish metabolism, and loss of comprehension.

THE BALANCE OF FIRE AND WATER IS VITAL.
NOT ENOUGH WATER AND THE POT BURNS.

BUT TOO MUCH WATER IN THE POT
OVERFLOWS AND PUTS OUT THE FIRE.

KAPHA (ka-fa) is the life force combining the water and earth elements. Kapha ("that which binds") is the composition of the cellular structure of our organs (structure) as well as the fluids which nourish and protect them (lubrication). The Kapha characteristics affecting the body include oily, cold, heavy, stable, dense, and smooth. Excessive Kapha force creates mucous buildup in the sinus, nasal, lung, and colon area. It affects the mind by causing rigidity, fixation, and inflexibility. Insufficient Kapha can produce a dry respiratory tract, burning stomach, and lack of concentration.

Changing Forces

The three life forces (Doshas) of Vata, Pitta, and Kapha are in dynamic motion, forever changing and balancing each other not only in human bodies but in all of life. The Doshas are the energies of life, the motion that makes life happen. When the Doshas are out of balance, they create disease.

The Doshas have a relationship to plant life. The flowers and leaves reaching into space and air are the plant's Vata force. The roots which store water in the depth of the earth is the plant's Kapha concentration. Resins, saps, spices, and the other essential oils of plant life are its Pitta. Human bodies rely on the life forces of plants to balance and harmonize our own concentrations of Vata, Pitta, and Kapha. To increase our Kapha force, for instance, we should eat root vegetables, milk and dairy products, and sedating herbs like Valerian. Vata forces can be increased by drinking herbal flowers like

Jasmine or eating dry grains. Pitta tendencies are increased when we consume hot, spicy foods like cayenne or concentrated protein like Bee Pollen.

BODY GOVERNANCE AND THE 5 ELEMENTS

Each of the five elements is concentrated in a region of the body and controls specific functions.

Ayurveda teaches us that we are made of the same elemental forces as the universe.

ELEMENT	CONTROL OF
Ether	**Brain** Nervous System
Air	**Nose, Chest** Respiration
Fire	**Upper Abdomen** Digestion Hormones
Water	**Urinary Tract** Lower Abdomen
Earth	**Lower Body** Excretion Stability

VATA

Ether, Air
All movement in the body and nerve impulses

Vata Activities of the Body

Cold: preservation and aliveness of the body
Light: movement, mobility, and flexibility
Dry: creates intercellular space

Mobile: all involuntary body impulses and air movement

Subtle: capillary & cellular breathing

Clear: represents creativity, perception, clarity and understanding

Astringent: represents respiration of the cells, circulating movement

Rough: rough skin, not sensitive or fluid, abrupt, variable

Dispersing: movement of nutrients

Causes of Vata Imbalances

Long hours of computer work, too much TV, chewing gum, excessive exercise, cold wind exposure, excessive travel, excessive movement, disorganized, undisciplined or irregular schedule, working at night, not enough sleep or poor sleeping habits, insufficient natural light, junk foods.

Vata Illnesses

Flatulence, forgetfulness, dryness, emphysema, all pain, spasms, rigidity, goose bumps, nervousness, muscle twitching, atrophy of muscles, impulsive behavior, osteoporosis, insomnia, babbling, sensory disorientation, confusion, emaciation, weakness, bloatedness, constipation, debility, stuttering, dizziness.

Emotional Imbalances

Insecurity, fear, anxiety, restlessness, confusion, indecision, secretiveness, sneakiness, changeable.

Best Diet for Vata

Summer: Cooked foods, primarily. Salads must be accompanied by lots of salad oil.

Winter: Soups, Immune Broth, stews, warm foods (well cooked), spices, many root vegetables and grains.

Sites of Vata

Colon, thighs, hips, ears, hands.

PITTA

Heat, Fire, Water
All change and transformation in the body

Pitta Activities of the body

Hot: creates stimulation of digestion, hunger, normalizes body temperature.

Sharp: clear communication, sharp memory, sharp pain, sharp words.

Oily: emulsifies, mixes, stimulates fire, transforms and regulates temperature.

Liquid: regulates and distributes the fire, assists digestion and assimilation.

Mobile: extends, stretches the warmth, circulation and temperature of the body.

Light: maintains the fire, glowing skin and hair, sharp vision.

Taste: sour, pungent. Sour strengthens digestive fire & stimulates digestion.

Pungent is found in the circulation and assists breakdown of sugars in the body.

Penetrating: enzymes penetrating into food, probing mind

Causes of Pitta Imbalances

Alcohol, drugs, hallucinogenic drugs, tobacco smoking, hot spicy foods, high exposure to the sun, competitive sports, excessive competition, sexual indulgence, and eating foods that are yellow, orange and red. It is important that Pittas drink plenty of water due to their natural high body heat.

Pitta Illnesses

Skin rashes, fevers, acid indigestion, gastritis, peptic ulcers, diarrhea, extreme thirst, excessive urination, hyperactivity, epileptic seizures, burning of the eyes, any yellow/red/orange discoloration of the skin, feces, urine and eyes, hepatitis, and all illnesses ending with "itis" (meaning inflammation).

Emotional imbalances

Judgement, hate, anger, jealousy, separation, recklessness, manipulation, division, excess bravery, slavery, intolerance, rivalry, egocentric.

Pitta represents all transformations of the body; hormonal changes, digestion and absorption. When Pitta is balanced, agni (digestive power) is in a perfect state.

Best diet for Pitta

Summer: Raw foods, cooling spices

Winter: Salads and warm foods with cooling herbs

Sites of Pitta

Small intestine, stomach, blood, liver, lymph, sweat glands.

KAPHA

Water, Earth
Muscles, all structure and lubrication of the body

Kapha Activities of the Body

Cool: maintains body temperature and slows metabolism.

Dense: all tissues.

Cloudy: lethargy, deep sleep, slow mind.

Slimy: lubrication of joints, slow, encourages relaxation & rest. All mucous membranes.

Liquid: controls all body secretions, distributes lubrication through joints. Lymph & circulation.

Oily: insulates skin, lubricates joints, insulates body.

Soft: protects the body, cushions.

Static: gives vigor, stability, security.

Thick: creates insulation through the body.

Heavy: building of tissue

Slow: movement is slow

Causes of Kapha Imbalances

Drinking with meals, too much sleep, not enough exercise, sweets, mucous forming foods, lethargy, cough, breathlessness, loss of appetite.

Kapha Illnesses

Edema, obesity, bronchial asthma, bronchitis, pneumonia, sinus congestion, hypertension, diabetes, hay fever, anorexia.

Emotional Imbalances

Not speaking the truth, hopelessness, hidden anger, envy, malice, insecurity, apathy, attachment, greed.

Best Diet for Kapha

Summer: Lots of salads with fresh spices

Winter: Warm foods with salads and spices

Sites of Kapha

Lungs, stomach, chest, pancreas, lymph, nose.

BODY TYPES

Individual Balance

For discovering your personal body type, see the Questionnaire in Chapter 14. Each of us is born with a unique balance of V-P-K that makes us who we are and determines our strengths and weaknesses. No two people are the same. There are said to be three pure types and seven mixed types (this type-ing is used for the sake of evaluation and treatment).

Compare this Ayurvedic view of individual variety to our present medical system where everyone is treated the same. For example, a person born with a high proportion of Pitta and small amounts of Vata and Kapha would be said to be a Pitta dominant individual. An individual with similar amounts of Vata and Pitta and very little Kapha is seen as a Vata-Pitta mix.

Due to climate, season, life stage, diet or lifestyle changes, over time an individual may get out of balance. If they gained 30 lbs., their V-P-K would change. They wouldn't feel "themselves" until they returned to the V-P-K combination they were born with. Ayurveda can help individuals discover their original balance and return to it.

VATA DOMINANT TYPE

An individual with a primarily Vata influence will exhibit many of the following characteristics: a thin-framed body, whether they are tall or short. Generally, "tall" is a man over 6 feet or a woman over 5 feet 8 inches. "Short" is a man 5 feet 5 inches or less and a woman 5 feet 3 inches or less. Their joints crack easily and irregularity is the rule, including possible protruding joints, bow legs, disproportionate bodies with long legs and short waist, scoliosis and uneven facial structure (i.e., deviated septum and crooked nose, etc.). Their body trunk will be out of proportion with their legs. If they do gain weight it will be around the middle. Their skin will have a tendency to be dry, rough and cool to the touch, and their skin coloration will be darker than the rest of their family. Hair may be dark, dry and kinky and prone to dandruff. Teeth are often crooked, protruded with spaces and tendency toward receded gums. Eyes can be small, dry, active, black or brown. Appetite is often variable or low, although they will often skip meals due to distractions and become ravenous, loading up their plate with more than they could possibly eat. Fingers and toes are long and thin with nails which are brittle and crack easily. If they become sick, pain and nervous disorders are likely. Thirst is variable, urine is irregular and scanty, and bowel movements are often gassy, dry, hard and constipated. Vatas walk fast, are physically active but expend their energy easily and may rely on caffeine, sugar and stimulants to continue. The mind is restless, active, curious and creative. Under stress they can become fearful, insecure and anxious. They change their mind easily, forget easily, yet have clear understanding and a good short term memory. They lose minerals easily and do not hold weight on the body unless their channels are obstructed. They are easily influenced and often dissatisfied in relationships. This body type shows up for many workshops and social events. They often dream about flying, running, jumping and fear. Sleep is difficult, interrupted and they can experience insomnia. Speech is fast, chaotic, impulsive; using incomplete sentences and often interrupting others. They are expressive and often talk with their hands. Money goes through their hands quickly as they spend impulsively. Their pulse is thready, feeble and erratic. Vata predominant types will vary greatly from one to another, but will share many of the above characteristics.

Balanced: Alert, friendly, loving, willing to serve, creative, forgiving, happy, joyful, and the life of the party.

Imbalanced: Extreme dryness, unclear, weight loss, anemia, weakness, tiredness, "spacy", chronic constipation, hyperactive, nervous, bodily functions impaired, low digestion, fatigue, impaired memory, respiratory disorders.

PITTA DOMINANT

An individual who is primarily Pitta will have a moderate frame, with a tendency towards being slender, that demonstrates good proportions. They can gain or lose weight relatively easily, have great appetites which require regular meals. Skin is often delicate, oily, burns easily, with a coppery or yellowish tone and is warm to touch. Freckles and moles are common with a tendency to acne. They perspire readily. Hair is soft, blond or red, greying early with a tendency to early thinning or balding. Fingers are well formed and proportional; nail beds have a pink appearance. Eyes are sharp penetrating gray, green, with a yellowish tint to the sclera (whites). If they become ill they will experience fever, inflammation and infection. Often thirsty. Bowel movements are soft, oily and loose, 3 times a day or more. Pittas enjoy moderate activity and love competition due to their aggressive nature. Intelligent and determined with a sharp memory, making excellent leaders, managers, in high positions with a high sense of responsibility. You can often tell a Pitta by their passion, high directed energy and commitment. Under stress they can be irritable, driving, angry and jealous. Pittas spend moderately and methodically. Dreams are fiery, passionate and colorful. Sleep is moderate and sound. Speech is sharp, clear, fluid but can be cutting and sarcastic. Pulse is strong and regular. All body functions concerned with heat, such as; functions of liver, spleen, hormonal changes, skin, small intestines, brain, digestion, assimilation, thirst, appetite and sight are associated with Pitta. Activities of fire in the mind, discrimination, perception, memory, decision making, bravery, desire, leadership, justification, manipulation, and knowledge.

Balanced: Cheerful, good digestion, able to eat anything, outrageous, courageous, pleasant, in charge, caring.

Imbalanced: Poor digestion, impaired vision, anger, demanding, irritable, oppressive, driven, irregular body temperature.

KAPHA DOMINANT

The pure Kapha is easy to recognize having large bodies on large frames. Hawaiians are a Kapha people with a skin that is thick, oily, cool to the touch, pale and white. Sweat is moderate. They have strong bodies, gain weight easily and must exercise to lose it. Hair is thick, oily, wavy with thick eyebrows and lashes. Teeth are strong, white, large and well formed. Eyes are big and attractive. Appetite is slow and steady, although they can easily skip meals without effect. If Kaphas become ill, congestion, excess mucous and water retention are common. They rarely experience thirst. Bowel movements are thick and oily and regular (once a day). Peaceful and content, moving slowly and wasting little energy. Endurance is good. Negative tendencies may be self centered-ness, greed and being overly sensitive. Kaphas are steady, loyal friends and employees. Slow to learn new things, they seldom forget anything once learned. Dreams are often romantic and involve water. Speech is slow and monotonous or melodious. They spend slowly, save easily and always have full cupboards. Pulse is slow and steady. Kapha's experience longevity of the cells, strength, stamina, stability, and a strong physiology. Kapha represents all structural aspects of the physical and solid parts of the body frame, physical growth, protection from heat, and lubrication of the joints.

Balanced: Strong, clear, ready, willing, open, healthy lungs, giving, caring, patient, understanding, happy, friendship, loyal, growth, grounded, sleeps easily, calm, centered, mental endurance, dignity.

Imbalanced: Obese, overweight, flabby, loose joints, impotent, insecure, jealous, greedy, introverted, excess mucous, secretive, couch potato.

THE 7 MIXED TYPES:
(V-P, V-K, P-V, K-V, P-K, K-P, AND V-P-K)

In India, where people largely marry into their own tribe or group, single Dosha types predominate. In the west we are a mixing pot because everyone marries as they wish and, therefore, mixed types predominate. Usually, in a mixed type, one Dosha will be dominant, with a second Dosha being a close second. For example, a Vata -Pitta person will have more and stronger Vata tendencies than Pitta. A Pitta-Vata person will have more Pitta qualities. Finally, there's the type called balanced tri-dosha (V-P-K), where no one type is predominant.

VATA-PITTAS - Thin like a pure Vata-type, quick moving, friendly, talkative, but more enterprising and sharper of intellect. Can be forgetful at times. They don't have the extremes of Vata, and are not as high-strung or irregular. Don't put on weight. Food is not particularly important to them, and they have stronger digestion. A greater tolerance to cold. They are more tolerant of noise and physical discomforts. They have the strong drive of Pitta with the imagination and creativity of a Vata-type. They are steadier, calmer, more confident than the pure Vata type. This type can easily fall into patterns of addiction and need stability. They love leisure activities, are creative, good speakers and have a good sense of humor.

PITTA-VATAS - are more of medium build with more musculature than V-Ps, their skin is more sensitive, and they are prone to infections. They're also quick in movement, have good stamina, are often assertive, with obvious intensity, but with a Vata-type's lightness. They have strong digestion and more regular elimination than V-P or V and become bloated more easily. This type loses weight easily. If they are under stress, they can react with fear or anger which can make them insecure, tense and hard driven. They love to eat, have a good memory and are fluid speakers. Too much heat can bother them. Intolerant to noises, love to talk, and to be in charge.

VATA-KAPHAS - This type is often hard to identify with a questionnaire due to the presence of opposites in many characteristics, and Vata's indecisiveness. They often have a thin Vata frame although can be neither fat nor thin. They are talkative with a Kapha-like relaxed, easygoing manner. They will be even-tempered unless stressed. Often quick and efficient, they are aware of their Kapha tendency to procrastinate. They desire to store up and save, and strongly dislike the cold. They can have slow or irregular digestion. They are very steady, loyal, committed and service oriented. This type can be confused with Pittas.

KAPHA-VATAS - are similar to a V-K but are more solidly built and slower moving. They are easier to please, even-tempered and even more relaxed that V-Ks, but with less enthusiasm. Have curly, thick hair. They tend to be athletic, with greater stamina. They may also have digestive irregularities, complain of cold, suffer mucous buildup, and can easily become depressed when not busy. They think more of others than of themselves.

PITTA-KAPHAS - are types with Pitta intensity in a strong Kapha body. Their skin is copper tone and they are more muscular than a K-type, and may be quite bulky. Their personality exhibits a K-type stability with Pitta force and a tendency toward anger and criticism. They are a good type for athletics, having energy and endurance. Always ready to take on a project. This type makes excellent entrepreneurs as money comes easily. They never miss a meal. They have Pitta-type digestion and Kapha-type resistance to disease. Food is their medicine. Prone to mucous and congestion in the lungs. They have direction and stability with strong stamina and drive.

KAPHA-PITTAS - are people who have a Kapha type structure, but more fat than a P-K type. They are rounder in the face and body, move more slowly, and are more relaxed than P-K's. They have a steady energy and even more endurance than P- or P-K type. They like exercise but are less motivated to do it than a P-K. When imbalanced they can put on weight easily and when balanced they easily lose excess weight. Money comes easily to them, and they know how to plan for the future. This type is dependable, loyal, and can take charge of any situation. Can be arrogant and unresponsive to criticism.

VATA-PITTA-KAPHAS - are the harder to describe, because they have equal amounts of each Dosha. They are the most balanced with a tendency to long life, good health and immunity. Any of the symptoms of any dosha imbalance can be present at any time. If they don't take care of themselves any dosha can go out of balance. Ayurvedic physicians say that these types are the most difficult to treat when they do get out of balance. This type can fit in almost anywhere, they adapt to situations easily. There are very few true V-P-K types. Many people who think they are V-P-K are usually a two-Dosha mixed-type.

CHAPTER 2

AROMATHERAPY

IN TODAY'S WORLD, many forms of treatments, both new and old, are available to bring greater vitality to our daily life. Aromatherapy is the art and science of using scent or aroma to beautify, rejuvenate, revitalize and heal the body. Aromatherapy is an important part of home health care because it puts the strongest concentration of herbal healing at your fingertips for rapid results. This ancient science goes back 3,500 years and was used in the Egyptian, Indian, Greek, Roman and Chinese civilizations to enhance health. The use of essential oils was an integral part of the medicinal system of each culture.

Aromatherapy uses aromatic plants, which contain volatile substances to support and maintain our health, allowing for a more enjoyable and pleasurable existence. No one enjoys being ill and, with aromatherapy, no one needs to be sick for long.

The essential oil of a plant is the most concentrated and healing part and contains many of the plants medicinal properties. The most common way to get the oil is through the distillation of plant material. Essential oils can be distilled from the seed, bark, fruit, leaves, sap, resins, flowers and roots of plants. Black pepper seed, cinnamon bark, orange skin, eucalyptus leaf, pine sap, frankincense resin, lavender flowers, and ginger root are classic examples of what can be distilled, each into a distinct oil containing special healing properties.

The essential oil is the active principle or life essence of the plant. "Oil" is really a misnomer (wrong naming) because it contains no vegetable oil and often has a consistency closer to rubbing alcohol. The natural chemicals that are extracted in distillation are composed of alcohols, aldehydes, cetones, terpenes, sesqueterpenes, ethers and esters. These natural chemicals possess healing abilities comparable to allopathic medicines. In fact, many pharmaceuticals are models of chemical constituents originally isolated from plants. These active ingredients have medicinal qualities such as being antiseptic, anti-viral, anti-spasmodic (calms muscles), aphrodisiac, carminative (helps digestion), diaphoretic (promotes sweating), expectorant (expels mucous), and diuretic, etc. They have profound effects on human physiology. When diluted by air or steam we can inhale them. When added to food or drink, they are consumed. When diluted in vegetable oil, cream or bath water, it is in contact with our skin.

Essential oils are highly concentrated and, therefore, should always be diluted. Essential oils can be directly absorbed through the skin, the gastrointestinal tract, and through the lung tissue causing powerful changes in the metabolism of all "entry" organs. After initial absorption, essential oils circulate through the blood and lymph, again being available for assimilation, until they are eventually eliminated through the lungs, skin, kidney, liver and gastrointestinal tract where they have additional therapeutic action on the "exit" organs.

When smelled, psychological and physical changes are instantly produced by directly stimulating the nerve pathways between the nose and the brain, stimulating the limbic system, which is our primitive brain where our memories, desires, and emotions are stored and accessed.

Daily, you are already using foods, medicines, shampoos, conditioners, perfumes, and skin products, which contain essential oils. To name a few: Spearmint Gum, Wintergreen Lifesavers, Vic's Vaporub, Campbell's soups, Snapple drinks, and Chanel #5 all contain "natural flavorings" (i.e., essential oils). Each plant has its own distinctive properties, which are held in the essential oils ready for our use.

Try trusting your "un-common" sense of smell if you feel drawn to an essential oil.

Trust your nose. Any oil, which you are attracted to, has a gift for you. They can be used to create a different atmosphere in your home. They are relatively inexpensive so you can experiment with different oils to see what effects you enjoy. Some will lift your spirits, some will create a sense of calm, others will improve your memory or awareness, etc.

Essential oils, when stored properly, have a shelf life of many years as opposed to herbs and spices which lose their potency in a matter of months. In some European countries, aromatherapy is prescribed by medical doctors and is part of the health care system, with many hospitals and practitioners prescribing the oils, and insurance paying their cost. You pick them up at the pharmacy.

Even though essential oils have been used for thousands of years, they have only recently returned to general awareness. The last twenty years have produced a renaissance in herbalism and its equal cousin, aromatherapy.

GUIDELINES OF ESSENTIAL OIL AMOUNTS TO BE USED IN VARIOUS APPLICATION METHODS

APPLICATION	FAVORITES
Bathing	
15-30 drops in bathwater.	Geranium, Lavender
Foot Bath	
15-20 drops per 2 quarts of water.	Peppermint, Eucalyptus, Tea Tree
Massage	
40-60 drops in 4 oz of carrier oil. For specific conditions: You may want to make it stronger; up to 60 drops per ounce.	Lavender, Rosemary Eucalyptus, Lemongrass
Compress	
3-6 drops in cup of water, absorbed into a wash cloth and applied to the affected area.	

Direct Inhalation
    2-3 drops per 8 oz. of   Rosemary, Eucalyptus
    boiling water in a bowl,
    place a towel over your
    head. Carefully inhale
    the steam for 3 minutes.

Facial Steam
    5 drops per cup of water.   Lavender, Rose

Candle Making
    40-60 drops per 8 oz. of wax.   Tangerine, Lemon

Body Wrap
    15 drops in 12 ounces   Juniper, Cypress
    of hot water. Soaked in
    cloth bandages (surgical sleeve)

Car Pottery Diffuser
    (A small clay ornament that   Bergamot, Peppermint
    will slowly disperse the oil's
    fragrance) 5 drops in pottery.

Bath Gels
    15 drops per 1 ounce.   Same as bath

Cooking
    1 drop=1 teaspoon of   All spice oils, i.e., Ginger,
    powdered herb in recipes.   Black Pepper, etc.

Douche
    1-2 drops per quart   Dhavana, Tea Tree
    of water.

Air Conditioner
    10-15 drops on filter.   Pine, Orange

Potpourri Pot
    3-10 drops in water.   Tangerine, Ylang Ylang

Toothpaste
    1 drop on toothbrush.   Fennel, Mint, Anise

Restful Sleep
    3 drops on pillow.   Lavender, Ylang Ylang

Liquid Cleanser
10 drops per ounce   Lemon, Orange, Pine
of liquid cleanser.

Pet Care Shampoo
15 drops per ounce   Pennyroyal, Eucalyptus,
of shampoo.   Cedarwood

Mouth Wash
10 drops per 4   Same as toothpaste
ounces of water.

Shampoo, Conditioner, Scalp Treatments
20 drops per 4   Chamomile, Lavender,
ounces of liquid.   Rosemary, Rosewood

Perfumes
100 drops per 1   Rose, Geranium, jojoba
ounce of alcohol,   Neroli, Lavender
oil or vegetable oil.

Deodorant
30 drops per 2 ounces   Bergamot, Tea Tree
of vegetable oil.

Meditation
1 drop of oil (mixed   Sandalwood, Elemi
into 1 drop of vegetable
oil) on third eye center
of forehead or in diffuser.

Clothes - Washing (for clothes line drying)
During final rinse put   Lavender, All Citrus
in 20 drops essential oil.

Clothes - Drying
Place 10 drops on a   Same
cotton ball or piece
of cloth in dryer 10
minutes before clothes
are done.

MINI MONOGRAPHS

Essential Oils, their Properties and Applications

* = Contraindicated for pregnancy   • = rare or exotic oils

*•ANGELICA - *"the archangel of healing"*; builds immunity, strengthens the hormone system; creates inner strength and bravery. (Bath, diffuser/spritzer/aroma lamp, inhalation, massage, perfume, tea)

ANISE - food and drink flavoring; helps asthma, coughs, colds, allergies, indigestion, lactation, and cramps; calming effect. (Bath, compress, food seasoning, inhalation, massage, tea)

*•BASIL {*the oil of Krishna*}- food seasoning; good for asthma, sinus, bronchitis, headaches, depression, and tension. (Bath, compress, diffuser/spritzer/aroma lamp, food seasoning, inhalation, massage, perfume, tea)

BAY - helpful in scalp dryness, respiratory problems, infections, indigestion; used extensively in food seasoning. (Food seasoning, inhalation, massage, perfume)

BENZOIN - preservative; useful for PMS, stress, wounds, softens scars, dry irritated skin, coughs, asthma, poor circulation. (Bath, compress, inhalation, massage, perfume)

BERGAMOT - used in Earl Gray tea; helpful for acne, fevers, infections, varicose veins and depression. (Bath, diffuser/spritzer/aroma lamp, inhalation, massage, perfume, tea)

BIRCH - " *smells like wintergreen"*; used for hair loss, mouth sores, insomnia, skin problems, anxiety. (Bath, inhalation, massage, tea)

BLACK PEPPER - *"great for seasoning foods"*; helps colds, toothache, indigestion, weight loss, gas, nausea. (Food seasoning, massage)

CAJEPUT - *"tea tree family"*, good for acne, wounds, infections, muscle pain, fluid retention, liver obstruction. (Bath, compress, diffuser/spritzer/aroma lamp, inhalation, massage)

*CALAMUS - used for treating asthma, sinusitis, fatigue, back pain. (Bath, compress, massage)

*CAMPHOR – asthma, bronchitis, nasal, sinus, congestion, acne, epilepsy, muscle spasms, hysteria. (Bath, compress, massage)

*CARAWAY – excellent in breads, sauces, and soups; helpful for indigestion, fluid retention, loss of memory. (Compress, food seasoning, massage)

CARDAMON – used in Lebanese coffee and cookies; detoxifies caffeine; opening to the heart; aids in indigestion, coughs, colds. (Bath, compress, food seasoning, inhalation, massage, perfume)

CARROT SEED– "*oil of the skin*"; tones and tightens skin; can assist in abscesses, boils, liver and gallbladder problems, colitis. (Massage, perfume)

*CEDARWOOD - "*the familiar smell of cedar closets*"; helpful in treating acne, oily skin and hair, bladder infection, eczema. (Bath, compress, diffuser/spritzer/aroma lamp, massage, perfume, tea)

•HIMALAYAN CEDARWOOD - " *scent of the Himalayas*"; creates clarity and connectedness; used in treating depression, urinary tract infection; respiration, congestion. (Bath, compress, diffuser/spritzer, inhalation, massage, perfume, tea)

•BLUE CHAMOMILE - "*The Blue Oil*" incredible anti-inflammatory and immune builder; used for burns, fever, skin irritation, menopause, migraine, stress, relaxation, and spasms. (Bath, compress, diffuser/spritzer/aroma lamp, inhalation, massage, perfume)

•GOLD CHAMOMILE - "*a children's oil*" because of its warm fruity smell; helpful for irritability, stress, fever, colic, indigestion, cramps, pain. (Bath, compress, diffuser/spritzer/aroma lamp, inhalation, massage, perfume, tea)

*•MORROCAN CHAMOMILE {absolute} - "*the smell is rich, warm and sweet*"; for acne, inflamed skin, bruises, burns. (Bath, compress, diffuser/spritzer/aroma lamp, massage, perfume)

*CINNAMON - " *the spice of life*"; adds warmth to perfume blends; aids in digestion, menopause, circulation, sore muscles, colds. (Bath, compress, diffuser/spritzer/aroma lamp, inhalation, massage, perfume, tea)

CITRONELLA - excellent bug repellent, good to add to pet shampoos; used as a deodorizer, disinfectant, antiseptic, stimulant, and purifier. (Bath, diffuser/spritzer/aroma lamp, massage)

CLARY SAGE - *"the woman's oil"*; helpful in PMS, menopause, frigidity, skin irritation, nervousness, infection; creates euphoria and relaxation. (Bath, compress, diffuser/spritzer/aroma lamp, inhalation, massage, perfume, tea)

*****CLOVE** - *"used by dentists for anesthesia"*; helpful with toothache, colds, cough, asthma, indigestion, vomiting, hiccups, low blood pressure. (Compress, diffuser/spritzer/aroma lamp, food seasoning, massage, perfume, tea)

CORIANDER - *"seed of cilantro"*; decongestant to liver, aphrodisiac; helpful in urinary infections, burns, skin irritation, indigestion, allergies. (Bath, compress, diffuser/spritzer/aroma lamp, inhalation, massage, perfume, tea)

CUBEB ~ has a light peppery smell; used for congestion, weight loss, indigestion, skin eruptions. (Compress, massage, perfume)

CUMIN - familiar Mideast seasoning; small amounts in perfume creates a sensual effect; excellent for the immune system, digestive, and carminative. (Bath, compress, food seasoning, massage, tea, perfume)

CYPRESS - *"oil to reduce all excesses in the body"*; excess bleeding, mucus, weight etc.; good for oily skin, nerves and muscle spasms; female rejuvenative; helpful in treating PMS and menopause. (Bath, compress, inhalation, tea, perfume)

•**CYPERUS** - distilled from a grass that grows wild in India. Woody, spicy, sweet; astringent, calming, and sedative. (Bath, compress, massage, perfume)

•**DHAVANA** - good for balancing the female cycle, reduces cysts and skin irritation; it is antiseptic, an aphrodisiac and calming. (Bath, compress, food seasoning, inhalation, massage)

DILL - add to salad dressing; helps with flatulence, muscle spasms, nervousness, vomiting and hiccups; reduces sex drive, promotes lactation. (Food seasoning, perfume, massage)

ELEMI - *"used in Europe for 500 years in salves and liniments;* " a freshener in perfumery; good for inflammation, wounds, cuts, excessive bleeding; expectorant. (Compress, inhalation, massage, perfume)

EUCALYPTUS - *"the respiratory oil"* excellent for asthma, bronchitis, colds, fevers, sinus, sore throats, diabetes; used in muscle and joint liniments. (Bath, inhalation, compress, massage, tea)

FENNEL - *"the breath freshener and digestant"*; the seed is often served at the end of East Indian meals; antiseptic, laxative, tonic; decongests liver; increases lactation; reduces hangover. (Compress, bath, inhalation, tea, massage)

FIR - *"the smell of the Christmas tree"*; refreshing, clean, uplifting; relieves muscle spasms, asthma, joint pain, and congestion. (Bath, inhalation, massage, compress)

FRANKINCENSE - *"used for over 5000 years;"* still burned in the Catholic Church for devotion and uplifting; for cuts, bruises, colds, sinusitis, mature skin, antiseptic, astringent. (Compress, massage, inhalation, perfume)

GERANIUM - *"an oil for women and children;"* helps maintain youthful skin; good for herpes simplex; anti-depressant, PMS, menopause, dermatitis, ringworm, shingles, ulcers, skin care, menopause. (Bath, compress, inhalation, massage, perfume)

GINGER - *"the Heating Oil"* digestive, expectorant, weight reduction, colds, migraines. (Bath, compress, inhalation, massage, perfume)

GRAPEFRUIT - lymphatic, congestion, diuretic, cellulite, anti-depressant. (Compress, bath, inhalation, massage)

*HYSSOP - *"mentioned 17 times in the Bible:"* an ingredient in Chartreuse liquor: use for fevers, high blood pressure, congestion, indigestion, wounds, confusion. (Bath, compress, diffuser/spritzer/aroma lamp, inhalation)

•IMMORTELLE - *"the dream oil"*, creates vivid lucid dreams; reduces scars, acne, immune deficiency, cramps, liver weakness, and colds. (Bath, compress, diffuser/spritzer/aroma lamp, inhalation)

*•JASMINE {*absolute*}~ *"queen of the night"*; relaxant, aphrodisiac; useful in hoarseness, depression, impotence. (Bath, compress, diffuser/spritzer/aroma lamp, massage, perfume)

•JATAMASI ~ *"the essential oil that Mary Magdalen anointed Jesus with at the Last Supper;"* calms the stomach, stimulant to male hormones, grounding; helps in menopausal symptoms; moisturizes skin; rejuvenative. (Bath, food seasoning, massage, perfume)

*JUNIPER BERRY - "mover of fluids"; useful for congestion, edema, acne, wounds, indigestion, joint pain, gout, urinary tract infection. (Bath, compress, diffuser/spritzer/aroma lamp, food seasoning, inhalation, massage, perfume, tea)

LAVENDER - "the universal oil"; brings balance to any condition; wonderful for children, skin care, burns, depression, headaches, tension, bites, stings, fatigue, fainting, congestion and more. (Bath, compress, diffuser/spritzer/aroma lamp, food seasoning, inhalation, massage, perfume, tea)

LEMON - "The refreshing and familiar fragrance is stimulating," creates clarity; useful in acne, indigestion, tiredness; used in many cleaning products. (Bath, compress, diffuser/spritzer/aroma lamp, food seasoning, massage, perfume, tea)

*LEMON BALM - "also known as Melissa"; important for the immune system; helps allergies, fevers, indigestion, nervousness, muscle spasms, insomnia. (Bath, compress, diffuser/spritzer/aroma lamp, inhalation, massage, perfume)

LEMON GRASS - "uplifting, anti-depressant"; aids digestion, headache, infection, muscle and joint pain, varicose veins. (Bath, diffuser/spritzer/aroma lamp, food seasoning, massage, perfume, tea)

LIME - "the after shave oil"; used extensively in men's toiletries; helpful in fever, nervousness, indigestion, tiredness, spasms, depression, infections. (Bath, diffuser/spritzer/aroma lamp, food seasoning, perfume, tea)

MANDARIN RED - "combined with orange makes a happy oil"; good for kids at bedtime, stretch marks, nervousness, tension, spasms. (Bath, compress, diffuser/spritzer/aroma lamp, food seasoning, massage)

*MARJORAM - "decreases sexual drive"; beneficial in arthritis, asthma, colds, constipation, tension, hysteria, insomnia, migraine. (Compress, food seasoning, massage)

*MYRRH - "one of the gifts of the Magi"; creates confidence and awareness; helpful in irregular periods, coughs, asthma, bronchitis, arthritis, skin care, rejuvenation, weight loss. (Bath, diffuser/spritzer/ aroma lamp, massage, perfume)

•MUSK FLORAL - "*a vegetable substitute for animal musk*"; excellent for aphrodisiac formulas, or as a base note for perfumes. (Bath, massage, perfume)

NIAOULI - "*tea tree family*"; especially effective in bacterial, yeast, viral and fungal infections; good for colds, flues, respiratory and urinary infections; joint and muscle pain. (Bath, compress, diffuser/ spritzer/aroma lamp, inhalation, massage, tea)

NUTMEG - stimulates brain activity, digestion, blood flow; grounding and strengthening. Good for toothache; aphrodisiac. (Food seasoning, massage, perfume)

ORANGE - from the orange skin; comforting and familiar, energizing and heart opening; used for cellulite, weak digestion, gingivitis, fever, sadness; also used for food flavoring in cakes and desserts. (Bath, diffuser/spritzer/aroma lamp, food seasoning, massage, perfume, tea)

•OUD - rarest and most expensive oil; creates a spirit connection between people; used to anoint the dead; aids transition; aura cleansing. (Perfume)

PALMAROSA - antiseptic, and cellular stimulant; good for wrinkles, dry skin, eczema; calming and uplifting. (Bath, compress, diffuser/ spritzer/aroma lamp, massage, perfume)

*PARSLEY - helpful in treating broken capillaries, circulation and fluid retention problems, abdominal or pelvic inflammation, swelling, stones, pain. (Compress, food seasoning, massage, tea)

PATCHOULI - grounding and calming, it can aid anxiety, depression, hypertension, apathy, wrinkles, and fluid retention. A noted rejuvinative, it is aphrodisiac and sedative. (Bath, compress, diffuser/spritzer/aroma lamp, massage, perfume)

*PENNYROYAL - good insect repellent for pets, added to shampoo. Some use in hysteria, nervousness, and headaches. (Bath, diffuser/spritzer/aroma lamp)

PEPPERMINT - excellent for headaches, fevers, coughs, tiredness, gum infections, nervousness, asthma. 1 drop = instant tea. (Bath, compress, diffuser/spritzer/aroma lamp, food seasoning, inhalation, massage, perfume, tea)

PETITGRAIN - Distilled from citrus leaves and branches; excellent for muscle spasms, inflammation, nervousness, poor memory, indigestion, pain, poor circulation; it is uplifting and calming. (Bath, compress, inhalation, massage, perfume)

•**ROSE- BULGARIAN OR TURKISH** - Many feel Bulgarian is the best. Turkish is more subtle; wonderful for insomnia; all roses have approximately the same medicinal properties. (Bath, compress, food seasoning, inhalation, massage, perfume, tea)

•**ROSE-INDIAN** - 1st. dist. - most rare; many people prefer the Indian Rose. All rose is highly prized in skin care for acne irritation, dryness and wrinkles. Rose is opening to the heart, reduces anger, decongests the liver. Helpful in PMS and menopause. (Bath, compress, food seasoning, inhalation, massage, perfume, tea)

*•**ROSE MOROCCAN** {absolute} - the Moroccan is warmer and sweeter; known rejuvenative, anti-depressant; regulates the menstrual period; aids digestion, fever, frigidity, and infection. (Bath, compress, inhalation, massage, perfume)

*•**ROSEMARY** - "*the health restorer*"; useful in sinus, lung congestion, colds, flu, joint and muscle pain, swelling, indigestion, mental fatigue, nervousness; enhances memory. (Bath, compress, diffuser/spritzer/aroma lamp, food seasoning, inhalation, massage, perfume, tea)

ROSEWOOD - grounding and connecting; antiseptic, relaxant, deodorizer; effective on dry skin and with infections. (Bath, compress, diffuser/spritzer/aroma lamp, massage)

***SAGE** (*Spanish*) - another women's oil; helpful with PMS, menopause, hot flashes, water retention, gum infections, wrinkles, hair loss and night sweats. (Bath, compress, massage, perfume)

SANDALWOOD - "*the spiritual oil of the Far East*"; helps with grounding, connection, and focus on personal growth; stimulating to the immune and endocrine systems; effective for infections, laryngitis (Bath, compress, diffuser/spritzer/aroma lamp, massage, perfume, tea)

•**SAFFRON** - extracted with vegetable oil; balancing to the nervous system because it calms the mind; useful for pain, spasm, irregular menopause, PMS, depression, asthma, infertility, impotence and enlarged liver.

TAGETES - "*English Marigold Oil*"; softens hardened tissues {calluses, scars, bunions, warts}; healing to skin irritations and wounds. (Compress, massage)

TANGERINE - "*children's oil*" - works well with gold chamomile and lavender, good for pregnant women because of its calming and uplifting qualities; aids in reducing tension, fear, sadness, insomnia, frigidity, digestive problems and PMS. (Bath, compress, diffuser/spritzer/ aroma lamp, food seasoning, massage, perfume)

TEA TREE - " *a first aid kit in a bottle*" with hundreds of uses; effective against fungus, yeast, virus, and bacterial infection. Helpful in bites, stings, acne, bronchitis and urinary infections. (Bath, compress, inhalation, massage, tea)

*****THYME, RED** - " *big red of essentials*"; #1 for infections including athletes foot, staphylococcus, respiratory, sinus, and urinary. Useful for missed periods, wounds, acne, arthritis. (Compress, diffuser/ spritzer/aroma lamp, food seasoning, massage, tea)

•**TRIFOLIA** - " *the traveler's oil*"; best known for relieving constipation when rubbed on the stomach; anti-fungal; warming, moisturizing. (Compress, diffuser/spritzer/aroma lamp, massage, perfume)

*****TUBEROSE** {absolute} - used in finest of perfumes; intensely strong and floral; anti-depressant, and mood elevator; helps focus on serving others. (Massage, perfume)

TUMERIC - immune builder; good for digestion, cough, arthritis, wounds, bruises, confusion, and anxiety. (Compress, food seasoning, massage, perfume)

VALERIAN ROOT - "*the pain killer*"; also used for insomnia, cough, headache, skin problems, colic, stress, and indigestion. (Bath, compress, food seasoning, massage, tea)

VANILLA {oleoresin} - a favorite food flavoring in drinks and desserts; used in perfumes for warmth and relaxation; helpful with anger, frustration, and tension. (Food seasoning, massage, perfume)

VETIVER - "*a grounding and balancing oil*"; helps with scatteredness, confusion, skin aging, depression, menopause, PMS, anorexia; a known aphrodisiac. (Bath, massage)

*****WINTERGREEN** - "*the icy hot liniment oil*"; stimulant with extensive use in liniments; assists with muscle and joint pain, sciatica, sore throat. (Compress, massage)

•**YARROW** - "*heal all*"; useful for fevers, bleeding, inflammation, ulcers, skin irritation, nose bleeds, headaches, and allergies; aids elimination; strengthens immune system. (Bath, compress, diffuser/spritzer/aroma lamp, inhalation, massage, perfume, tea)

YLANG YLANG - "*flower of the Philippines*"; aphrodisiac, antiseptic, sedative; helpful for frigidity, depression, insomnia, oily skin, and headaches. (Bath, compress, diffuser, massage, perfume)

CHAPTER 3

PREGNANCY

*Once again, as the Miracle
of Life occurs, our Divinity beckons.*

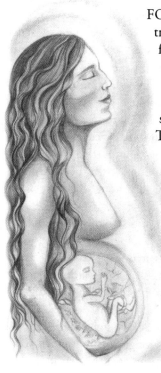

FOR MANY YEARS, birth has been treated as a dis-ease by the medical profession in this country, while in many other countries it remains a natural occurrence. Many indigenous women give birth and then get up, wash themselves, and continue with their duties. This is a stoic example from the opposite extreme, called for by harsh environments and urgent survival needs. Ideally, after giving birth, mother and child will bond. The being who has been inside for nine months can now become reassured that he is still connected, even though he is now outside of the mother. He must adjust to the new feeling of gravity, air, touch, sounds, feeding; a whole new world. The mother can take this time to reflect on the great gift which she has received, the opportunity to guide another soul into adulthood and the mutual growth, learning and expansion that the relationship can bring.

Fortunately, the attitudes of the medical profession have swung back toward more of a "hands off" stance in the birth process. More women are requesting natural childbirth and have come to see the birth experience as a strengthening process and a blessing. A woman's pregnancy cycle can be empowering. A woman who enters her pregnancy with a healthy, positive attitude begins to trust her body and can have an easy time with her pregnancy and birth.

Pregnancy is a Kapha process and yet Ayurveda continues to recognize different metabolic body types and their specific lifestyle and dietary needs. The expectant mother will add 30-50 pounds of Kapha tissue. The goodness and purity of the food should be of the highest quality. Urges to sleep more and cravings to eat more should be seen as a natural part of pregnancy. Vata will crave more rich and oily foods such as yogurt, ghee, cheeses and nut butters. Pittas will crave more proteins and Kapha types will be attracted to sweets and starches. Listen to your cravings within reason.

In today's busy western society, women have become very active in the world and it is essential to plan having babies in the midst of a career. Bringing a new life into the world is a twenty year commitment. Due to the speed of our lifestyle and the immense changes that are occurring within society, I encourage you to be conscious about bringing new life into the world. We are in need of a new generation of beings who are strong and self-sufficient, yet responsible and ready to make a difference. This requires tremendous commitment from the parents. Unloved children, left to be taught and cared for by the public schools, day care and sitters will only add to the problems of a troubled society.

When planning a baby, it is best to avoid smoking or a smoking environment. Start by consulting with a practitioner about your health and your partner. Both partners may need to make health changes in preparation for conception. Begin a healthy diet that works for your body types, and often an internal cleansing program can be helpful before planning to conceive.

Babies have awareness, in the womb, of thoughts and feelings. They can even register conversations through the abdominal wall. Unwanted babies may create miscarriage unless it is their karma to be born with that unwanted feeling. A woman's stresses are passed into the baby. Anything which the mother experiences, the fetus experiences also. Therefore, try not to conceive during a time when your life is "rocky", or when your relationship with your husband is challenged. Often women think that having a baby will solve their marriage problems, however, this can make things worse. Others may think that this is the way to hold on to a relationship. When necessary, go to counseling sessions and work any major problems out before attempting to conceive. Sometimes babies "just happen" and then there is nothing to do except adjust your life to their coming by taking positive steps forward.

During the months of pregnancy, it is good to develop communication with the baby by singing, reading, meditating, chanting and talking. Also read books which educate you about the miracle of pregnancy. Become #1 in your life. Take the best care you can of yourself and maintain a healthy attitude towards the world. Keep good relationships and clear communications with all people, especially with your husband or partner. When life challenges come about, hold your tummy, communicate with your baby, let it know that this situation will pass and that the best is yet to come.

"Choose" a support team during your pregnancy and for your birthing. You need to feel *very good* about anyone involved in the process. Do not accept any practitioner with whom you do not feel good about; it is important to like them. You need to be able to communicate your needs, wants and desires to this support team. It is important that you feel totally free to express yourself, and that your interaction with others comes from a comfortable place for you and for them. This is possible when you clearly know that you have choices in your life. Do not sacrifice yourself by feeling obligated to have people at the birth because *they* want to; only invite those whom *you* want.

HOME BIRTH

When possible, have your baby at home in your own personal environment, surrounded by the things you love and where you can be more comfortable and at ease. Many certified nurse midwives and some doctors are available for home births. Today, there are also wonderful birth centers in many hospitals, which have birthing rooms where family members can be part of this miraculous event. Seek only highly qualified, caring, sensitive and professional people for the birth of your baby. Speak to other women who have had an easy, wonderful birth. Go to people who give you the time you deserve and always make sure that the people, environment and circumstances are exactly as you want them. A birth center is a closer step to a home birth, yet provides fast access to emergency facilities and personnel, if needed.

My preference is to work with a midwife or a sensitive, caring female doctor. A woman understands the female body better than any male. Man would have to give birth to truly understand. There are, however, many men who are sensitive, very caring, and excellent physicians. When choosing a male doctor, look for these qualities always remembering that you and your baby deserve the very best.

Birthing centers are a wonderful option available today that provide a home environment, allowing you to bring personal belongings from home. Many of these centers also have facilities for an underwater birth.

REBIRTHING

We each carry within us the memory of our own birth. Our birth could have been traumatic, induced, drugged, or difficult. This would be part of our cellular memory and locked up within our unconscious. We tend to repeat patterns. If our birth was dominated by fear (i.e., our mother was afraid, or people attending the birth were anxious, or adrenaline was flowing from mother to baby), then these old feelings may come up as we approach our own giving birth. In the rebirthing experience you relive the birth process from the perspective of your now mature understanding, instead of the viewpoint of a baby. We can now let go of those feelings because we see that they were unnecessary. We survived and everyone involved did the best they could. Ayurveda says that we chose our parents and birth experiences for the learning opportunities they bring. We cannot learn unless we revisit the past. It is recommended that expectant mothers (and even fathers) go through one or more rebirthing treatments to come to terms with your own birth memories. Transforming your own birth memories will assist the experience of your baby's birth, making it the relaxed and joyous occasion that it is.

BROTHERS AND SISTERS

If you have other children, include them in the pregnancy and birth process. Let them massage and talk to the baby through your belly. Read positive stories of angels and fairies to them and to your unborn. If they are involved they will not feel resentment, but instead, will feel joined with the new baby. Do not tell them that the stork brings the baby. Tell them how you and daddy asked God for a baby and he sent this special one to grow inside of you. Education about your pregnancy is important for your younger children and there are many wonderful books on the subject.

BIRTH

During the birth, you can use specific essential oils to help you concentrate and focus, and other essential oils to assist with relaxation and feeling connected. Learn breathwork and other techniques which assist you in this experience. Massage your belly and your body everyday, using a mild essential oil mixture. Coconut oil and cocoa butter are excellent for prevention of stretch marks. When showering rub the nipples with a wash cloth or a loofa to toughen them in preparation for breast-feeding.

NURSING

Babies who are breast-fed have a stronger bonding with the mother; it provides a feeling of safety in the world as well as strengthens their immune system. Many experts say that breast-feeding is preferable to inoculation and without the risk of reactions. Breast feeding also makes it easier and convenient for mother and baby to travel. No carrying around of formulas, washing bottles and sterilizing. Your baby does not have to suck on plastic. The breast is ready at all times. Your extra milk can even be frozen and is then available for the times when you are gone. The baby can receive this wonderful nutrition from momma's body even when she is away. Humans are the only mammals who allow other animals milk or man-made formulas into their young ones. Cow's milk has much more fat than human milk and creates excessive growth. Goat's milk is closer in content and may be better if human milk is not possible. When my husband and I adopted, we went out and bought a milk goat and she became part of the family.

Nursing on demand is good as long as you have long feedings. Nurse for at least 1/2 hour to 45 minutes. This should be a very relaxing time, so create that for yourself and your new baby. First time mothers can become tense, nervous, jumpy and excited. Women who have had other children take time for themselves and their baby making it a pleasurable and blissful experience. It is good to create a feeding schedule, although the baby often creates its own, with a little help from mother. If baby is always hungry and never satisfied, the mother's milk could be deficient of certain nutrients. Green vegetables and herbs are important for healthy milk; cows get their milk from grass, which provides green chlorophyll. Train your baby to sleep through the night without feeding. This gives the mother and baby's digestive tract a rest.

When you are nursing, anything that your baby needs is provided through your milk. When the baby has a problem such as colic or rash, take time to look at your diet and what you are putting into your body. Take out anything in your diet that can be aggravating the baby. If you eat chocolate the baby can get a rash; if you eat cabbage the baby can have gas; or if you drink coffee, the baby won't go to sleep. Everything is shared, even your emotions. Even if you adopt a baby you can breast feed with the help of herbs (explained later) and a devise called "lactaid" which allows formula or donated mothers milk to be fed to baby from a small feeding bag draped over the neck and through a small diameter tube placed on your nipple. The stimulation of these feedings will trigger production of your own milk (1-2 months). This device can also be used for women who have insufficient milk flow.

PROTECTION

Many ancient cultures believe on keeping the baby's head covered for forty days to allow the soul to integrate into the child's body. Part of this tradition is for protection from the sun, wind or cold. It is best to avoid loud, chaotic, busy places for the first few months, such as malls and loud shopping areas.

The newborn child enters the world in a state of pure light and begins to experience separation from its higher source according to how much care is provided by everyone around him or her. Parents who live in a higher state of consciousness can help maintain this illuminated state in the young ones by the example in which they live.

RETURNING TO WORK

When possible, work at home. Start your own business or assist other mothers in taking care of young ones. Some women must return to work. If this is the case for you, again, find someone with whom you feel confident about caring for your baby. It is possible to extract your milk and freeze it for the next day's feedings. In the computer age, many more mothers can log on and work at home.

In many European countries, the government supplements the mother's income for one year in support of the mother and child. In other cultures, grandmothers and family are very involved for the first few years of the child's life to assist and support its growth. In this culture, very few women today have the privilege of staying home and being a full time mother, and the very fabric of the family heritage is becoming lost. Our culture has forgotten how to honor the mother.

MASSAGE

Take care of your baby. Massage and stretch their limbs. This can be learned from books. I recommend, "Loving Hands" by Frederick Leboyer; a life changing book. Essential oils can be added to the massage oil to relax and soothe your baby. Babies respond quickly to just a few drops of essential oil in your massage mixture. Massage your belly and your body everyday, using a mild essential oil mixture. Coconut oil and cocoa butter are excellent for prevention of stretch marks. When showering, rub the nipples with a wash cloth or a loofa to toughen them in preparation for breast-feeding.

TEETHING

Teething can often be an exciting time in a baby's life. Do not use synthetic creams or any which are loaded with sugar and chemical gels. Orris root or powder, frozen carrot or fruit can be a natural relief for the baby's gums. The health food stores have many homeopathic and herbal remedies (these are later discussed on pages 56 & 57). Crying, irritability, crankiness, and even fevers are naturally part of the uncomfortable process. These light fevers need not be suppressed with medicine or become a cause for alarm.

CRYING

When a baby cries for no apparent reason, it might be appropriate to allow it to cry as long as you know you've done everything appropriate. A good healthy cry can be 5-10 minutes long. Often they just want attention and want to see what you will do. They are beginning to test their limits. Shortly after birth, you will learn about the different kinds of cries. High-pitched cries are often pain and distress. A vigorous cry will make them sleep better.

POSSIBLE CONDITIONS DURING PREGNANCY

Backaches	Warm compress, bath, chiropractic care, massage, exercise.
Bleeding gums	Floss, regular dental check -ups, rinse mouth with essential oils.
Constipation	Eat roughage foods, plenty of fruit and vegetables, whole grains, flax seeds, phyllome, exercise.
Dizziness	Use essential oils for pregnancy, rest, meditate.
Heart burn	Food combining; eat cooling not hot foods.
Hemorrhoids	Eat fresh salads, plenty of fluids (herbal teas and juices.)

Insomnia	Breathing, meditation, massage shoulders, head and neck before sleep, use calming and soothing essential oils, drink relaxing teas.
Leg cramps	Foods high in calcium such as greens, sesame seeds, massage, and warm baths with essential oils.
Mood Swings	Meditate, breathing exercises, prayers, walks, B Vitamins.
Morning sickness	Equal amounts of Chamomile and Fennel tea (Pitta), Ginger and Fennel tea (Vata and Kapha), B vitamins, whole grains.
Nasal congestion	Vitamin C, inhalation with essential oils, nose drops, vaporizer at night, walks.
Sciatica	Massage, acupressure, warm bath.
Soreness of ribs	Essential oil compresses, yoga.
Stretch marks	Oil belly every day, use essential oils with cocoa butter, foods high in Vitamins A and E.
Swelling, Edema	Cut out fried and processed foods, allergic foods, salt, take baths with essential oils, exercise, and walk.
Varicose Veins	Walk, exercise, essential oil baths, massage legs regularly, elevate legs when possible.

Recommended Herbs

Alfalfa: PK-V+
Oat straw: VP-K+
Black hawthorn: PK-V+
Dandelion: PK-V+
Ginger: VK-P+
Strawberry: PK-V+
Blessed thistle: PV-K+

Chamomile: VK-Po
Red Raspberry: PK-V+
Nettles: PK-V+
Rose Flowers: PKV=
Lavender: PK-Vo
Ashwagandha: VK-P+
Chayavanprash Jelly: VKP+

Slippery Elm: PV-P+
Parsley: VK-P+
Cilantro: VK-Po
**MaterniTea: VKP

Rose Petal: VKP=
Coriander: VKP=
Licorice: VP-K+

** Product of UniTea Herbs, Colorado

HERBS TO AVOID DURING PREGNANCY

Bitter Herbs (cleansing)

Chaparral
Gentian
Barberry
Balmony
Blue Flag
Buchu Leaves
Calumba
Chicory
Culnos Root
Eyebright
Golden Thread
Indigo
Mandrake
Oregon Grape
Passion Flower
Primrose
Yarrow
Cascara Sagarada

Pau d'Arco
Peony
Peruvian Bark
Poke Root
Rhubarb
Rue
Senna
Stone Root
Vervain
Tansy
Tarragon
Wahoo
White Poplar
Willow Bark
Worm Seed
Violet
Yellow Dock

Tonic Herbs to avoid

Bibhitaki
Gotu Kola
Guggul

Jasmine Flowers
Neem
Punarnava

Pungent Herbs to Avoid

Root Bark
Pennyroyal oil
Goldenseal
Barberry
Bayberry

Mugwort
Bitter Root
Self Heal
Shepherd's Purse
Squaw Vine

Comfrey
Garlic
Hot Spices
Anise
Arnica
Basil
Tulse
Buchu Leaves
Calamus
Camphor
Caraway
Betony Wood
Cayenne
Cloves
Aibels
Savory
Onion
Turmeric
Watercress
Wild Carrots
Yellow Dock
Yerba Mate

Stillingia
Galangal
Gravel Root
Ground Ivy
Hops
Horehound
Hyssop
Marjoram
Mormon Tea
Ephedra
Motherwort
Oregon
Paprika
Parsley
Sage
Sassafras
Thyme
Valerian
White Pine
Witch Hazel
Yerba Santa

Always consult with an herbalist when herb is not listed anywhere above. When there is a medicinal need for the above herbs, consult a Health Practitioner.

ESSENTIAL OILS TO AVOID DURING PREGNANCY

Angelica, Anise Seed, Basil, Camphor, Cedarwood, Champa, Citronella, Hyssop, Jasmine, Juniper Berry, Lemon Balm, Lovage, Marjoram, Melissa, Mustard, Myrrh, Pennyroyal, Peppermint, Rosemary, Sage, Savory, Spanish Thyme, Tarragon, Thyme, and Wintergreen.

PRODUCTS TO AVOID DURING PREGNANCY

Alka Seltzer	Tylenol	Pepto Bismol	Maalox
Antihistamines	Rolaids	Insect Sprays	Estrogen
Cough Medicine	Antibiotics	Household Chemicals	
Datril	Tobacco	Aspirin	

RECIPES FOR HEALTH CARE

Afterbirth

Shatavari & milk, rice milk, or soy milk	Restores vitality
Lady Mantle	Restores vitality
Raspberry Leaves	Toner
Shepherd's Purse	Bleeding
Ghee	Vitality
Wheat grass/Barley green	Promotes milk porduction

Baby Oil

Formula #1

Primrose Oil	50 drops
Jojoba Oil	3 drops
Wheat Germ Oil	10 drops
Almond Oil	2 tsp.

Formula #2

Hazelnut Oil	80%
Wheat Germ Oil	20%
Neroli essential oil	1 drop

Baths for Relaxation - For Mother

Chamomile	10 drops
Tangerine	2 drops
Lavender	3 drops
Geranium	2 drops

Breast Feeding

Fennel	2 drops
Jasmine	2 drops
Base Oil	1 oz.

Circulation - For Mother

Rose	3 drops

Clary Sage	2 drops
Lavender	2 drops
Base Oil	2 oz.

Cracked Nipples

Rose	4 drops
Lemon	2 drops
Vegetable Oil 2 Tbs.	

Earache - For Baby

Lavender	1 drop
Cajeput	1 drop
Olive Oil	1 Tbs.

Edema Foot Bath - For Mother

Lavender	10 drops
Cypress	3 drops
Juniper Berry	3 drops
Patchouli	2 drops
Water	1 quart

Hospital Oil - For Mother

Rosewood	Equal amounts
Lavender	Water in spray bottle. Spray around your bed and in the hospital room.

Inflammation - For Mother

Blue Chamomile	Equal amounts
Lavender	Equal amounts
Base Oil	Sunflower Oil

Insufficient Engorgement

Geranium	2 drops
Peppermint	2 drops
Vegetable Oil	2 Tbs.

Labor

Chamomile	Calming
Comfrey	Helps with tearing
Cloves	Take two weeks before giving first birth; increases contraction. Take 1 tsp. of clove per cup of boiling water. Steep for 15 minutes.
Sage	Good for infections

Two weeks before labor

Drink clove tea	1/2 tsp. clove tea - 1 cup water

Massage

Roman Chamomile	5 drops
Rose	2 drops
Neroli	2 drops
Almond Oil	2 oz.

Milk Flow

Fennel	Excellent. Prevents colic.
Hops	
Blessed Thistle	
Galangal	
Shatavari	

Use the above herbs to make an herbal blend.

Nose Bleed

Cypress	5 drops
Lavender	5 drops
Water	1 cup

Mix essential oils into water completely. Soak cloth in water. Place compress on nose, holding head back.

Postpartum

Clary Sage	2 drops
Neroli	3 drops
Bergamot	3 drops
Vegetable Oil	1 oz.

Preparing for Childbirth

Nutmeg	3 drops
Sage	2 drops
Neroli	1 drop
Almond Oil	4-5 tsp.

Massage blend on belly.

Stitches

| Nettles, comfrey, oat straw | In equal amounts |

Make herbal blend (or use tincture) and use with compress over area.

Stop Milk Flow

Massage breasts with sage oil:

| Sage Essential Oil | 10 drops |
| Vegetable Oil | 1 oz. |

Do once per day for one week.

Teething

Chamomile	3 drops
Yarrow	3 drops
Lavender	3 drops
Vegetable Oil	1 Tbs.

Toothache - For Baby

Peppermint	1 drop
Clove	1 drop
Vegetable Oil	1 tbs.

Varicose Veins

Cypress	5 drops
Juniper Berry	5 drops
Lemongrass	5 drops
Vegetable Oil	2 oz.

CHAPTER 4

CHILDREN'S HEALTH & CHILDHOOD ILLNESSES

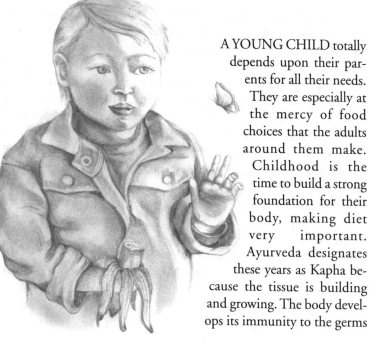

A YOUNG CHILD totally depends upon their parents for all their needs. They are especially at the mercy of food choices that the adults around them make. Childhood is the time to build a strong foundation for their body, making diet very important. Ayurveda designates these years as Kapha because the tissue is building and growing. The body develops its immunity to the germs and it learns to adjust to the surrounding environment. Our spirit uses this time to integrate slowly into the physical body. At the end of this time our spirit is fully capable of expressing itself and pursuing its purpose in life.

Many childhood illnesses, such as mumps, measles and chicken pox, are important for strengthening the ability of the immune system to fight other dis-eases in later years. Any of these illnesses, when contracted as an adult can be very dangerous. Many experts feel that immunizations weaken the resistance of the child, disrupting the immune system and causing other problems later on (possibly arthritis, cancer, multiple sclerosis, etc.). Children are more sensitive than adults. They respond readily to homeopathics, herbs and essential oils. Supporting their immune system with these natural therapeutics, rather than suppressing it with drugs, will pay dividends later. A fever is not only a symptom of infection, but also one of the body's defense mechanisms to combat. Germs do not thrive at higher temperatures. If you suppress a fever with aspirin or Tylenol, you miss this benefit. A fever that gets dangerously high can be lowered with a cool bath or a rub down with lavender, chamomile and water on a damp washcloth.

Affection and touch are important components of the child's development and is of primary importance in a child's life. Often we take for granted that our children know that they are loved. With the efforts that we make for them and the amount of time we spend providing for them, we assume that they know that we do all this because we love them. A young child lacks maturity and experience and will have no awareness of what parenthood is all about until later on in life. They need touch, affection and communication to "know" that they are loved. There are simple ways to express your love daily. Especially in the morning and at night. When they are on the verge of the dream state, their deep subconscious takes in your touch, words and tone of voice. When the child comes home with a story or a picture and mom or dad is rushing around making dinner, we often say, "not now, I am busy", and the child feels unloved, not understood and rejected.

Those magic moments occur daily and are an opportunity for the parents to take time to be with the child, praising them. Just be present and understanding. This break in rushing around allows us to acknowledge what is important. Breathe and become centered.

If your child asks you, "what's wrong mom?" its important for their development that you do not pass them off with "oh, nothing". Their feelings of intuition are a very important guide in their development. They do know that something is going on. Honor that sense within them by acknowledging that something is up (appropriate to their age and maturity), and how you are feeling about it. Acknowledging that "knowing" helps them learn to trust their intuition.

Touch, kisses and hugs are another way to reinforce that the child is loved. All primates (and man is one) spend several hours a day grooming each other. This intimate touch reduces stress, creates group unity and an individual sense of belonging. It increases immunity, accelerates growth in infants and lowers aggressive tendencies. Since humans don't have hair that hides fleas, massage, hugging, touching, hand games, and even wrestling may be the most appropriate way for us to connect with each other. A short massage and a bath with essential oils before bed will ensure relaxation and a restful sleep as well as assist with prevention of other illnesses.

DIET

Unfortunately, a natural diet in today's school system and in our society is not encouraged nor supported. Children are exposed to a large amount of sugar and processed foods with debilitating consequences to their system, causing tooth decay and hyperactivity, to name a couple. Do not make a fuss yourself about sugar; just keep the amount you add very low - from birth on. White sugar can be very addictive to a child's palate. Find other ways to satisfy the sugar craving by using healthy items. A sugar craving is often an indication of a lack of minerals and chlorophyll in their body. The health food stores have many fruits and treats that are sugar-free. Fructose is better than white sugar and you can find many cookies made with fruit juices. Remember, even honey, fruit sugar, natural sugars, and maple syrups should be a small part of the diet even though they are natural.

Bottled juices have more sugar than fresh pressed due to the fact that the boiling process concentrates the sugar. Freshly made juices contain enzymes and vitamins that bottled juices do not. Dilute the juice with herbal teas such as peppermint, hibiscus, chamomile, rosehips, ginger, and cinnamon. These herbs will add vitamins and minerals to the juice mixture and assist in digestion. Use equal amounts of tea with equal amounts of juice. Drinking this mixture can be beneficial to adults also, as well as a good way to take any medication. Remember, babies should drink mother's milk and water only. Babies fed fruit juices develop early cavities in their new undeveloped teeth.

Substitute fresh fruits and nuts for snacks. Dry fruits are best soaked overnight or blended into sauces or purees. Celery sticks and nut butters are good also.

Do not make a big deal about natural foods. Simply serve good foods and do not make the child feel that he "is different" (you must eat it too). If you don't want a child to eat something, do not have it in the house. If they get birthday cake at school occasionally, allow it. It is what you do most of the time that matters. Some children love vegetables and love vegetarian foods while others have a great dislike for them. When you have a child that does not like vegetables, grate them into spaghetti sauce and serve with pasta, rice, in a spread, into chili, omelets, etc. - when it is all together it does not show. In their sandwiches you can also cut up small pieces of vegetables and mix in with the spreads and nut butters. You can add vegetables and spices to shakes, nut milks, soups, and dips with chips. Children love chips. Chinese foods, noodles, garnishes, stews and samosas are other good ways to eat vegetables. Become creative! My husband, Bryan, makes a tasty zucchini pancake. Sauté fine cut onions, spinach and vegetables, add refried beans, and serve in burritos with avocados and mild salsa.

The market is flooded with sodas that are detrimental to health and very addictive. They contain large amounts of sugar, caffeine, and phosphoric acid. NutriSweet breaks down into several substances which are dangerous to humans and restricted by the EPA (Environmental Protection Agency) (including formaldehyde), yet has somehow received the Food and Drug Administration's approval (I'm sure big money wasn't a factor). It has been implicated in epileptic seizures and its use is cautioned by many pilot organizations. Look at all the foods this substance is now in! The health food stores have many sodas that, in large amounts, can be as bad as coke. Become aware. Find a good brand of health food drink that your child likes and provide it as an *occasional* treat.

A great educational experience for your child is to provide this demonstration: when they lose a tooth, have them place the tooth overnight in a glass of cola. The tooth will be mostly dissolved by morning. When they look for their tooth, or at what remains of it, explain that their teeth are part of their bone tissue, therefore, this decay would also occur in their bones when drinking too much soft drinks. This is better than the Tooth Fairy story.

Fruits, vegetables and whole grains should be approximately 75% of a child's diet. This provides the child with important minerals and vitamins to create a strong foundation. Milk and yogurt can be important, as long as the child does not develop an allergy towards them.

There is a lot of controversy about eating meat today, yet I believe that it is an individual decision. If you do eat meat it is best that it is antibiotic and pesticide free. Often cows are given growth hormones that affect and interfere with the child's growth. The grains they are fed contain pesticides and herbicides. Meat is a great source of protein, yet is hard to digest. Children do best with turkey or fish. When preparing meat it is another opportunity to add vegetables to the meal. The young children love hamburgers and to this mixture you can add small pieces of grated or chopped celery, beets, carrots and any other vegetable you may desire. If a history of meat consumption is a part of your genetic heritage, your child may be healthier if you include some meat in their diet. I would not urge a Hindu to be a meat eater or an Eskimo to be a vegetarian. Native Eskimos ate a natural diet with an attitude of gratefulness to the Mother Earth. Modern Eskimos who eat imported "white man's" food are often disconnected from natural resources, and suffer many modern diseases.

Healthy attitudes and a natural diet contribute to the creation of a society in which individuals are strong and who trust themselves. A natural diet and lifestyle create positive, energetic individuals and allow for a connection to their own true nature.

DISCIPLINE

Today we have a generation based on guilt and fear due to too much blame, harsh punishment, and unforgiveness. Children need discipline and rules of good behavior taught to them. Yet in the process it is also important that they have self-worth and self-respect. Children learn by imitation, therefore, you are truly their teachers. If we want respect, we must give it. This follows in every quality and virtue. A child who is beaten would only know how to beat others; they pass on what they have been taught or modeled. Negative reinforcement will only create negative behavior and a lack of self-worth. Every thought and every word has an effect on the physical body. Be firm and clear, yet keep the love intact. Good communication is a function of love. Never tell a child that they were wrong or bad. Instead, say that they made a mistake. Ask them how they would do it differently the next time.

"Time out" can be a very good experience as a correction. It can be a useful and constructive time for the child, and gives them time to reflect. Make them a special pillow and then let them beat on it or some stuffed animals. Shred old rags or old clothes. Let them pound nails with a hammer. Another type of discipline would be for the child to run around the outside of the house; they use up their energy and are then ready to relax, listen and alter inappropriate behavior. Remember, the only true discipline is self-discipline. Punishment produces rebellion and resentment. Teach children to tell the truth because they will feel better about themselves, not because they may be punished.

I went to pick up my two-year-old grandson from preschool. The children had been throwing pretzels during lunchtime. When I walked into the classroom, four of them were on "time out" and each child was in a different corner of the room. Each child's body postures demonstrated a feeling of shame, lack of self-worth and self-respect. They had evidently been told that "they were bad" in addition to being given "time out". I believe these feelings were locked into their tissue and this may be where rebellion begins. A better way to handle it may have been to have them run around the playground three times, then talk to them as a group about the sacredness of food, its shortage in some parts of the world, and show them pictures of starving children. Explain the benefits of order and the drawbacks of anarchy.

It is best not to hit a child when you are angry with them. The American Indians said that it only drove the bad into them. Calm yourself. Take a breath. Speak to them calmly and let them know how their behavior was inappropriate. Ask questions rather than accuse them. You might ask, "What would happen if everyone behaved that way"? or "what were you feeling?" Often their answer is, "I don't know". You might respond, "I understand, but if you did know, what would your feeling be"? Support them in sharing their feelings. Ask if a more appropriate expression would produce a happier outcome.

Children are a reflection of their environment as they learn by imitation. Watch them and you will see an aspect of yourself. Often they are a product of our habits. They are constantly observing the behaviors of others. Be that which you want them to be. We can demand respect, but it will not always be given. We can earn respect and then it comes without struggle.

TELEVISION AND COMPUTERS

Both can be educational and informative yet, with this medium, the child is looking outside of himself for stimulation and answers, receiving quick information and finding themselves outside of the experience. They are unable to experience the Self in this manner. Cut down the programs they watch to one hour per day, at most, and be selective of what they see. Television is passive entertainment. Let them learn and entertain themselves with crafts, arts, games, conversation, etc.

Computers should be used for doing homework or for finding information. Long hours of computer games will stifle their creativity and stiffen their muscles. Observe their postures. They both isolate the child and it can become an escape from their real life, allowing them to live in a world of make believe and often of violence. Let a small amount of computer games be a reward for accomplishment (completing homework or chores).

SHOULD I IMMUNIZE MY CHILD?

Every decision a parent makes regarding their child's health should be made after reviewing all the risks and benefits involved. Unfortunately, the people we trust and turn to for advice on this topic have an agenda and routinely are un-informed themselves. They are often incredulous that you question the status quo. They will often tell you that there is no risk to immunization; that they are perfectly safe. If you persist in questioning the procedure, doctors may threaten to dismiss you as a patient, school officials may bar your child from classes, social services may threaten to cut benefits, and insurance coverage may be dropped.

Here is information that may help you decide:

1. Many millions of children are immunized and suffer no apparent harm. However, many health professionals believe that these immunizations interfere with our immune systems and contribute to later auto-immune diseases which have been increasing in the last part of this century when mass immunization practices began (Cancer, MS, MD, Arthritis, Chronic Fatigue, Epstein Barr, etc.).

2. The immunization injections contain live bacteria, live viruses, chicken embryo, monkey kidney, calf serum, undetected animal viruses, formaldehyde, embalming fluid, mercury (deadly toxin), and aluminum (a neuro-toxin). The manufacturers do not guarantee that they are safe or effective. During a four year span, an estimated 340,000 adverse reactions and 7,000 deaths occurred as a result of vaccinations. An adverse reaction can include fevers, uncontrolled high pitch screaming, seizures, paralysis, brain damage, rashes, voice changes, diarrhea, projectile vomiting, and death.

3. Vaccine manufacturers have lobbied to be protected from responsibility for the injuries that their products cause. A government fund was created but it has already paid out $522,000,000 in claims, with thousands more claims pending with an estimated liability of $1.7 BILLION for pre-1988 damages. Claims take as long as ten years to be processed and most are denied. The majority of those who are disabled are never compensated and rely on medical plans and social services for assistance.

4. The risk of future illnesses or immediate injury and death to your child "might" be overlooked if the benefits outweighed them. However, immunization doesn't appear to protect you from the disease and may even give it to you. For instance, of the 2,720 cases of measles reported in Ohio during 1989, 72% occurred in children who were vaccinated and pre-

sumed protected. In the medical journal, Clinical Infectious Diseases, (February, 1992, pp. 568-579), a study concluded that every case of polio in the United States since 1980 was caused by the vaccine. Lancet, the prestigious British medical journal reported (October 12, 1991) that children given a measles vaccine died in significantly higher numbers of common childhood diseases than children who did not receive the vaccine.

5. If you allow your child to be vaccinated, they will receive their first at birth, followed by six more at two months, five vaccinations at four months, and four more vaccinations at six months, with a total of 32 vaccinations by the time the child enters first grade. Our "normal" immune response is built up in stages via multiple mild sicknesses fought on the battle sites on our peripheral defenses. These immunizations are injected directly into the muscles of young and defenseless bodies.

6. Our country is the most thoroughly immunized in the world. In most countries, immunizations are optional. Here, they are enforced by the school systems, our social services, and our medical system. Parents who refuse to immunize their child are scolded, ridiculed, threatened, and harassed to force compliance. Yet, with all these vaccinations, our infant mortality rate is twenty-third in the world, worse than some third world countries! In 1950, before mass immunization, we were rated third best in the world. If immunizations are so great, why is our country so sick? If they are so safe and effective, why do they hide the facts, give us misinformation, and attempt to force vaccinations on us?

If you decide not to immunize your child, be prepared to be attacked and harassed by everyone from your mother-in-law to your family doctor. In order to withstand pressure from the family, doctors and school administrators, you need more information than I can give here. Purchase the book, Immunization Theory vs. Reality, by Neil Z. Miller, New Atlantean Press, P.O. Box 9638-925, Santa Fe, NM 87504.

I have not immunized either of my children nor am I immunized. My children and I are healthy. We have traveled all over the world without being bothered. Yet, in every school my children entered, I was told they must be immunized. When I objected, eventually I was given an exemption form, sometimes a religious exemption form. Occasionally, I was also required to get a letter from my minister verifying that it was against our religious principles. There are exemptions if you seek them. You may even have to join (as a subterfuge) the Church of Christian Science or the Universal Life Church (Modesto, California). There are also homeopathic immunizations that are safe. If this should be your choice, as soon as the decision is made, go to your county office and obtain a form that can be notarized by your Minister. Whatever you decide, I bless you and wish you luck.

CHILDREN'S ILLNESSES

Homeopathic medicines often work better for children than herbs due to their minute dosages. When using herbs, dilute them or give with fruit juices. Homeopathics are taken without any liquid.

Allergies	Alum cepa, Arsenican. For sneezing with burning, Arcenicum.
Bed Wetting	Arsenium, Causticen, Equisetan, Pulsatilla, Corn silk tea (1 tsp. per cup)
Bladder Infection	Apis, Berberry (when accompanied with pain in kidneys)
Boils	Apis, Arnica
Bronchitis	Aconite, Antimonium
Chicken Pox	Aconite Apis, Belladonna. Use in first stages.
Cold and Flu	Aconite, arsenium
Constipation	Nux Vomica. Very hard dry stool, Alumina.
Cradle Cap	Sulphur. Use 1 tbs. of lemon essential oil in 1 tbs. of almond oil.
Diaper Rash	Sulphur, ciarrihea arcenicum
Diarrhea	Arcenicum (with burning)

Ear Aches	Belladonna, Chamomile, Bellas cal cort Belladonna. For both early and recurring stages, Aconite.
Fever	Yarrow aconite, Chamomilla,
Headaches	Aconite, Belladonna
Immunization Side Effects	Apis (swelling; Belladonna (high fever); Hepar (when site is not healing).
Insect Bites	Lavender Oil
Lice	Lycopodium, skin lapsorumium. Use Lice Free essential oil blend for head Lice: Part hair with comb, apply to scalp, continue pulling all over. Prevention - add 20 drops to shampoo.
Measles	Acoulte Apis, Belladonna (with fever)
Medicines	Avoid baby aspirins. Use alcohol bath instead.
Pin Worms	Neem Enema, Cina
Pink Eye	Aconite - with discharge Argenitum
Poison Ivy	Phystox. Essential oil of tea tree.
Runny Nose	Arsenicum
Stomach Pain	Acoulte
Sunburn	Utica - Urens
Teething	Chamomille, Aconite, Impetigo, Antimonium
Tonsillitis	Barium Carb. Hepar Sulph yellow discharge
Vomiting	Antimonium. For gas & bloating, cycopodium
Warts	Thuja. Use essential oil of tagetes - apply on wart 3 times a day.
Whooping Cough	Antimonium tart

CHAPTER 5

YOUNG ADULTHOOD

TEEN YEARS

THE TEEN YEARS can be the most exciting and yet challenging time for parents. It is a time to be available, but not hold them too close. During these years they are in search of their individuality and an adversarial relationship is easy, but non-productive. Adolescence comes with a strong development of will, and forces a need to express themselves in the world. It is tough to stay in their confidence, support them, and yet provide guidance while gradually releasing them to their full self-reliance.

The age can bring uncertainty and awkwardness. The young adult begins to assert himself or herself, often rebelling and only wanting to do what they want. It is a time to test the world and their upbringing. This is the beginning of the Pitta lifecycle, a time when their bodies are transformed by rising hormone levels, turning their little bodies into well formed, vital adults. (This is also time for a good supplement therapy.) For some, acne occurs, creating problems with self-esteem. Acne is a metabolic imbalance, created by a lack of balance between the dietary intake of lipids (fats) and the body's capacity for assimilation. Because of poor breakdown due to too much heat in the body (created by hormonal changes), the fat deposits in the pores of the skin, which results in acne. Flax seed oils in tablet form are very beneficial. Vitamin E and vitamin A are excellent regulators and a Pitta reducing diet helps. At this age it is particularly difficult to work with their diet due to peer pressure and life "on the run". A good supplementation program is about all you can do sometimes.

Teens like to eat what they want, when they want. It is hard for them to "hear" anything related to a healthy diet. This is a time for parents to become their friend and to open your heart to them with patience and understanding. Many teens become more rebellious to demands from parents, but they can take some individual responsibility in creating a healthy diet and lifestyle for themselves. Support them by allowing them to help you in the kitchen. Take them to health food stores and fresh food markets and let them purchase foods that they would like to eat and/or prepare. Poor diet has a price; good diet has a reward. Let them know that they can trade their acne for a healthier eating pattern.

Also, as parents, be honest about your own experiences as a teenager. Health is not just about food, but also about healthy relationships, healthy finances, healthy communications, etc. This will allow them to see that you had similar problems yet were able to overcome them. Support them by being open and honest about these years. Don't pretend to have never experimented with drugs or had sex. If they see you as human and hear about your teen experiences, it will allow them to see your humanity. If they can feel safe to share their experiences with you, you become their confidant and advisor instead of an outsider, out of touch and unapproachable.

Many young females experience guilt, shame, and are uncomfortable with their menstrual cycle. This is a time to give support and closeness. A special celebration or ritual can be created to honor their menstrual cycle as it holds great strength, power, and creativity. The ceremony can be done with other females, rituals, prayers, and blessings, which gives the young woman a chance to know and understand the sacredness of life. It is a time to instill a profound reverence and respect for her ability to create life and to welcome the ancient feminine wisdom.

The same can be done for a young adult male entering puberty; the right of passage to manhood. Gather with friends in ritual for the young male to understand his focus and his responsibility for his role in relationships, family, society and the world. There are many good books available on this subject.

Peer Pressure

Teenagers need to look a certain way because of a desire to be accepted, to be the same, not wanting to be different. During these years, females especially become concerned with their weight, becoming anxious and skipping meals. Tell them that exercise + calories = weight change. To lose weight, exercise more. Your metabolism burns hotter (more calories) when stimulated by activity. A couch potato can gain weight just by looking at food. An athlete can eat anything and just burn it up. Good protein powder shakes, soy protein milks and rice milks all provide nutrition and are yet low in calories. One good healthy meal a day may be all you will be able to encourage them to do, which is usually dinner. To be especially effective, use all the secrets available from the previous chapter.

Alcohol and Drugs

These become great temptations because of peer pressure. With my teenagers, from early on, I allowed them to have parties at home, making very serious rules about drinking. I did not approve of drinking, but my feeling was that given the fact that they were probably going to drink anyway, it would be better for them to do it at home where they were safe and where they were supervised. The rule was that anyone who drinks does not drive home. Anyone can spend the night if they call home and inform their parents. Over the years no one got hurt, a few kids threw up, and at times my house was a big pajama party. My kids learned their tolerance and discovered moderation. Providing a safe space for them to experiment creates trust in you and in them. The more you fear their behavior, the more they will act it out. Drug problems are often the result of emotions that they are holding onto and not expressing.

In questioning over 100 teenagers and young adults, many expressed that they would have liked to have seen their parents "walk their talk," in everything that they expected of their children. Many parents want their children to behave in certain ways, yet they do things that they advised their children not to do. The teenagers see the hypocrisy in this. Our children are our best mirrors. "I saw my parents drink and drive lots of times" was often stated.

Teens and Sex

It is with great joy that my husband and I give couples detailed anatomy (i.e., how to find the G spot), take them through processes to shed the guilt and negative images, and offer them new perspectives to the spiritual experience that sacred sex can be. We urge parents to expand their sexual awareness by reading books, listening to tapes, or attending seminars. When you are comfortable with your own sexuality, you can truly be available to your child's questions about this great mystery. Teens can be embarrassed by their peers if they don't know about these things. They will truly appreciate having a parent who can give them up-to-date, enlightened information from a place of comfort. Unwanted pregnancy, sexual disease, and date rape are just a few of the problems that can be prevented through information and awareness.
Speak to them about the gift of being in a relationship, and how sexuality can be the ultimate ecstatic experience of love. This experience can bring awareness and healing. Make them aware of protection and safety.

YOUNG ADULTS AND HEALTH

Everyone comes to this earth to re-member and to fulfill his or her purpose in life. In Ayurveda, we call this purpose "Dharma". Dharma means virtue, attribute, and a course of conduct or disposition. Ayurveda believes that if we do not discover and accomplish our purpose, we must return again and incarnate to complete it. When we have completed any unfinished business (Karma) and have achieved enlightenment, we can choose not to return to the earth plane. One way that we can be lead towards discovering our purpose is by paying attention to what we enjoy, what we are attracted to or get excited about, or have a passion for. We will know our passion because we will get up early eager to do it and stay up late working on it. We would do it for free because it gives us such joy.

Many people of all ages feel a lack of purpose. A good friend of mine, Sandy Levy, works with people all over the world assisting them in finding their purpose. She always says, "When everyone on the planet is doing their purpose, there will be no sickness, unhappiness, crime or war. Everyone will be too busy doing what they love. We will truly have peace on earth." Her workshop involves a series of interactive processes through which each individual, young or old, will discover their purpose and exactly what form it will take in their life. When you are on purpose, your immune system more easily repels any sickness. Health is automatic.

Many young adults may not go to college and they begin floating in life without direction. Eventually, they will find themselves because life's experiences will slowly guide them on their way. We have created a society that does not offer the true support or guidance for young people to discover themselves. In times past, a young adult could become an apprentice to experience a trade or profession. Under the guidance of an experienced tradesman they could discover if the trade was for them. This is where a person could offer their gift that they had mastered to an interested youth.

In the past, young people worked in the family business, helping to support the family unit and gaining work experience. "Smith and Sons" illustrates this concept. When was the last time you saw an "and Sons" business? The tendency in young people is to search for freedom. But this unencumbered freedom is empty and lacks connection. If you discovered your purpose, could you really be free to do anything except embrace it? The price of freedom is responsibility (the ability to respond appropriately). Running away from your home, looking to get far away from family beliefs and traditions may look like freedom, but it is not. People run because the family structure did not provide that which they were looking for. They leave home empty, unsure of themselves. They begin to travel, looking for answers and working jobs with very little pay, stuck in survival. When you are lost in survival, accidents, injuries and sickness happen more frequently because you are not "connected" (to self, purpose, family, society, and spirit). Lack of connection may be the only disease there is.

It can be helpful that while in this questioning and searching period of life, that appropriate herbs and good nutrition are available. When you are under stress, you need nutritional support the most. A common problem with young people and health is their "rough and ready" approach. They will read about a concept within "health", such as raw foods, fasting, macrobiotic, strict vegetarianism, fruitarianism, and breatharianism and attempt to eat in that way without really understanding the concept and understanding the need for a transition diet. Often they go to the health food store and think the prices are too outrageous. Then they attempt to be a vegetarian with vegetables from Safe Way. Or they start a fast the day after they ate at McDonalds without any colon cleansing, drinking city water, while working a job. There are many ways to get in trouble, trying to be healthy. A little bit of knowledge can be dangerous.

COLLEGE YEARS

Most people who start college come straight from high school and are in that Pitta stage with lots of vitality, and a strong digestive system. It is easy to forget how sacred our body is and to take the physical body for granted, abuse it or mistreat it. The only time one pays attention to health is when we feel discomfort or pain. Even then, it is easy to ignore or suppress the symptoms (taking aspirin). Pay attention to your body. The minor things can be treated become ma- way of saying, nore a smoke investigate. before they jor. Pain is nature's "danger". You don't ig- alarm when it goes off. You

Going away from home to college is different for each individual. The Pitta type knows what they want and has an easier time with this new experience. Their focus is clear and they go into college with goals, which helps make the transition easier. Their knowing attitude allows them to move forward with surety and excitement, rather than getting caught up in distractions. For most individuals, going to college can be uncertain, but for the Pitta person the new energy and excitement makes the transition easier than for any other type.

The Vata type has a harder time because this personality likes change, but not too many changes. Too much new energy makes them spacey and ungrounded. They can be unsure of where they are going and the many choices available can create more uncertainty. It is easy for them to go into confusion and become scattered. They can change their major many times and constantly question their path. Even when they graduate, they won't be sure what to do. They will do best in areas that utilize their creativity.

Kapha's don't like change. Their home is their stability and anchor. They have the hardest time adjusting to college, and it is easy for them to get homesick. Many Kapha individuals end up back home without completing college, or transfer to a local college that they can commute to from home. Those that go away to college, stay in their dorms a lot, sleep long hours, going out only for meals and classes. They often pick a major early and stay with it.

For all types, at first, the excitement of a new life, new friends, new classes and a new sense of freedom is exhilarating. At last, no curfews or house rules and no one to tell you what to do or how to do it. You are making your own decisions and doing what you want. Shortly, all of this new excitement wears out. Having the responsibility of budgeting your own money, keeping a checkbook, paying bills, and keeping your grades up for grants or scholarships is sobering. The large campus and classrooms (filled with up to 300 students) produces its own stress. You realize you are now only a single person in the middle of a small scholastic city and that to remain here you are going to have to apply yourself, budget your finances, and be responsible.

Being away from home and your family, who have always been there to give you support and encouragement, can become overwhelming. At some point you start missing what you could not wait to get away from - Home! Cafeteria food becomes boring and mom or dad's cooking becomes something to dream about. They will really appreciate their family on their visits home.

To make it through school, the student must become confident and develop a plan of action that keeps them in touch with their Higher Self. Follow your passion towards your goal in life and that which brings you joy. The circumstances of life will be easier if you listen to your inner needs and communicate them to your peers and teachers. Most problems have their root in fear and non-communication. If you plan, schedule and follow through you can maintain a state of wellbeing during this stressful time. Good nutrition, the amount of sleep you get, good study habits, doing things that give you passion, and activities that are relaxing can all contribute to getting through the college years.

Monitoring your health is important because you are now responsible for yourself. In some cases, you may be paying for your medical care. But in any case, sickness interferes with your goals.

With all your new freedom, the temptation for drugs and alcohol can show up. Staying up late, parties and dating will all be vying for your limited time. As a young adult, if you choose to experience drugs or alcohol, be observant. Do you really enjoy the effect? How do you feel the next day? How is your concentration? Is it worth it? Are you willing to suffer the legal consequences if you get caught? Does it really add to who you are?

Cafeteria eating will offer many unhealthy choices. Unlimited amounts of soft drinks, desserts, fried foods, ice cream, milk and meats. All of which should be eaten in small quantities, if at all. There will be other more healthy choices that you can try to eat more of. Vegetables, fruits, grains, fish, legumes (beans) can be chosen more often and in greater amounts. Romaine and red leaf lettuce and other vegetables can often be picked out of a salad that contains largely iceberg lettuce (no nutrition). Meals and snacks purchased off campus can be healthy. A small refrigerator and hot plate in your room makes a small but complete kitchen where you can choose healthy additives to the cafeteria diet. Vitamins and minerals are your domain and herb tea bags can be carried to the cafeteria and made there.

I won't tell you to have or not have these experiences because everything has its use... and its abuse. People say that every culture had its mind-altering substances. But, historically, their uses were for inner searching, religious experiences or social bonding. Are you seeking to "get wasted" or are you searching for a "connection"?

Notice your usage patterns; do you have a drink or does the drink have you?

HERBS & ESSENTIAL OILS FOR COLLEGE STUDENTS

Aloe Vera (VPK=)	Antifungal, antibacterial, antiviral. Has laxative properties, soothes stomach irritation when taken internally, enhances burn and wound healing
Ashwagandha (VK-P+)	Tonic energizer, memory, muscular energy, nerve exhaustion, insomnia
Bilberry	Night blindness, visual disorders, anxiety
Borage (PK-V+)	Courage, uplifts a heavy heart, adrenal tonic, gland balancer
Brahmi (essential oil) (VPK-)	Clarity and ease
Chamomile (VP-Ko)	Soothes stress, anxiety, helps with sleepless nights, indigestion
Clove (KV-P+)	For toothaches, place drop of essential oil on gums
Echinacea (PK-V+)	Infections, cuts, wounds, improves digestion, regulates menses
Eyebright (PK-V+)	Eyestrain, minor irritation, allergies, watery and itchy eyes
Feverfew (PKV+)	Headaches, migraines, muscle tension, pain, menstrual problems, arthritis
Garlic (VK-P+)	Colds, flu, any disease or infection, enhances the immune system, improves circulation, lowers blood pressure
Goldenseal (PK-V+)	Infections, cuts, wounds
Ginger (VK-P+)	Motion sickness, nausea, vomiting, circulation, fever, indigestion

Ginkgo Biloba	Mental clarity, circulation, depression, headaches, memory, ringing in the ears, asthma, eczema, leg cramps
Ginseng (V-KPo)	Memory, increases energy, immune system enhancement, stress, strengthens adrenals
Gotu Kola (VPK=)	Mental clarity, strengthens nerves, decreases fatigue and depression, poor appetite, sleep disorders
Fennel (VPK=)	Abdominal pain, gas, flatulence, gastrointestinal tract spasms, indigestion, abscesses, PMS, hangover
ImmuniTea (VP-K+) (UniTea Herbs)	Colds, Flu, maintains healthy immune system
Mental ClariTea (VP-K+) (UniTea Herbs)	Helps with stress during finals
Peppermint Tea (PK-Vo)	Energy booster, digestion, headache
PuriTea (UniTea Herbs)	Detoxes, cleanses, purifies the blood
Rosemary (KV-P+)	Mental clarity, headaches, menstrual cramps, high and low blood pressure, digestion, circulation, dandruff
St. John's Wort (PK-V+)	Depression, insomnia, arthritis, viral infections, nerve pain (do not take with other anti-depressants)
Tea Tree (VPK=)	Disinfects and heals all wounds/ skin conditions, acne, athlete's foot, abscess, dandruff, candida, insect bites, herpes

Skullcap (PK-Vo)	Headache, anxiety, insomnia, fatigue, muscle cramps, stress, pain
Valerian (VK-P+)	Insomnia, anxiety, stress, calms muscle spasms, alleviates menstrual cramps, dysmenorrhea, migraine, flatulence
Yogi Tea (VK-P+)	Energy, aliveness, connection

ESSENTIAL OIL BLENDS FOR VARIOUS APPLICATION METHODS

(See Chapter 2)

Mental Clarity Blend
Basil
Eucalyptus
Camphor
Lemon
Lemongrass
Orange
Lemon

Relaxation Blend
Sandalwood
Geranium
Tangerine
Lavender
Chamomile (any)

Headache Free Blend
An Earth Essentials Florida product - see Resource List in back of book.

DIFFUSE OILS: In your room on an aroma therapy ring on a light bulb.

DO: Self massage per chapter 12.

AVOID: Caffeine, black tea, and excess soda.

CONTRIBUTED BY CHARISMA BYSTROM, SWEDEN (15 YEARS OLD)

"It's easy to become depressed and feel confused while having an active mind with lots of fantasy and looking for ego gratification such as sweet pop drinks, cigarettes, and alcohol. Find ways to channel these feelings; do gymnastics, exercise, yoga, bike ride, rollerblade, draw, paint, read, go bowling, t'ai chi, take walks with friends, and release emotions to a good friend."

CONTRIBUTED BY SAGE, LIGHT MILLER'S YOUNG ADULT APPRENTICE

"Life is a constant transformation. In America, the "young adult" is usually expected to complete a course of schooling or some other training structure to secure a good financial lifestyle. As I watched many friends enter this "main stream" lifestyle with little true passion, I decided to explore more options in a free-flowing, adventurous path more conducive to my creativity. I quickly found that there are many challenges to any path we choose. It is a very awesome thing to meet the challenges between freedom and discipline.

The first lesson I experienced is that surrendering to a healthy mind-body-spirit is a choice that will undeniably change everything that surrounds you for the better. Eating right is a good way to begin. There are often questions about finding a new way to eat that still satisfy taste, and are cost and time efficient. I found my information from a variety of sources, from the ages of 19 to 23.

Most people have vast misconceptions of what healthy eating entails. At first, it seems difficult to sift through all the information and define a new and individual diet, yet it is actually a very enlightening, exciting, and ongoing experience. For example, start looking at the ingredients in most packaged and grocery store foods and ask yourself...How do these ingredients effect my body? Here are some things to watch out for: food colorings, preservatives, high fructose syrups, carbonated drinks, processed flours, hydrogenated oils, most gelatin is made from pig hooves, high salt content, iodized salt, MSG, caffeine, sugar and syrup based juices (fruit is sweet enough on its own,) fried foods, synthetics, pesticides (organic food is best,) high fat content, chemicals (not often listed,) hormones (mostly in meat that is not free range,) meat, dairy and eggs from animals that have been fed meat and harmful foods and are treated cruelly, processed cheese, and spreads, etc. These are only a few of the destructive ingredients that modern society regularly consumes. Eventually, these toxins will build up in the body, setting up imbalances as well as probable future health problems that may be painful and costly.

Stated simply – we are natural beings meant to eat natural foods. Try eating foods that are fresh, natural, and cultural, home cooked or from a health food restaurant, fresh squeezed fruits and juices, and natural energy boosters. By eating more natural foods, I believe my mind is clearer and more creative, and I have discovered one of the real meanings of independence.

When I was 18-19 and on my own, it was easy to survive on fast and convenient food, yet I did not even know my options. Now that I have experienced a new variety of foods for the last four-and-one-half years, I would never eat my old way again. There are ways to eat tasty, healthy foods that save time and money. These are some ideas that my friends and I have used:

TASTE: Invest in a health food cookbook, have fun home cooking with a variety of natural herbs, use alternatives found in health food stores, check out juice bars and healthy restaurants, meet health conscious people and learn how to cook from them, research how other cultures cook, they often have mastered healthy tasteful food. (I had never eaten Thai or Indian food before I was twenty, now they are my favorites.)

TRADE: Don't be shy to offer a trade or skill for food. For example, I sing for a local health food restaurant for a good meal and tips. Also, I may have a friend cook me dinner in trade for a back rub. Sometimes, I will cook my friend healthy dinners in trade for music lessons.

SHOPPING: Search out a good food co-op or natural health food store that offers lower prices for large bulk orders. It is usually a fun, casual environment that is rich in knowledge from other health conscious people. Try buying inexpensive staple foods in large quantities like rice, millet, couscous, quinoa, beans, oats, lentils, peas, potatoes, dried fruits, nuts, and flours. When you shop, basically, look at prices closely and buy more of what is cost efficient. I have friends that either work part-time or stay in close contact with local organic farms and get a lot of veggies for free. Some people enjoy working at health food stores and get discounts on all groceries.

Eat what is available in the environment. For example, I live in Florida and usually handpick citrus, papaya, and mangos. A lot of people go fishing here as well. It is not hard to buy a few seeds or plants to grow in pots or to plant a small garden. As I started meeting people of like mind, we often organized potluck dinners where everyone would bring something healthy to eat (great fun, good source of new food ideas). Also, look at what else you spend money on. Could you make health more of a priority in your spending?

SAVE TIME: Start by observing where you spend most of your time such as watching far too much television, going to the bar or coffee house, sleeping for too long, having long meaningless conversations, etc. Become aware. Then PRIORITIZE. Place your health before anything else.

Cook large portions of healthy foods that you like (such as burritos or pasta, or pasta sauce), store in your freezer or refrigerator, and when in a hurry you simply heat the food and have a very nutritious, efficient meal. I almost always take my daily food with me in a backpack (some people use coolers). Pack all your un-spoilable foods the night before. When I have absolutely no time to cook and nothing prepared, I stop at my local health restaurant and get an inexpensive meal to go. There are also so many new quick foods available at health food stores like veggie burgers, tofu dogs, and organic dried soups (just add water). It only takes ten minutes to steam fresh vegetables. I like to make quick sandwiches with hummus spreads or fresh ground nut butters. Leftovers are completely underrated: I often cook a beautiful tasty meal for dinner and then have it for lunch the next day. For breakfast there are organic pancake mixes, oats, quinoa, or granola. Fresh fruits and vegetables are so fast and simple.

Even though this modern society is faster paced, it is very important to take time, chew your food well, and be in the moment when you are eating. This is vital for digestion and nutritional absorption. Time is not something that controls me; it is a tool that I use to organize what I want to experience within the cycles of the universe.

One thing that I have learned (and apprenticing with Light has reinforced) is that it takes experience to master anything. There is always more to learn. The most useful and beautiful thing about Ayurveda is that it shows people how to understand their specific body type. I am just now beginning to comprehend that health is not only a matter of going to the health food store, avoiding harmful substances, meditating, singing once in a while, bike riding, and occasionally referring to my herb book. I am learning how to restore and maintain balance within every aspect of my life, and this is the way to freedom. Keep asking questions and be gentle and know the truth is available. I have always imagined what the world would be like if more people chose a path which was more harmonic with themselves, others, and nature. Now is the time to choose this awareness. One of the lessons in this eternal song called life is, "*Knoweth Thyself*!"

CHAPTER 6

MATURITY AND THE AGING PROCESS

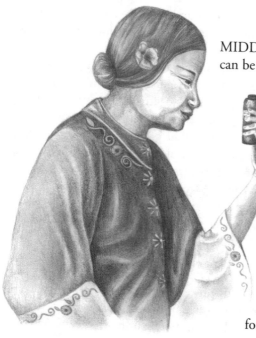

MIDDLE AND OLD AGE can be one of the highest experiences of a human being's life. By this time you have had many experiences in the world, have overcome many challenges and gained much awareness. Wisdom is our strength and our gift. Native people often looked to a council of elders for guidance. Instead of living out life in a retirement center, you can be a source of wisdom to the young. This cycle of life can be filled with joy and well being, especially when feeling healthy and strong.

Ayurveda acknowledges that this cycle has Vata qualities. This is a time when we begin to lose bone mass and our skin dries and wrinkles. This common sense science of Ayurveda offers us ways to extend and prolong life. As we become more of the Vata forces operating on us, we can counter them appropriately and postpone the effects of aging. We can begin by examining our thoughts and attitudes. Our thoughts can be one of the main causes of our aging process. Fear of becoming old and ill will be manifested in our bodies. "As we think, so shall we become". Our thoughts create our reality and this can be proven by scientists. In Deepak Chopra's book, "Quantum Healing", he relates that scientists documented how a selected group of retirees reversed the aging process in all measured parameters by simply reliving an enjoyable part of their past for two weeks. By beginning to change our thinking, we can age gracefully. As the individual becomes the observer of his own life and begins to take a different point of view relative to situations and actions that no longer works for them, health begins to happen. The knowledge of the universe is ours and when we take the time to tap into that source of knowing, we have an opportunity to slow down aging.

There are many scientific studies that prove that our thoughts affect our physical bodies, therefore, our thinking must also have a response on our aging process. Negative thoughts, confusing thoughts, and fear-based thoughts, which usually have nothing to do with the present moment, are all present at this time. Aging begins to happen because the physical body can no longer keep up with all that is going on. Our bodies are made of the same components as the universe. When we are aging and dying, we are missing the life force that is available to us through this process. As we let go of old beliefs that no longer serve our life, we begin to slow down the process of aging. Our thinking process is forever interfering with our physical body. The immune system has to integrate into our body over a billion cells every heart beat, and our thoughts are forever interfering with this process.

Our organs are created to live over 300 years when given the right nourishment. As we become older, our hormone and enzyme production, assimilation, and transportation of nutrients slow down. The mirrors that we have of old age are people taking pills, in wheel chairs, hospitals, retirement homes, arthritic joints and many other problems. One needs to begin to examine their nutrition and the concept of eating foods for the lifecycle that they are in and that are the most appropriate for the body's composition. This requires not only paying attention to the physical body, but also looking at the quality of life we are living and begin to treat it as a disease.

To age gracefully into a beautiful mature life, one must begin to take things a step at a time. Bring to each breath a sense of awareness of the body that is mediating between the mind and the body, stimulating the body with aliveness, joy and the possibility of reaching out to unlimited potentials, following the law of its true nature.

STRESS

As we allow the illusion of this existence to become real in our life, we become the prisoners of our own life. We become the stress created by our own ego mind and take on the belief system of the mass consciousness that is the core domain at this time on earth. As we buy into the belief that life is stressful, we begin to forget our true nature which is Divine and lose sight of what we came here to do.

Stress creates a short circuit in our physical body caused by becoming absorbed in the everyday reality. The individual's negative thought puts them out of context with the true essence of their being. When we begin to live in the world with a sense of trust and detachment to the outcome rather than pushing for our desires and wants, we begin to become free of stress.

When we push for our desires, wants, and point of view and having to be right, we become consumed by these thoughts and stress takes over, losing our true sense of being. This curbs aliveness in the tissue. This does not mean we need to become meek or dormant in life, it simply means that we speak from a state of consciousness of trust and alignment with the outcome. You begin to see the perfection of the experience, to be attuned to the will of the universe and the lesson. This form of thinking is freeing and brings forth to the individual a stress-free life and a glimpse of peace. It is in the letting go that we receive our gifts.

As we approach the year 2000, our fast paced life presents us with overwhelming choices and challenges, as well as opportunities for stress at any given moment. Fortunately, there is a wide range of measures covered in this book which can help with stress reduction and prevention.

MENOPAUSE

The pharmaceutical industry has created a "disease" out of a normal aging process. Many languages don't even have a word for menopause because, historically, the transition produced few effects or discomfort. It was a reward, a freedom. We have been programmed and it has become part of our belief system that we will suffer horribly without estrogen therapy.

For most women at this time of life, their children are grown and have left the "nest". This brings a new sense of freedom for the mature female. Whenever possible, this is a time to explore what is next for this wise woman ready to give to herself, becoming a radiant light that gives her wisdom to the world.

The opportunity is for a woman to begin to rediscover herself after years of managing a household and raising children. A time for her to find this treasure that she accumulated through raising a family. As we begin to mature, our body is no longer growing and we need less quantity and more quality. Our food supply today is filled with chemicals that are detrimental to our health. As our bodies get older, our elimination system becomes less effective. We fare much better without these toxic burdens by eating organic foods.

A woman who understands and sees this concept begins to take care of herself and to maintain her youth and her vitality by feeding her physical body the ingredients needed for the estrogen level in her body. Normally in a healthy woman, the adrenals pick up the job of the ovaries. In this society we often suffer from adrenal insufficiency due to stress. Weak adrenals and poor nutrition produce menopause symptoms. The Divine Mother Earth has blessed us with many plants to nourish and replenish ourselves through the process of rebuilding our adrenals and smoothing the transition.

Possible changes that a woman experiences during this turbulent period can be dryness, sweats, anxiety, heart palpitation, sleep disturbances, headache, lack of sexual desire, fatigue, weight gain, gas and bloatedness. None of these are necessary if you take care of yourself. Begin to educate yourself by reading books to learn the natural approach to this process. Take time to meditate, address any anger or fear based thoughts, and participate in activities that reduce stress. Begin breathing exercises, center your focus on yourself, and listen to the power within. As you are able to take care of yourself, you are able to enter into these years with ease. You may even become a teacher; an example of what is possible during this wonderful transition.

HERBAL ALLIES FOR MENOPAUSE

Note: V=Vata (Air)   P=Pitta (Fire)   K=Kapha (Water & Earth)

ALFALFA (Medicago Sativa):
Extremely nourishing herb (caution: may increase hemorrhaging); good for all tissues of the body, rich in calcium and magnesium. PK-V+

ALOE VERA GEL (Spp.):
Specific for maintaining youthfulness of the reproductive organs. VPK=

ASHWAGANDHA (Withania Somnifera):
Tonic; rejuvenator. The ginseng of Indian medicine. Lack of sleep; sexual debility. Excellent for the mind. VK-P+

BHRINGARAJ (Elicipta Alba):
Chinese name - Han Lian Cao. Prevents gray hair; very high in minerals. Highly astringent and rejuvenescent herb. VPK=

BLACK COHOSH (Cimifuga Racemosa):
Helps regulate menstruation, especially good for relieving cramps. Clinically proven to be effective for relieving menopausal problems such as hot flashes. PK-V+

BORAGE (Borago Officinallis):
Helps build all tissues of the female organs. Slows down the aging process. PK-V+

CINNAMON (Cinnamon Zeylanicum):
Excellent for blood circulation; good for erratic periods. VK-P+

DAMIANA (Tunerra Aphrocisiacia):
Sexual vitality stimulant. K-VoP+

DANDELION (Taraxacum Off.):
Rich in plant hormones; high in minerals. Especially nourishes the liver. PK-V+

DHAVANA:
Excellent for any female disturbance; cancer prevention; yeast infection. VPK-

DONG QUAI, DANG GUI, TANG KUEI
(Angelica Sinensis): Supports estrogen production. Most commonly used around the world for female problems. VK-P+

DEVILS CLAW (Oplo Nax Horridum):
Helpful for hot flashes; sore joints; diabetes (stabilizes blood sugar). PK-V+

FALSE UNICORN (Chamaelirium Luteum):
A profound ovarian and uterine tonic. Excellent for women who flood during menopausal years. VK-P+

FENUGREEK (Trigonella Fornumgracoum):
Improves digestion; nourishes glands; balances blood sugar. VK-P+

FLAX SEED (Linum Usitatissium):
Increases production of hormones. An excellent laxative. V-KoP+

GARDEN SAGE (Sage Off):
Excellent for hot flashes, emotional swings and menstrual cramps. KV-P+

GERANIUM - ROSE (Palargonium Ordoran):
Balances the hormones. A cooling herb. PK-V+

GINGER ROOT:
As a tea, warms and nourishes the entire pelvis. VK-P+

GINSENG (Pawas Quonque Folium):
Balances the hormones, and helps relieve menopausal problems. V-PKo (except for PK in excess)

GOKSHURA (Tribulusterrestis):
Increases female vitality. Excellent for kidney and bladder problems. VP-Ko

GOTU KOLA (Hydiocotlye Asiatica):
Rich in minerals. Excellent for the mind. A rejuvinative herb. (Do not take with an overactive thyroid.) VPK=

GROUNDSEL (Senecio Vulgaris):
Helps with nausea. (Use only flowers and leaves in tincture.) PK-V+

HOPS (Humulus Lupulus):
Excellent sedative. Helps produce estrogen. PK-V+

HORSETAIL (Equisetum Armense):
Helps reverse osteoporosis; reduces bloating and fatigue. High in minerals. PK-V+

JASMINE FLOWERS (Jasminun Glawdiforum):
Uterine cleanser. Increases love and compassion; helps the mind become more receptive. PK-V+

JATAMASI (Aroka Rasemosa):
Hormone balancer; high phytoestrogen. VK-P+

LADY MANTLE (Alchemilla Vulgaris):
Nourishes the uterus; excellent for flooding. VPK

LICORICE (Glycyerhita Glabia):
Hormone balancer; anti-inflammatory. VP-K+

LIFE ROOT / GOLDEN RAGWORT
(Senecio Auteus): Female regulator; use in small doses for two weeks. VP_K+

LOTUS SEED (Nelumbo Nucifera):
Calms the mind and gives spiritual understanding. An astringent. Excellent for flooding. Heals and prevents tumors; a sexual stimulant. PV-K+

MOTHERWORT (Leonorius Cardiaca):
Eases stress, anxiety and insomnia. Menstrual regulator. PK-V+

NETTLES (Uridica Dioice, Urtica Urens):
Immune system supporter; strengthens bones; helps prevent cancer. Rehydrates vaginal tissue. PK-V+

OATSTRAW (Avena Sativo):
Stabilizes blood sugar; helps blood vessels be more elastic; nourishes the nerves. VK-P+

PRIMROSE (Primula Vulgaris):
Increases estrogen production; balances hormones. PK-V+

RED CLOVER (Trifolium Protense):
Cancer curative; blood purifier; calms anxiety and increases energy. PK-V+

REHMANNIA (Rehmannia Glutimosa):
Good for irregular menstruation; helps lubricate tissue; increases vitality. PV-K+

RED RASPBERRY LEAF (Rubus Spp.):
Hormone balancer; relieves menstrual cramps; regulates cycle. Astringent. PK-V+

ROSE FLOWERS (Rosa Spp.):
Female tonic; menstrual regulator; relaxant and coolant. VPK=

SAFFRON (Crocus Sativus):
Regulates cycle. Promotes tissue growth and vitality. VPK=

SARSAPARILLA (Similax Spp.):
Supports progesterone; sexual stimulant; rejuvenates the female organs. VP-Ko

SAW PALMETTO (Serenoa Serrulata):
Tonic; sexual stimulant. Prevents atrophy of ovaries, vaginal and bladder tissues. V-PK+

SHATAVARI / TIAN MEN DONG (Asparagus Raeemosus):
One of the best female tonics. Rejuvenates all female organs. Excellent for stiff joints. PV-K+

SHEPHERD'S PURSE (Capsella Bursapastoris):
Good for flooding. Astringent. PK-V+

SKUNK WEED (Syumplocarpus Foetidus):
Nerve relaxant; helps with cramps. VPK-

SNAKE WEED / BISTORD ROOT
(Polygonum Historia): Anti-inflammatory; strong astringent; helps with flooding and spotting. PK-V+

SWEET BRIAR (Rosa Camina):
Tonic; regulates the cycle. VPK+

TRIKATU (Ayurvedic Formula):
(Ginger, Black Pepper, Pippallo) - Strengthens and energizes female organs. VK-P+

VALERIAN (Valeriana Spp.):
Helps with cramps, pain, and for grounding. An excellent relaxant. Mixes well with magnesium. VK-P+

VETIVER (Viteria Zizanoid):
Helps exhausted female energies; keeps you grounded and from going out of control. Helps sagging skin and stretch marks. VP-K+

VITEX / CHASTEBERRY (Vitex Agnius-Castus):
Pituitary support; hormone stimulant. (Caution: lowers sex drive in men.) VPK-

CHAPTER 7

THE CAUSES OF ILLNESS

THIS BOOK IS CHOCK FULL of fixes for common health problems, but we all know that prevention is better than cure. We "prevent" having to rebuild our car engines by changing the oil every 3,000 miles; much cheaper. Our medical system is full of expensive high priced "fixes" (i.e. triple bypass surgery) when simple health practices (i.e. good heath) would "prevent" heart attacks. A close look at the causes of illness could take some of the mystery out of "why we get sick?" The following is a partial list that will cover the major causes, although other causes may be factors.

POOR DIET: Our country's food supply is grown on soil which has been farmed for up to 300 years. Certain crops can deplete the soil in just a few years (i.e. tobacco). We have been able to maintain production (but not nutrient content) by using fertilizers which stimulate growth but don't add nutrients.

Alternative Choice: Eat organic foods raised on farms which organically build their soil. Increased demand will create more supply and lower the price.

ENVIRONMENT: We have created a dangerous chemical environment and support an under-regulated chemical industry. 2,000,000,000 (BILLION) pounds of pesticide are sprayed on our food and water supplies. In addition, we are using millions of pounds of herbicides and fungicides. We even pay pest control people to spray our yards and inside our homes. Big money politics keeps these poisons legal, many pesticides which we still allow were banned in Israel, where the breast cancer rates have dropped dramatically. Even the banned chemicals (DDT) are still produced here, shipped to Mexico, etc. and used on crops which are transported back to this country. As well, two-thirds of our water supply is contaminated.

Alternative Choices: (a) Buy organic foods (you vote with your money for what you want more of in the world); (b) Buy mountain spring water or use a water purification system; (c) Do not spray your yard or home - save money - find healthy alternatives.

OVERCONSUMPTION: Most of us overeat and over consume. Two-thirds of Americans are overweight. Many diseases are caused by excesses; excess salt = hypertension and hardening of the arteries; excess fat = heart disease; excess alcohol = liver disease; excess sugar = hypoglycemia and diabetes. Laboratory animals who are fed less calories live longer than those fed on amounts comparable to the average American.

Alternative Choice: Eat less. Chew more. Stop eating before you are full. Eat a light breakfast consisting of fruit and whole grains. Skip high caloric deserts, opt for more fruit.

OVER PROCESSING OF FOOD: Over ONE BILLION pounds of food additives are added to our foods each year - that is over five pounds per person per year. Food coloring (red dye #2), preservatives (nitrates, BHT), taste enhancers (MSG), and many more dangerous chemicals have become part of our food supply. Overcooking, freezing, bleaching, canning, packaging, milling, refining, fast foods, and hydrogenation all remove nutrients from food and contribute to illness. Over 50% of all meals are eaten away from home in restaurants.

Alternative Choices: Prepare foods at home. Avoid processed and refined foods, eat whole fresh, organic food. Season your own foods. Buy a cook book.

ILLNESSES CAUSED BY MEDICAL MISTAKES: When you turn yourself over to doctors trained to treat illness with drugs and surgery, several unfortunate occurrences may happen: botched or unnecessary surgeries and complications, contra-indicated medications given for wrong conditions, adverse reactions caused by drug mixtures, allergic and anaphylactic shock reactions, injuries, illnesses and deaths caused by radiation and chemotherapy treatments. All of these account for one-third of hospital admissions.

Alternative Choices: Seek alternative practitioners for all but emergency care, including herbalists, chiropractors, natural M.D.'s, osteopaths, massage therapists, etc. Take control of your own health, read books, get second opinions, and don't trust anyone just because they have a degree.

LACK OF PURPOSE: When we are out of touch with our higher self and when we feel separated from God and love, our metabolism, immune system, and thoughts are all operating at a lower, slower frequency. We are more susceptible to illness. Illness can be a "distraction" from our discomfort. When we discover our talents (things which we do well and which give us joy), we can offer them in service to humanity. The joy and connection which purpose creates increases our immune response, dispels illness and negativity and produces health.

Alternative Choice: Search out your purpose and find the appropriate form to express it.

FAILURE OF THE MIND-BODY CONNECTION: This would include the making of poor choices in diet, lifestyle, and getting caught up in negative thinking. Alternative choices in diet and lifestyle are listed above. Negative thinking produces stress, anger, shame and fear. These emotions disrupt our metabolism, digestion and immune function and age us. Thoughts and the feelings they produce are a primordial cause of disease; toxins, deficiencies, etc. only supply fuel to the fire of negative thought patterns which are destructive down to the organ, tissue, cellular and chemistry level.

Thoughts of separation block the healing and regenerating force of divine intelligence. Auto-immune disease is what is making us sick today. Our bodies are attacking themselves. Arthritis, MS, cancer, and heart disease are caused by defects in our immune system. This is the result of unconscious thoughts; no being would "consciously" destroy self. A darkness, a blockage, a forgetting takes place at all levels, "as above, so below". A light, an opening, an awakening reveals the deepest truth of our divinity and begins the process of deactivating our self-destructive thoughts.

Attitudinal healing is when a stronger thought of higher vibratory rate deactivates a negative thought which has been embraced in the cellular chemistry at the DNA level. Tarpana is an Ayurvedic ceremony which transforms our fear based unforgiving thoughts to recognition of innocence and love. Meditation is an Ayurvedic practice of letting go of the world's thoughts and merging with the universal mind. Mantra is the Ayurvedic science of using primordial sound to raise the vibratory nature of the body into resonance with the cosmos.

Using these tools we can rebuild our bodies, heal any disease process, rejuvenate ourselves, and become unaffected by the disharmony of the world. We can "dwell in the world, but be not of it". Our identification is with things eternal, universal, and unchanging. Meditation and mantra are like safe harbors where, daily, our ships (bodies) can return after excursions into the turbulence, to rest, repair, and restock. Peaceful thoughts and harmonious resonance are what sustain us.

Deepak Chopra tells the story of researchers who were studying heart disease in a population of rabbits fed high cholesterol diets. Only one group showed no incidence of coronary heart disease and it was discovered that the only difference in the groups care was that the attendant feeding this group took time to stroke each rabbit every day. Love and affection created an enzyme that dissolved cholesterol. Ayurveda gives us tools to do this with ourselves. Healing is already within us. We just need to release it. No poison can harm us when we are connected to source, and no diet can heal us if our chemistry is bound up with self destructive thoughts.

Alternative Choices: Connection to purpose, run with a positive and supportive crowd, read positive books.

Conclusion

Information is power. Knowledge creates the opportunity for change. To be free of illness requires taking personal responsibility for our choices. Wellness is a possibility but you must act. Many of your new choices will cost you money in the short run (natural foods, herbs, supplements, natural physicians), but they will save you in the long run. Health cost savings, less lost time from work, and reduced medication costs can drop health insurance premiums. Save money by eating at home, growing some of your own food and experiencing greater productivity by doing your purpose.

PHYSICAL IMBALANCES

Physical illness can come about due to environment, diet, lack of exercise, and contagious dis-ease. As has been explained previously, it is important for each body type to create a routine which works with their schedule. It is extremely important to do this in order to reap the benefits of good health, endurance, agility, flexibility and strength.

Lack of Exercise

The history of exercise goes back thousands of years. In the third century B.C., Bhramin physicians practised natural therapeutics which was a main ingredient for perfect health. Daily exercise is an act of taking responsibility for your physical health. Yoga originated in India with many postures modeled after the stretches of animals, while Tai Chi in China had their therapeutic motions prescribed by priests for pain relief and other ailments. The ancient Greeks had temples of healing and their God, "Aessculapius" had shrines built for healing.

Lack of exercise does more than weaken our muscles and make us flabby. Muscle movement is what clears out our lymphatic (waste removal) system. Without movement, lymph stagnates like a slow flowing swamp. The cells are surrounded by waste and toxins and they begin to suffer.

Exercise causes calcium and minerals to be stored in the bones for future use. We are prone to osteoporosis later in life if we do not maintain our exercise. Two-thirds of our metabolism takes place in our muscular system (after digestion). If our muscles are weak, this translates as low metabolism and lowered immune system. All things are connected and exercise is directly connected to metabolic and immune health.

Environment

Today, throughout the world there are illnesses which have never been known before. We pollute our waters using chemicals and pesticides which we know very little about. We call ourselves civilized. Yet many of the ways in which we treat our environment is bringing forth many types of illnesses.

Vikriti (imbalances in the body) can only happen when the immune system is weakened. Humankind's immune systems are becoming more and more depressed, thereby allowing illnesses to manifest. We poison ourselves by eating foods which are chemically altered, as well as being surrounded by environmental pollutants from air, water and the food supply.

Our environment is increasingly overwhelmed by many chemicals; from foods grown with fertilizers, pesticides, herbicides, plastics, oil spills, toxic dumping, and industrial pollutants. We have taken the earth for granted. As inhabitants of this earth, we should each take responsibility to care for this planet, respect the earth once again, and become its caretakers. It is time to accept responsibility for the gift that has been given to us by The Earth Mother.

When there is no listening and there is a lack of cooperation, an imbalance occurs. We have collectively forgotten the natural laws of nature and have replaced them with industry and commerce. Disharmony does not only affect some individuals, it has an effect on all inhabitants of the planet. With the growing use of pesticides, herbicides and chemicals of all types, we continue to pollute in ever greater amounts. What we put in the air, water and earth becomes part of the food chain. The higher you are on the food chain, the more concentrated toxins become. We are at the top. We will suffer effects first and the strongest.

When each individual begins to understand that we are no different than the universe, healing can begin within ourselves. We can then begin healing our families, communities, and the world. As we individually achieve balance we will be given the steps to heal our environment. When we feel good, we have more energy and this creates a sense of clarity and guidance that we will be able to apply to the elemental forces on this earth. The state of our perfect health will assist us in discovering how to begin to do the same with the environment.

When we open ourselves to receive guidance our pranic sheath is strengthened. We will be able to fight the dis-eases of today. Many of the dis-eases we have in our world represents the condition of our state of mind and our values. Change our mind about our values, take the necessary action, and the world will be changed.

We must begin to tap other resources besides nuclear and fossil fuels and find better ways to handle our waste products. We are reaching a peak, and it is time for us to pay attention, set new priorities with consideration for the Whole, and take charge.

- Everything that we need to know has been given and the time has come for us to begin applying the laws.
- Eat low on the food chain. Vegetarians live longer.
- Buy organic. Support the organic farmers and merchants. We vote with our dollars. If you buy inorganics, you are voting for more chemicals in the earth, air and water..
- Travel less, share rides, buy more fuel efficient cars, refrigerators, water heaters, etc. Use less electricity.
- Prepare your own food. Then you know what you are eating and voting for.
- Recycle. Use less.

The same way we need to clean our external environment (nature), we need to periodically clean our internal environment. Pancha Karma is a seasonal house cleaning of all the body systems to get rid of Ama and Vikriti (more later).

Diet

It seems that many people beyond the age of 40 experience one disease after another. It may be diabetes, high blood pressure, rheumatism, arthritis, asthma, heart disease, or cancer. Yet, most of this disease can be prevented with diet. Unfortunately, very few people are interested in paying attention to what they consume. Mostly they only seek out the pleasure they get to experience through their taste buds by eating foods prepared by others, i.e., Baskin Robbins 31 flavors, Heinz 57 varieties, Kentucky Fried Chicken, 17 Herbs & Spices, etc.

Charak - The ancient physician, said, "The life of all living things is food; complexion, clarity, voice, growth, strength and the intelligence are all established in food".

He also said, "One must not *even* take light and easily digestible food in excess of bodily requirements or after the appetite has been satisfied. Foods that are hard to digest should not be taken every day but when eaten, they should be a small part of the meal. Excessive poor quality food is the cause of more Vikriti (imbalance, dis-ease) than environment or contagions. In later chapters we will learn more about correct use of food. Basically, we should eat to live. . . NOT live to eat!!

Contagious Diseases

If we take time to build our immune systems, contagious dis-eases cannot enter, because the body is strong. A balanced system resists dis-ease. We have 3 types of immunity; Passive, Active and Innate.

Passive immunity involves the transference of antibody (defense) mechanisms from mother to child, while still in the womb (via placenta) or during lactation. This presents a good reason not to be born in a test tube, instead to be breast fed as long as possible, by as many women as possible. For a brief period of time (1950-1990) breast feeding was discouraged by a combination of scientific arrogance and formula company propaganda (advertising). We can assume that many people raised during this era lack some passive immunity.

Active or Acquired immunity comes from being exposed to and surviving a virus or bacterial infection, by which process the body develops a specific immunity to that organism. You get measles, mumps, or chicken pox, you get sick, you recover, and you never get it again...even if exposed. Mothers used to take their well children to visit friends or relatives with chicken pox - to get it over with. They say garbage men never get sick because they handle everyone's germs. So don't isolate yourself. The American Indian population suffered horrible losses (90%) from common diseases (mumps, measles) that had been bred in the unsanitary conditions of medieval Europe, then transported 3,000 miles to an isolated people.

Innate immunity is activated when you are exposed to an organism for which you have no passive or acquired immunity. Your defense is based on your general health. Immune strength, speed of immune reaction, and reserve energies are all important. A person whose health is compromised by nutritional deficiencies, emotional or mental stress, allergies, addictions, or exposure to elemental extremes will suffer more and take longer to construct an immune response to an invading organism than a person in good health.

Doshic imbalances will increase stresses and slow your immune response. We are all born with strengths and weaknesses. Another translation of Dosha is "fault" or "Crack" (like an earthquake fault). Doshic imbalances open the cracks (weakness) in our constitution. That is where AMA (waste) can be deposited or disease can settle. Disease loves waste. You find more bacteria in a swamp than in a mountain stream. Staying in balance seals up your faults and keeps waste and disease out. If you are born with a strong constitution, the Doshas can increase to any extent with no symptoms. If your constitution has it's weaknesses and your Dosha's are out of balance you will surely have symptoms.

In conclusion, the best way to keep free from contagious disease is to keep your Doshas balanced, eat a natural, organic nutrient rich diet and keep your life on purpose.

EMOTIONAL IMBALANCES

Negative Emotions

All negative emotions come from the same place as positive emotions; the mind. Our thoughts come from the interpretation of our own experiences. Since both positive and negative thoughts come from the same place, it must be a matter of training to cancel thoughts that do not produce the results we desire. We came to this earth to heal, to remember, to grow, and to expand. Louise Hays, in her book, shows us how emotional dis-eases attack the different parts of our body, while corrective thoughts (affirmations) can produce positive results.

Relationships

Relationships are where we act out our unforgiven thoughts, guilts and unexpressed emotions. Everyone in the world is in some relationship with co-workers, friends, love interests or family. When the mind is in a Rajasic or Tamasic state of mind, there is a tendency for relationships to cause stress, entanglement, or ill health. In order to have health, one must have harmony in relationships. Whatever we did not work out in our childhood, we continue to work out in our present day relationships. We will attract in present time those people who are similar or will re-act similarly to the people whom we struggled with in our youth. It is not what happens in the relationship that we can transform, it is our thoughts and feelings about the happenings. What we think they mean is what we can examine. When we look at relationships as a learning experience, it is easier to let go of expectations and negative emotions.

Keep a diary of your inner most thoughts regarding your work relationships, love relationships, and other support relationships. This can be insightful. It offers the opportunity of examining your thoughts to see if they serve or harm. Are they Rajasic thoughts of control and domination, Tamasic thoughts of fear, resignation and isolation, or Sattvic thoughts of compassion.

Ayurveda says the way out of this illusory mess is to take back all of the projections about yourself and others. To ground yourself in that which is true. When you can see the innocence of your brother and sister knowing that they are stuck in the same illusion, knowing that they have been lost behind a mask in the cycle of guilt and attack, you can open yourself to compassion and take back the thoughts you have about this crazy illusion. Forgiving them provides the possibility of forgiving yourself. They are as innocent as you are. You both have been lost in Maya and a deeper truth leads to the way home. We are all one. We are Cosmic Intelligence.

ADDICTIONS

Definition: Any substance, use or behavior which is detrimental to realizing the True Self; usually requiring repetition, with the emphasis in acquiring a momentary sensation, experience, feeling or thrill rooted in the senses.

Addictions are the cause of many imbalances leading to dis-ease and self destruction. In the west we are not only inclined to alcohol, tobacco and coffee, but also junk food, drugs, allopathic medicine, and thrills (adrenaline). This is because our society is based on fear. We are afraid of getting close to our true self, expressing feelings, and speaking our truth. It is easier to cover up and hide our feelings behind addictive behavior. The way out of this is to begin to express ourselves and to create freedom from our anxiety and depression.

Alcohol

Alcoholism is not the same as drunkenness. A person may get drunk once in a while but that does not make them an alcoholic. Some people drink to get comfortable in order to socialize, to experiment, to show off. Yet an alcoholic drinks because they must, some people even dislike it, yet they are dependent upon it.

Alcohol is a depressant, affecting the control center of the brain so an intoxicated person may behave in ways that are usually re-strained by self-control. They are likely to be disoriented and con-fused. Prolonged drinking leads to serious effects like delusion, trem-ors, mental confusion, liver damage, etc. Treatment of alcoholism includes care of the physical body as well as of the emotions. Alco-holism can promote weight gain or loss, depending on the body type, and causes sleep disturbances, accelerates fear and anger. All addictions are detrimental to health. Alcoholism triggers psycho-logical-physiological problems which create a greater craving for more alcohol.

Ayurveda tends to see alcoholism as a dis-ease of the mind and emotions; a failure of intellect, a loss of Dharmic path. A person who is "on purpose" will not fall into addictions.

Kaphas tend to handle alcohol best, Pittas should use modera-tion or abstain, and Vatas can benefit from a small serving of wine before dinner to increase appetite.

Food Addictions

When we eat the same foods every day we can become addicted, to the allergic response our body has to the food. In our culture people often become addicted to the allergic reaction that their body produces in response to milk (or dairy). Adult humans sometimes find themselves drinking 4-8 glasses a day of a food especially formulated for growing baby cows. They say, "I love milk, when I get tired it gives me energy". A more accurate description might be, "My body craves the substance I am addicted to. When my energy level drops, drinking milk stimulates my immune system to mobilize (adrenals). I feel a surge of energy as my body prepares to defend itself". The body accustoms itself to cycles of craving and satisfying that craving; much like a cigarette smoker or crack addict. Suspect anything you crave or eat repetitively. The foods we ate frequently in childhood sometimes seem most desirable. To change the pattern of our diet takes time and mental strength (determination).

Today our diets are in the hands of commercial interests and advertisers. Foods can be medicine or poison. In order to have good health, pay careful attention to your diet. Keeping a diet diary can clue you in to repetitive eating patterns. Eating is usually so automatic. Daily use of the Diary allows you to see exactly what you are eating and how often. Also, if any undesirable symptoms are associated with the food, i.e., peanut butter at 3 pm; headache at 4 pm.

Tobacco

It is a dangerous narcotic, more addictive than cocaine. The Native Americans originally used wild tobacco at a meeting or gathering to take members on a spiritual journey. This is due to its hallucinogenic effect when used occasionally. It was a crime against the tribe to smoke habitually because you were not able to join the group in the hallucinatory experience. Habitual use kills the hallucinogenic effect.

Many tobacco companies have added additional nicotine to make it more addictive. They also add a variety of other substances for various effects including; clary sage because it is euphoric, menthol from mint because it is cooling, and salt peter to cause the cigarette to continue to burn even when not being puffed on. Salt peter had been used in the manufacture of gun powder and added to food of military personnel to decrease libido (fearful of homosexuality). Because of these additives, cancer rates in smokers are much higher in the U.S.A. than in Europe (no additives). Thousands of deaths occur each year due to fires caused by cigarettes which continue to burn when a smoker has fallen asleep. Smoking will be worse for Vata and Pitta and can be better tolerated by Kapha.

Ayurveda does not recommend regular tobacco use, but uses many herbal smoking mixtures in treatments.

Coffee

The United States ranks highest for the consumption of coffee. Americans drink over 500 million cups daily. Other leading countries are Brazil, France, Great Britain, Italy, Japan and West Germany. The average person drinks for the stimulating effect it produces. There are people who drink up to 20+ cups per day.

This drink causes insomnia, weakens adrenals, creates heart problems, peptic ulcers and weakens the pancreas. The cerebral vessels are constricted by caffeine.

Always work to cut down your intake of coffee. Cardamom and coriander can be added to the blend as an antidote to the caffeine. Kaphas are the only type which do well with small amounts of coffee.

In General

Vatas are more addicted to pain killers, Pittas become addicted to substances that fuel aggressive behavior, and Kaphas become addicted to food and substances which isolate them (such as marijuana and downers).

CHAPTER 8

HEALTHY EATING

HISTORICALLY, MAN HAS USED SPICES not only for flavoring, but also for the preservation of foods (due to lack of refrigeration), and as an aid to digestion. Spices are strong and can kill bacteria. Dried cloves, peppers, caraway, and cinnamon, when added to food, will make it last longer. Spices stimulate gastric and intestinal enzymes for cleaner and more efficient digestion.

In many parts of the world, the same foods are eaten at every meal. A variety of spices give a different taste to each meal. Variety and pleasing taste make for better enjoyment and digestion.

Parasites are also discouraged by such spices as onion, garlic, cloves, and pepper. Many experts feel that parasites are a major drain on our health, even in first world countries. Spiced foods don't just produce good tastes, but also makes good sense. Hot spices should be eaten in moderation because when abused, they can produce ulcers or irritation in the stomach, usually for Pittas.

Cooking with fresh spices gives us the opportunity to add more green into our diet with the benefit of additional vitamins and minerals.

SPICES FOR COOKING

Vata	Pitta	Kapha
Cilantro	Fennel	Cilantro
Basil	Parsley	Peppermint
Ginger	Dandelion	Ginger
Fennel	Borage	Basil
Rosemary	Violet leaves (in salads)	Dill
Dill	Sweet Onion	Garlic
Garlic	Cilantro	Sage
Turmeric	Dill	Turmeric
Marjoram	Coriander	Oregano
Oregano	Lemongrass	Marjoram
Nutmeg	Lemon Peel	Nutmeg
Bay	Turmeric	Bay
Cardamon	Saffron	Cardamon
Coriander	Rosewater	Coriander
Saffron	Black Pepper	Saffron
	(moderation)	
All Spice		All Spice
Anise Seed		Rosewater
Rosewater		Juniperberries
Juniper Berries		Anise Seed
Black Pepper		Black Pepper

PREPARING FOODS

When cooking food it is best to slow cook and keep the food well covered in order to maintain the nutritional value of the food. Do not use large amounts of oil in cooking. Food that is cooked slowly and well covered while cooking is easier to digest. Your average westerner does not have the enzymes to digest raw food. When food is cooked it is easier on the digestive fire. While raw food does have more enzymes and more life force, the average person does not have adequate digestive power to break down the food. Raw foods are best for reducing and cleansing diets due to their lightness. It is usually recommended that fruit is best when eaten raw. However, when someone is in a high Vata condition, it is recommended that they cook fruits. Most grains are best cooked, although when sprouted they are easily digested, and at this stage they become a vegetable and are no longer so starchy. When building tissue, starch is important.

Cooking is an art! A personal experience of enjoyment! A gift to people you love! Always enter the kitchen free of negative thoughts, clean hands, a clean apron, and a tidy work area. Never fight, be in a bad mood, or have negative thoughts while cooking. We are energetic beings and our energy is added to the food which is being prepared. Chanting, positive affirmation, or singing are positive energies which we can bring to the food preparation. Listen to the vibrations of the vegetable. When you listen, they will be guiding you as to how they want to be prepared. Always use stainless steel or good quality cast iron pots and pans. Stay away from aluminium or teflon.

Equipment to have in the kitchen:

- A good wok
- Wood lids for pots
- Steam basket
- A pressure cooker
- Good cast iron skillet
- Good stainless steel knives.
- Plastic cutting boards for meat (to prevent bacterial contamination)

Always keep your equipment handy in a clean and well organised kitchen as this provides an easy and enjoyable environment to work in. When cooking Ayurvedically, it is good to have a cookbook or take a cooking class. "The Ayurvedic Cookbook" by Amanda Morningstar is a great cookbook. Her other book, "Ayurvedic Cooking For Westerners" is full of eastern recipes. Not everyone is ready for Indian foods all the time, especially when beginning a new diet. Include a variety of other forms of food preparation, such as Thai, Chinese, or Macrobiotic while keeping the Ayurvedic principals. We are a multi-cultural society and the average American is afraid of Indian food because it is foreign to them, and always think of this type of food as "hot". Slowly, you can transition into a full Ayurvedic Indian cooking lifestyle. The market is flooded with good cookbooks and once the Ayurvedic energies of food is understood, they can be adapted to many recipes. For those times when one has a busy schedule, it is good to create a menu for the week. Use a shopping list to avoid numerous runs to the store, and always buy certain foods in bulk, like grains and nuts. If possible, always use foods which are in season. In the tropics, sometimes foods will need to be stored in the refrigerator, even grains, nuts, etc.

Whenever you can, use spring or purified good water or boil your water before cooking to remove chlorine.

As you go through this chapter, recognize that food has its own balance and energy. Many forms of energy can be seen as we learn to prepare them. We need warm food to keep alive and to keep our fire burning. When we lose our fire, we become ill and weak. Too much cold food takes away the fire. When eating, it is important to experience all tastes and energies for the body to feel satisfied.

The way we eat is a reflection of the condition in which we live our life. The way the food is presented on the table and plate creates an important vibration that we take into our bodies.

Springtime - We have all the greens and fresh herbs peaking out, unfolding and opening. It is a good time to introduce greens and fresh herbs and to begin to modify our diets. The dandelions or the young mustards can be added to soup or for quick sautéing. Now work to reduce salt intake and stay away from fermented foods or pickles and as the summer approaches, add a bit of raw foods (it is important to know the doshic condition at this time).

Summer – Many more fruits and vegetables are available at their peak growth. The foods which grow in this season have more active, expansive energy, more Vata. Salads can be served more frequently. Vatas should still maintain their oil intake while eating in the summer. Begin to cook simple meals, prepare foods that are tasty, and plan dinners in the park with friends and families. It is a good time for outdoor parties and barbecues. Fruit gelatin with melon would be a great addition.

Autumn - The tubers and root vegetables are ready for harvest. We begin to slow down and our energies become more inward. We start feeling the season changes with the onset of cold, dry winds. Start preparing yourself for winter, building the immune system with squashes, apples, oranges, onions, cabbage, and turnips which provide good physical nourishment. Many of these harvested crops will last through the winter by drying, canning, pickling, freezing or storing them in a food cellar.

Winter - The strong winds start moving in and snow covers parts of the northern hemisphere during the winter season. As this inward movement deepens, eating cooked foods prepared with a variety of spices is recommended. A time for warm, nourishing, bountiful homemade soups, stews and casseroles. More oil can be added for all doshas to keep the body warm. Other helpful additions to a winter diet are salt, fermented foods, more grains, wheat breads, jams, roasted nuts and nut butters. It is the time to clean and burn the excess nutrition built up during the summer months.

When preparing foods, keep the visuals in mind; color is a form of energy decorating your plate to stimulate the appetite.

Lime and lemons - A slice of citrus can add a sour touch to the plate which helps with breaking down foods, increases digestion, stimulates the liver and gastric juices. This is especially good to serve with fish.

Green Foods - Chard, cabbage, spinach, broccoli, green onions and scallions are calming, helps with detoxifying effects.

Yellow Foods - Millet and squashes are good for the stomach and spleen.

Red Foods - Beets and berries stimulate the heart and blood circulation.

Orange Foods - Carrots, sweet potatoes and yams help build the immune system.

White Foods - Potatoes, rice, and barley help the lungs and intestines.

Currently, Americans eat 50-60% of all foods in restaurants. Restaurant eating should be left for special occasions. Microwaves devitalize food, altering the molecular vibrations. Gas stoves are better than electric stoves for cooking. For my busy clients I always recommend a crockpot as its easy, slow cooking is healthful and makes food available throughout the day. They can prepare it before they go to sleep or before they go to work. It is one of our western conveniences. It does not take a lot of attention and space and all kinds of food can be cooked in it. When the food is prepared overnight in slow cookers, it is ready for the next day and the food can also be taken to work.

FOOD COMBINING

Food combining is very important for good digestion, weight reduction, and for the prevention of cellulite. Avoid eating protein and starches together, i.e. meats with potatoes. Proteins such as meat and dairy products should be eaten with non-starchy vegetables. No fruit with proteins. Fruits and starchy veggies are best not mixed. Grains mix well with all vegetables, nuts mix with green vegetables, citrus fruits or sour fruits; starchy vegetables like squashes and potatoes mix best with green vegetables.

It takes different enzymes to digest different types of foods. Proteins call for hydrochloric acid and pepsin to be released on the stomach contents for an acid protein digestion (clearing proteins into amino acids). Starch digestion begins in the mouth (with ptyalin from the saliva) and will continue in the stomach if no acid is released. This is why proteins and starches are more efficiently digested separately. This is important in sick, weak, or persons with poor digestive fire. Healthy people need not pay as much attention to "food separation". Beans and grains are a natural combination of starches and proteins. For healthy people, restricting fluid intake with meals and eating fruits separately is usually adequate.

When looking to have more efficient digestion it is best to follow this rule:

Never drink with your meals with the exception of milk unless an herbal therapy drink has been recommended. This weakens digestion and creates fermentation (gas). When too much liquid is eaten at mealtime, this dilutes digestive enzymes. Example: If you set your washing machine for a small load with the proper amount of detergent, at a low water level, then someone comes and raises the water level too high, your clothes are not going to come out clean. You don't mix white and colored clothes when you wash. It can be the same with starches and proteins.

Always eat when you are hungry. Stop to think if you are are hungry, or are you feeling empty or anxious? You could be covering up your feelings with food.

Vata: Needs to eat more often. Their blood sugar drops easily and it is not good for them to go long periods without food. Snacking is important to them.

Pitta: Needs to have regular solid food. They require a large meal in the middle of the day and it is important that they eat at least three full meals per day.

Kapha: Can get by with one or two meals per day. Eat the largest meal in the middle of the day and a light meal at night. Snacking is not good for them.

Never exercise after a heavy meal unless it is a mild walk; it is best to wait a couple of hours after a meal for other forms of exercise. Sex should be avoided immediately before or after a meal. Never watch television while eating. Smoking disturbs the digestion. Do not go to sleep immediately after a large meal. Small amounts of wine (4 oz.) is best before mealtime to stimulate appetite; especially good for Vatas. Desserts are usually best as a snack apart from a regular meal. It is usually too much food and the sweetness interferes with protein digestion (causing putrification).

THE ART OF CHEWING

When we improve the quality of the food we eat, we must also change our chewing habits. Chewing is especially important when eating for health, as it is the first step of internal transformation. Our manner of eating is an indication of our intuitive understanding.

Digestion begins as soon as food enters the mouth. If food is chewed to a liquid state, the body's assimilation functions are enhanced because the stomach is not overworked and the intestines can absorb more efficiently. Chewing causes a strong secretion of saliva, which decreases the formation of mucus and helps prevent over-eating. Proper chewing releases locked-in nutrients and promotes smooth digestion.

The foremost rule is complete mastication. Chew food to a liquid until it practically swallows itself. When chewing food, separate the liquids by using the tongue and cheek linings. Swallow the liquids and continue to chew the remaining solids. This is essential so we can properly assimilate what we eat. The human jaw is unique in its ability to operate in all directions, especially in a sideways grinding motion. Twenty-eight of our teeth are designed to act as "grinders". Increase the amount of side-to-side chewing.

Chewing enables us to distinguish refined or fake food from real food. If processed food is held in the mouth, its additives create an unnatural odor and unpleasant after-taste which rises into the nasal passage. Most people have therefore developed the unconscious habit of chewing food near the back of the mouth and swallowing before this happens. Real food becomes sweeter and tastier as it is chewed and mixed thoroughly with saliva. Relaxed chewing facilitates the full enjoyment of the whole spectrum of tastes and aromas found in natural food. Enjoy every morsel, savoring its flavor until it is swallowed.

The teeth are related to the spinal vertebrae and are directly correlated to the central nervous system. Therefore, chewing has a massaging effect upon the whole body. Proper chewing develops facial muscles and stimulates the cerebrospinal fluids, thus improving will and memory. Do not eat when tired, angry or worried. Do not think or talk about unpleasant subjects during mealtime. Maintain proper posture by keeping your back erect when eating to facilitate long, deep breathing. Take small bites, eat slowly and chew with intent. Use this time for meditation and gratitude. If you have already made the transition to whole foods, conscious chewing will heighten your awareness even more.

Food should be eaten as fresh as possible or freshly cooked or juiced. Always buy organic when available. It is best to stay away from foods grown with pesticides or inorganic fertilizers. Eat as much fresh fruit and vegetables as possible.

RESTAURANT EATING

In the west, many people eat 50% or more of their meals out, due to busy schedules and fast lifestyles. Restaurant eating is a convenience, and is part of day-to-day survival for some people. The quality of food at a restaurant could never replace that of home cooking. The person who is preparing the food is not able to connect with the people who eat in his restaurant. That is not to say that there are no conscientious chefs. Generally, restaurants buy large quantities of food and quality is not a priority, unless you go to a small gourmet food restaurant and pay the price. The $50-$100 that you pay for a truly fine meal can go a long way towards shopping in a health food store.

Fine ethnic foods often are better than just plain American cooking. Chinese, Indian, Korean, Thai, Japanese, Vietnamese, Greek, Italian and Mexican foods use plenty of fresh vegetables, spices, beans, rice, guacamole, fresh cilantro and freshly made sauces. More and more restaurant owners and chefs are realizing the transformation that is taking place concerning food consciousness, especially in this part of the world. A willingness to serve makes it possible for restaurants to make substitutions for specific foods that a person is unable to eat and will accommodate "off the menu" requests (i.e. no MSG or please add extra basil).

Always stay away from restaurants that prepare foods with microwaves, use lard, or MSG (especially found in Chinese cooking). Visit and support health food restaurants. They are often conscientious and have as much organic food as possible. Fast food restaurants are not recommended, yet in today's busy times, sometimes we must use them. *Wendy's* has a Pita sandwich with shredded veggies and romaine lettuce. *Subway* offers a veggie burger, and *The Harvest* carries sweet potatoes and many vegetarian dishes. Even in *McDonald's* you can choose a fish burger or charbroiled chicken sandwich over a Big Mac. Remember, we vote with our money. Whatever you buy, you are asking for more of the same.

Always stay away from busy, crowded restaurants. The idea of dining out is to have time for yourself, free from preparation and clean up. Questions to ask at the restaurant:

- Do you have filtered water?
- Are the vegetables fresh?
- Do you have romaine lettuce?
- Do you fry, boil or bake?
- Do you use lard or vegetable oil?

- Do you use whole grains?
- Do you carry herbal teas?
- Is there preservatives in the salad bar?
- Do you have honey?
- Do you have vegetarian food on the menu?

Vata does well with any place that has warm soups and vegetables. Pitta does well with Thai and Chinese foods. Kapha does well with salads and all vegetable dishes.

CHEMICALS IN OUR FOOD SUPPLY

Food Additives to Avoid As Unsafe or Poorly Tested

Artificial Colorings

Blue #1	Artificial coloring used in beverages, candy, baked goods.
Blue #2	Used in pet food, beverages, candy. Causes brain tumors in rats.
Citrus Red #2	Coloring of skin of some Florida oranges only. Causes cancer.
Green #3	Used in candy, beverages. May cause bladder cancer in rats.
Red #3	Coloring of cherries in fruit cocktail, candy, baked goods. Causes thyroid tumors in rats.
Yellow #6	Beverages, sausage, baked goods, candy, gelatin. Causes tumors in tested animal's adrenals and kidneys. Dye often contaminated with carcinogens.
Brominated Vegetable Oil	Emulsifier, clouding agent -Used in soft drinks. Builds up in fat residues.
Butylated Hydroxyanisole (BHA)	Antioxidant - Cereals, chewing gum, potato chips, oils, etc. Caused cancer in rats.

Butylated Hydroxy-toluene (BHT)	Antioxidant - Cereals, chewing gum, potato chips, oils, etc. May cause cancer.
Caffeine	Stimulant - Coffee, tea, cocoa (natural); soft drinks (additive). May cause miscarriages or birth defects - avoid if pregnant. May trigger Fibrocystic breast disease.
Propyl Gallate	Antioxidant - Vegetable oil, meat products, potato sticks, chicken soup base, chewing gum. Suggestions of causing cancer.
Quinine	Flavoring - Tonic water, quinine water, bitter lemon. Could cause birth defects - pregnant women should avoid.
Saccharin	Synthetic sweetener - "Diet" products. There is repeated evidence it causes cancer.
Salt (Sodium Chloride)	Flavoring - Most processed foods: soup, potato chips, crackers. In 1977, the FDA proposed a ban (not acted upon). Excess use of it has proved to cause high blood pressure, heart attack and stroke.
Sodium Nitrite, Sodium Nitrate	Coloring, flavoring - Preservative Bacon, ham, frankfurters, luncheon meats, smoked fish, corned beef.
Sugar (Sucrose)	Sweetener - Table sugar, sweetened foods. Suggested "cause" of many modern health problems.
Sulfur Dioxide, Sodium Bisulfite	Preservative, bleach - Dried fruit, wine, processed potatoes. Has caused 12 deaths from allergic reactions. Asthmatics should avoid. Destroys vitamin B1.

FOODS TO USE WITH CAUTION DUE TO POOR TESTING OR OVERUSE

Artificial Colorings

Red #40	Soda pop, candy, gelatin desserts, pastry, pet food, sausage. Poor testing.
Yellow #5	Gelatin dessert, candy, pet food, baked goods. Allergic reactions (especially aspirin sensitive people).
Artificial Flavoring	Soda pop, candy, breakfast cereals, gelatin desserts; many others. Hyperactivity.
Aspartame	Artificial sweetener - Drink mixes, gelatin desserts, other foods. Breaks down into banned toxic and carcino-genic causing chemicals. Many docu-mented adverse reactions, including seizures. Not recommended by airline pilot organizations because of incidents.
Carrageenan	Thickening, stabilizing agent - Ice cream, jelly, chocolate milk, infant formula. Needs more testing; may harm intestines.
Corn Syrup	Sweetener, thickener - Candy, toppings, syrups, snack foods, imitation dairy foods. No nutrition, only calories.
Dextrose (Glucose, Corn Sugar)	Sweetener, coloring agent - Bread, caramel, soda pop, cookies, & many other foods. Empty calories; we get too much sugar.
Hydrogenated Vegetable Oil	Source of oil or fat - Margarine; many processed foods. Most Americans get too much oil.
Hydrolyzed Vegetable Protein	Flavor enhancer - (HVP) Instant soups, frankfurters, sauce mixes, beef stew. Contains MSG.

Invert Sugar	Sweetener - Candy, soft drinks; many other foods. Empty calories.
Monosodium Glutamate	Flavor enhancer - (MSG) Soup, seafood, poultry, cheese, sauces, stews; many others. Kills brain cells in rats. Causes tingling sensation in sensitive adults.
Phosphoric Acid; Phosphates	Acidulant, chelating agent, buffer, emulsifier, nutrient, discoloration inhibitor - Baked goods, cheese, powdered foods, cured meat, soda pop, breakfast cereals, dehydrated potatoes. May contribute to osteoporosis.

*This information was distilled from a poster created by Center for the Public Interest and is available from CSPI; 1875 Connecticut Ave., N.W., #300; Washington DC 20009.

THE ROLE OF VEGETARIANISM AND THE VARIOUS CLASSES OF DIETS

Life is sacred and there are karmic (cause & effect) consequences for taking life. We bless our food in thanks for the exchange of energy as we consume other organisms, animals and plants. It is generally thought that the lower you eat on the food chain, the better off you are; that there are less consequences for eating a plant than an animal. Certainly, in these times with environmental toxins progressively building up in the higher part of the food chain, this is true. Plants will have small amounts of lead and mercury. Cows who eat plants will have more. People who eat steak will have the most.

Without entering into the debate of whether man should be vegetarian or not, we have listed in this book foods from both animal and vegetable sources for their specific nutrients.

Classes of Diets

| Cannibals | People who eat people. Reviled of all civilizations. Outlawed internationally. |

| Omnivores | Those who consume everything, both animal and vegetable. |
| Carnivores | Those who eat only flesh. The Eskimo in his natural habitat would by necessity fall into this category, living in reverence of the animals who sustain them, blessing each creature who sacrifices so that he may live. |

It is possible to eat animals and still have a spiritual connection with nature. I wonder, if the average westerner had to personally kill and butcher their cows, sheep and chickens, would they eat as much? We are so distanced from the meat industry that children are sometimes shocked to discover that hamburger is made from those cute cows, and that a drumstick was walking around as the leg of a live chicken.

Ova Lacto Vegetarians

Eat eggs, dairy products, and vegetables. It is possible to take no life if you eat unfertilized eggs. This diet is a firm step toward the bottom of the food chain and yet includes enough animal protein for most metabolic types.

Lacto Vegetarians

Eat dairy products and vegetables. This diet is a definite choice not to take animal life and cultivates a more peaceful beingness.

Vegans

Feel that the slavery of dairy animals is wrong. They get their protein exclusively from nuts, seeds, beans and grains. They are true vegetarians.

Fruitarians

Believe that even killing plants involves some karma and so they only eat what drops from the tree, saving the seeds for planting. Both veganism and fruitaranism should be approached through a transition diet and systematic cleansing (colon, lungs, kidneys, skin, liver).

If you have not cultivated peacefulness within yourself, you will not do well on this diet.

Breatharians

Only saints need apply. Beings who know the true source of their sustenance can exist on only water and air.

Whatever diet you choose for yourself, let the decision come from the heart. Read and learn about your diet and listen to your body. Trust and don't judge other's for their choices.

SHOPPING FOR HEALTHY, NATURAL FOODS

Many of the supermarkets today carry a variety of natural foods and organic products. May I suggest that you begin to read the labels because many packaged foods contain undesirable chemicals. Avoid irradiated foods - there is no life force remaining in them! Try an experiment with some irradiated fruit - place it in your refrigerator and see how long it will last before beginning to decay. It can be months! This suggests that there is very little life force, if any, left in the product, therefore, can provide no nutrients nor life force to you when eaten.

The word "natural" can be used on anything today, it does not mean organic or pure. A product can be grown with herbicides and pesticides, but because it may contain a small substance of natural food it can be labeled "natural". This word has been abused and misused. Only reputable companies in the health food industry have specific labeling; know and ask questions about the foods you purchase.

There are many foods containing sugars such as sucrose, dextrose, maltose, corn syrup and these ingredients are labeled as natural. These sugars are of poor quality and weaken the pancreas and digestive process.

The health food industry gained some popularity in early 1960 with many bulk foods, grains, and herbs. It has now become one of America's largest growing industries with chain stores, fancy packaging, and attractive labels. Be Aware! Many of the original stores were food co-ops which are slowly disappearing. Yet, in many metropolitan areas food co-ops are available if you search them out, so

I suggest supporting them and any business that provides natural bulk foods. Food co-ops save money and keeps food costs down. It can be a joy to experience a quality health food establishment. Look for them in your area.

Support natural organic products, natural foods, and natural food stores. Remember to use a variety of fruits, vegetables, and whole grains. When using the same foods over and over again, we become sensitive to them. Rotate your foods!

"Take back your freedom, my friend", says Tom Phiefer of UniTea Herbs in Boulder, Colorado. We vote with our dollars! The more we buy, the more of those products we get. When we support companies that are producing foods which do not benefit the well being of humanity, we are part of the oppression of human beings. Many products are the result of cheap child labor in third world countries. Politically, when we purchase these items, we are contributing to the subjugation of women and children.

As you travel a healthy journey, there are new and exciting ways of eating available to you. It can be an adventure and an ongoing experience which provides many rewards.

FOOD ITEM	SUGGESTED HEALTHY REPLACEMENT
Coke, Pepsi, Sodas	Natural colas, Ginger Blast, Blue Sky, fruit juices, herb teas
Margarine	Ghee
Iodized Salt	Sea Salt
Soy Sauce	Braggs Amino Acids
Refined Sugar	Sucanat, Stevia, honey, maple syrup, rice syrup, pure cane sugar
Chocolate	Carob
Beef	Veggie burgers, free range chicken/turkey/eggs, organic meats are the best if you are consuming meat products
Refined Flower	Whole grains

Coffee	Pero, roasted dandelion, Caffix, herbal teas
Wheat (when allergic)	Quinoa, spelt, amaranth (they make excellent breads), rice, barley, rye, sprouts, possibly bread without yeast

Many people have become lactose intolerant and developed many kinds of allergies due to the conditions of our dairy farms.

Dairy	Soy products
Milk	Soy milk, rice milk
Yogurt	Soy yogurt, amazaki
Cheese	Soy cheese, tofu
Ice Cream	Rice Dream, Toffutti, Soy Ice Cream

CHAPTER 9

WHY DO I NEED VITAMINS AND MINERALS?

VITAMINS ARE ORGANIC chemical compounds found in food in small amounts that are essential to our health and wellbeing. Without them we suffer deficiency symptoms and can die. They were first discovered when sailors spent long months on sea voyages without fresh fruits and vegetables and developed "scurvy". This deficiency disease, caused by the lack of vitamin C, created muscular weakness, bone weakness, ulceration of the mouth, gum disease, loss of teeth, lowered immune response and death. Whole navies were laid low and battles were lost because the crews did not have the strength to man the ships. The British discovered that lime juice put into kegs and rationed daily prevented the problem (which is how they got the nickname, "Limeys").

When rice and wheat were first milled to remove the vitamin rich outer layers, producing a white product, the people who could afford this refined product (the rich) came down with "berry berri", a disease caused by a B vitamin deficiency. Symptoms included nerve loss, muscle weakness, tingling and numbness.

Children fed a diet low in vitamin D developed curved legs from weak flexible bones. This is a deficiency disease called "rickets".

Lack of minerals can also cause deficiency diseases. In areas of iodine deficient soil, a swelling of the throat (thyroid) called goitre develops.

At first, these diseases were mysterious. No one understood their cause. Scientific exploration led to discoveries of individual vitamins and further experimentation showed what the least amount that a person could ingest without deficiency disease symptoms. Any less and illness occurred. Based on this, the Food and Drug Administration set up the MDRs (Minimum Daily Requirements). Some scientists objected to a scale of measurement so close to the edge of disease, so the FDA came out with the RDAs (Recommended Daily Allowance) which are somewhat higher. Many health experts agree that these amounts are still too low for maximum health benefits, and the population may suffer from a multitude of autoimmune symptoms. For instance, the RDA for vitamin C is 100 mg., while many doctors recommend 1,000-2,000 mg. per day for prevention. Nobel Prize winner, Dr. Linus Pauling (the discoverer of vitamin C) took 10,000-16,000 mg. of vitamin C for years to prove that it was safe.

So, Why Should I Take Vitamin and Mineral Supplements?

1. Our food supply is grown on increasingly deficient soil and is lacking in the nutrition it once had, and we develop deficiencies even eating three meals per day.

2. Our food supply is grown with herbicides, pesticides, and nitrogen fertilizers which stimulate growth in deficient soil. These chemical residues are harmful to our metabolism, creating need for more vitamins.

3. Smoking, second-hand smoke, and air pollution are harmful and create nutritional deficiencies. Water pollution creates more need.

4. Mental, physical and emotional stress causes deficiencies in our bodies.

5. The table salt that we use has been stripped of its minerals (and they are sold back to us as mineral supplements), the grains we eat have been milled and bleached, which removes minerals. The sugar we eat is stripped and bleached of minerals. It actually takes vitamins and minerals from other sources to process this food through our metabolism.

6. Cooling, freezing, and canning removes some vitamins and minerals.

We may not be experiencing disease symptoms such as scurvy, pellagra, rickets, or goitres, but health experts agree that many of the modern diseases of lowered immune function are caused by vitamin and mineral deficiencies.

Symptom and Diseases Caused By, or Affected By, Deficiencies Include:

Tiredness
Allergies
Colds and flu
Bad breath
Bad gums and teeth
Sore joints and muscles
Poor eyesight and loss
  of night vision
Kidney stones
Hair loss
Menopause symptoms

Heart disease, arteriosclerosis
Cancer
MS, MD, Scleroderma
Cold sores
Osteoporosis
Arthritis
Varicose veins
Headaches
PMS
Hypoglycemia
Diabetes

Taking supplements can never replace the need for a good diet. It is highly recommended that you try to get your nutrients from an improved diet of whole food.

How Can I Get More Vitamins and Minerals in My Diet?

1. Eat seaweed; high in all minerals and trace minerals.

2. Eat organic food grown on organic rich soil.

3. Eat unprocessed, fresh foods and juices.

4. Eat sea salt that has not been stripped of minerals.

5. Use honey, maple syrup, and whole sugar (sucanat products) instead of white sugar.

6. Eat whole grains.

7. If you eat meat, eat organic, free range, or wild (venison) meat. The organs, which are high in nutrients, (kidney, liver, brains, ovaries, testes, intestines, stomach and pancreas, etc.), are the best for you. Cook the joints and bones in soup to get the minerals. Indigenous peoples and carnivorous animals always eat the whole animal, not just the steaks (muscle meat).

8. Grow your own vegetables organically and feed them richly with kelp, compost, etc.

9. Raise your own animals; chickens, rabbits, and fish, if possible. Feed them well.

10. Chew your food thoroughly and use good food combining to get the most out of your food. Most people only digest 20-30% of what they eat because of poor digestion. Good health is not only a matter of what you eat, but also what you digest and assimilate.

Even if you do all of this you may still need vitamin supplementation because it can take several months or even years to overcome and correct a nutritional deficiency.

Always take your supplements with food. Only a few should be taken alone. Many vitamins are made from food. They are concentrates or derivatives from foods. If you eat them with food your enzymes will break them down more easily. Fat soluble vitamins (vitamins A, D, E, F) are best eaten with oils or fat. Water-soluble vitamins (B, C) are best eaten with vegetables or fruits. Mistakenly, people sometimes treat supplements like pharmaceuticals, afraid to take more than 1 or two; yet supplements are concentrated nutrients, and should be taken in the sufficient quantities to rebuild the body. When purchasing vitamin supplements, always choose *quality* products even though they cost more. Vitamins are *not* all the same! Educate yourself.

AYURVEDIC VITAMIN CHART

VITAMIN A

Stress, Depleted or Low Immune

Utilized in the Body	Helps night vision, increases hair growth, strengthens all bone tissues, and balances all tissue linings.
Deficiencies	Allergies, split ends of hair shafts, loss of smell, dry skin, susceptibility to frequent colds, tooth decay.
Functions	Builds and strengthens immune system to fight infections; assists with aging process; prevents senility.
Synthetic	Acetate or palmitate
Toxicity	300,000 IU
R.D.A.	5,000 IU with no special health problems; therapeutic dosage up to 100,000 IU with specific problems (i.e., acute infection, candidiasis).
Fat Soluble	Animal sources
Water Soluble	Vegetable sources
Depleted By	Stress; overwork
VATA	Fish, Liver, Eggs, Milk, Yogurt, Carrots, Spinach, Red Pepper, Winter Squash, Sweet Potatoes, Yams, Mangos, Soaked Seaweed
PITTA	Milk, Cottage Cheese, Fresh Water Fish (liver oil), Kale, Collard Greens, Turmeric, Lemongrass, Mangos, Cabbage, Raspberry Leaf, Dandelion, Mints, Cilantro, Spirulina, Dark Leafy Greens
KAPHA	Buttermilk, Milk, Lemongrass, Parsley, Spinach, Mangos, Nettle, Mints,

| | Dry Seaweed, Paprika, Sage, Cayenne, Chickweed, Kelp, Turmeric |
| Sources of Beta Carotene | Beta-carotene is a vegetable sourced precursor (can be made into) which must be converted by the liver into vitamin A at a ratio of 2 to 1 (i.e., 20,000 IU beta-carotene = 10,000 IU of vitamin A). |

NOTE: The dosages of Vitamin A mentioned above regarding illnesses are often significantly higher than the maintenance dose. The elevated amounts are not recommended for more than one month unless prescribed by a physician who understands vitamins. There have been a few reported cases of toxicity with long term use. A death has been reported from eating polar bear liver.

B-VITAMINS

B-vitamins work together as a complex and are often sold together in varying amounts or in equivalents (50 mg. each). If you take an isolated B vitamin, it can create a deficiency of other B's so always take a balanced B-complex tablet also (i.e., B-1000 mg. and B-complex 100 mg.

| Depleted By | Smoking or second hand smoke, medication, antibiotics |

VITAMIN B-1 — THIAMINE

Metabolism

Utilized in the Body	Brain, ears, eyes, heart, muscle tissue, liver
Deficiencies	Gastrointestinal problems, anger, irritability, muscle tone, numbness, nervousness of hands and feet, stabilizes appetite
Functions	Builds blood, assists with strengthening all tissue; circulation; assists digestion; nerves; stabilizes appetite

Synthetic	Thiamine hydrochloride; Thiamine mononitrate
R.D.A.	1.4 mg. Therapeutic dosage up to 240 mg.
Toxicity	No known oral toxicity
Water Soluble	
Depleted By	Alcohol, coffee, sugar
<u>VATA</u>	Asparagus, Shatavari (Asparagus), Citrus, Garlic, Black Strap Molasses, Seaweed (Nori, Kelp), Catnip, Watercress, Rice Bran
<u>PITTA</u>	Cauliflower, Kale, Barley Grass, Seaweed, Asparagus, Dandelion, Red Clover, Raspberry Leaf, Catnip
<u>KAPHA</u>	Cauliflower, Kale, Citrus, Spirulina, Garlic, Ghee, Asparagus, Brewer's Yeast, Dandelion, Red Clover, Raspberry Leaf, Watercress, Rice Bran, Yeast

VITAMIN B-2 — RIBOFLAVIN
Emotional Balance, Blood

Utilized in the Body	Brain, nervous system, intestinal tract, epithelia tissue, spleen, liver
Deficiencies	Red bulging eyes, canker sores, nausea, weak digestion, sore cracked tongue, early gray hair, wrinkles
Functions	Metabolizes fat; assists functioning of antibodies and red blood cells; assists normal breathing patterns
Synthetic	Riboflavin
Toxicity	None known
R.D.A.	1.6 mg. Therapeutic Dosage: Up to 900 mg.
Water Soluble	

Depleted By	Hot flashes, crying jags, antibiotics, tranquilizers
<u>VATA</u>	Raspberry Leaves, Catnip, Hops, Dulse, Currants, Watercress, Rosehips, Ginseng, Mushrooms, Organ Meats, Black Strap Molasses, Parsley, Dulse, Fenugreek, Rice Bran
<u>PITTA</u>	Brussel Sprouts, Red Clover, Raspberry Leaves, Alfalfa, Yarrow, Sago Palm, Steamed Onions, Legumes, Dandelions, Yellow Dock, Rice Bran
<u>KAPHA</u>	Nettles, Red Clover, Peppermint, Rosehips, Beans, Beet Greens, Asparagus, Shatavari, Legumes, Parsley, Dandelions, Fenugreek, Yellow Dock, Yeast

VITAMIN B-3 — NIACIN, NIACINAMIDE, NICOTIC ACID

Anxiety, Depression, Cholesterol, Heart pressure

Utilized in the Body	Brain, gastrointestinal, nervous system, liver, skin, circulation, cholesterol, dilates blood vessels
Deficiencies	Skin problems, depression, nervous disorders, headaches, cold feet and hands, liver disorder, muscle weakness
Functions	Balances cholesterol levels; metabolizes carbohydrates; balances hormones and hormone production; dilation of blood vessels, increases appetite; enhances energy levels; assists circulation, blood flow and lymph movement.
Synthetic	Nicotinic Acid, Niacin, Niacinamide
R.D.A.	6.6 mg. Therapeutic Dosage: Up to 300 mg.

Toxicity	200 mg. in some people
Water Soluble	
Depleted By	Fatigue, digestion abnormalities
VATA	Rice Bran, Burdock Root, Hops, Slippery Elm, Asparagus, Bee Pollen, Licorice, Rice Syrup, Organ Meats, Eggs, Avocados
PITTA	Slippery Elm, Spirulina, Echinacea, Cabbage, Red Clover, Licorice, Nettles, Rice Syrup, Milk, Rice Bran, Potatoes, Burdock Root, Hops, Raspberry Leaf, Sunflower Seeds, Organ Meat, Lean Meat, Eggs, Avocado, Sunflower Seeds, Lean Meats, Peanuts
KAPHA	Spirulina, Bee Pollen, Nettles, Parsley, Potatoes, Burdock Root, Hops, Raspberry Leaf, Prunes

Note: Niacin in amounts greater than 100 mg. will cause skin flushing (redness and tingling).

This property has been used in detox programs in combination with extended sauna (2-3 hours) at lowered temperatures (150 degrees) to promote elimination of toxins via the skin. Increasing amounts must be taken each day to elicit this response as body tolerance increases.

VITAMIN B-4 — CHOLINE

Utilized in the Body	Brain, hair, gallbladder, kidneys, liver, thymus, liver/bile production, endocrine system, urinary tract, balances cholesterol
Deficiencies	Ulcers, heart disorders, high blood pressure, kidney problems, stomach ulcers, intestinal bleeding, liver/gall bladder disorders, poor assimilation of fats

Functions	Works together with inositol; a basic constituent of lecithin; cell growth, emulsifies fat (cholesterol)
Synthetic:	Choline bitartrade or Biotin
Toxicity:	None known
R.D.A.:	None established. Therapeutic dosage: Up to 1,500
Water Soluble	
Depleted By	Alcohol; fried foods
VATA	Egg Yolk, Organ Meats, Wheat Bran, Wheat Germ, Liver
PITTA	Soybeans, Green Leafy Vegetables, Lecithin
KAPHA	Brewer's Yeast, Soybeans, Green Leafy Vegetables

VITAMIN B-5 — PANTOTHENIC ACID

Muscle Spasms, Allergies, Adrenal Insufficiency & Assists Body in Producing Cortisone

Utilized in the Body	Fat metabolism, aids in breaking down proteins, adrenal support, brain tissue, digestive system, musculoskeletal system, epithelia tissue, endocrine system (particularly the adrenal glands)
Deficiencies	Constipation, duodenal ulcers, eczema, hypoglycemia, kidney disorders, hair loss, infections, sensitivity to gluten, auto accident injuries, muscle spasms, allergies, adrenal insufficiency, pain, muscle spasms, inflammation, vomiting, menstrual cramps, skin disorders, frequent colds
Functions	Assists in producing cortisone; assists muscle healing; antibody production;

	assimilation of vitamins; stops muscle spasms
Synthetic	Calcium pantothenate
Toxicity	10,000 - 20,000 mg.
R.D.A.	10 mg.
	Therapeutic Dosage: Up to 1,000 mg.
Water Soluble	
Depleted By	Stress, overwork, not enough self-care, muscle injury, accident, shock, trauma
VATA	Rice Bran, Organ Meats, Egg Yolk, Liver, Molasses, Royal Jelly, Wheat Bran, Wheat Germ
PITTA	Green Vegetables, Legumes, Soybeans, Peanuts, Whole Grains
KAPHA	Green Vegetables, Legumes, Soybeans, Royal Jelly, Brewers Yeast, Whole Grains

Highest source is yeast and rice bran syrup.

VITAMIN B-6 — PYRIDOXINE

Immune System, Skin, Herpes Sores, Cancer Preventative

Utilized in the Body	Circulation, muscles, nerves, skin, immune system
Deficiencies	Anemia, skin problems (acne), kidney/bladder disorders, nervousness, nausea, vomiting, arthritis, depression, menstrual cramps, dizziness, herpes sores, canker sores, arthritis, frequent infections, anger, fear, A.D.D.
Functions	Alleviates nausea, antibody formation, digestion (hydrochloric acid produc-tion), weight control, assists in balancing sodium and potassium, cancer preventa-

	tive, increases immune function, improves complexion, prevention of cancer
Synthetic	Pyridoxine hydrochloride
R.D.A	2 - 100 mg. Therapeutic Dosage: Up to 1,800 mg.
Toxicity	None known
Water Soluble	
Depleted By	Constipation, fasting, oral contraceptives, radiation, heart problems
VATA	Fish, Turnip, Cooked Spinach, Green Pepper, Organ Meats, Black Strap Molasses - unrefined, Wheat Germ, Carrots, Banana, Avocado
PITTA	Broccoli, Kale, Bananas, Leafy Greens, Peanuts
KAPHA	Fish, Spinach, Green Pepper, Leafy Green Vegetables

VITAMIN B-7 — BIOTIN

(Also known as Vitamin H)

Utilized in the Body	Brain, hair, skin, muscular tissue, bone tissue
Deficiencies	Glandular disorders, dry hair, dry skin, dandruff, split ends, weak tissue, MS, insomnia, early gray hair
Functions	Aids in recovery from fatigue; assists cell oxidation; metabolism of proteins, fats & sugars; nerves; antiseptic; assists antibody formation, assists assimilation of vitamins
Synthetic	Biotin
Toxicity	No oral toxicity
R.D.A.	30 - 300 mg. Therapeutic Dosage: Up to 450 mcg.

Water Soluble

Depleted By   Shock, trauma

VATA   Liver, Sardines, Whole Grains,
                     Beef, Fruits, Nuts, Eggs

PITTA   Unpolished Rice, Legumes,
                     Whole Grains, Fruits, Milk

KAPHA   Legumes, Whole Grains, Fruits,
                     Basmati Rice

VITAMIN B-8 — INOSITOL

Utilized in
the Body   Brain, heart, kidneys, liver, muscle, hair,
                     skin, bones, endocrine system, muscular
                     system, assists choline & biotin

Deficiencies   Hypertension, constipation, eczema, eye
                     disorders, hair loss, skin disorders, weak
                     bones, cystitis

Functions   Calming effects, cholesterol reduction,
                     prevents eczema, promotes hair growth,
                     skin improvement, mental clarity
                     and strength

Toxicity   None known

R.D.A.   Unknown.
                     Therapeutic Dosage: 100 - 1,000 mg.

Water Soluble

Depleted By   Fried foods; excess fat

VATA   Black Strap Molasses - unrefined, Whole
                     Grains, Nuts, Citrus, Organic Meats -
                     Liver, Lecithin, Wheat Germ

PITTA   Milk, Whole Grains, Cabbage

KAPHA   Citrus, Whole Grains, Brewers Yeast,
                     Raisins

VITAMIN B-9 — FOLIC ACID

Healthy Bones, Calm Nerves, Flexibility of Tissues, Adrenal Insufficiency

Utilized in the Body	Endocrine, urinary tract, epithelia tissue (skin), blood, hair
Deficiencies	Canker sores, nervousness, anxiety, fatigue, depression, early gray hair, allergies, anemia, edema, mental depression, overweight, infertility, muscle spasms
Functions	Relieves muscle spasms, production of hydrochloric acid, assists milk produc tion, improved appetite, protein metabo lism, formation of red blood cells, adrenal and pituitary enhancement, strong bones, pain reliever, division of body cells, hydrochloric acid production, red blood cell production
Synthetic	Pleroylglutamic Acid
Toxicity	None known
R.D.A.	4 mcg. Therapeutic Dosage: Up to 4,000 mcg.
Water Soluble	
Depleted By	Stress; accident; overwork
VATA	Catnip, Comfrey, Dark Green Veg- etables, Root Vegetables, Salmon, Sage, Mushrooms, Nuts, Asparagus, Cilantro
PITTA	Greens, Plantain, Chickweed, Pepper- mint, Kale, Broccoli, Milk, Nettles, Alfalfa, Asparagus, Legumes, Parsley
KAPHA	Nettles, Alfalfa, Parsley, Sage, Chick- weed, Broccoli, Kale, Beet Greens, Dark Green Vegetables, Oysters, Root Veg- etables, Catnip, Asparagus, Legumes

VITAMIN B-12 — CYANOCOHALAMIN

Utilized in the Body	All cells, nervous system, brain, circulation
Deficiencies	Anemia, brain damage, poor appetite (anorexia), neuritis, Chronic Fatigue, general weakness, speech difficulties, irritability, stuttering, anemia, hypoglycemia, fatigue
Functions	Increases appetite, blood cell formation, relieves depression, promotes longevity, memory, increases energy, promotes growth in children; pituitary function; balances nervous system; relaxes tissue
Synthetic	Cannot be synthetically made
Toxicity	None
R.D.A.	6 mcg. Therapeutic Dosage: 10 - 1,000 mcg.
Water Soluble	
Depleted By	Stress; poor diet
VATA	Pork, Cheese, Lamb, Banana, Comfrey, Catnip, Concord Grapes, Cheese, Eggs, Seaweeds (Kelp, Dulse), Liver, Wheat Germ
PITTA	Freshwater Fish, Milk, Banana, Alfalfa, Catnip, Miso, Sunflower Seeds, Milk
KAPHA	Freshwater Fish, Kelp, Peanuts, Alfalfa, Miso

VITAMIN B-13 — CALCIUM ORATE

Utilized in the Body	All cell production
Deficiencies	Cancer, Multiple Sclerosis, aging, muscle weakness, early aging, degenerative disorders

Functions	Essential for biosynthesis of nucleic acid, cell rejuvenation, pregnancy, hormone production
Synthetic	Cannot be synthetically made
Toxicity	No known toxicity
R.D.A.	None established
Water Soluble	
VATA	Brown Rice, Laetrile (Apple Seeds), Grape Seeds, Nuts/Seeds, Wheatgrass, Pink Lentils-well cooked, Root Vegetables, Yogurt, Curdled Milk, Rejuvelac, Liquid Whey
PITTA	Sunflower Seeds, Laetrile (Apple Seeds), Grape Seeds, Legumes, Nuts/Seeds-(diet/dosha specific), Wheatgrass, Liquid Whey
KAPHA	Brewer's Yeast, PumpkinSeeds, Sesame Seeds, Laetrile (Apple Seeds), Grape Seeds, Lentils, Legumes, Nuts/Seeds-(diet/dosha specific)

VITAMIN B-15 — CALCIUM PANGAMETE

Utilized in the Body	Kidneys, immune organs, nerves, urinary tract
Deficiencies	Heart disorders, glandular disorders
Functions	Aids in recovery from fatigue; cell oxygenation; fat, protein and sugar metabolism; endocrine system; lubrication of glands, cell regeneration
Synthetic	Pangamic acid
Toxicity	600 mg.
R.D.A.	None established; possibly 50 mg. Therapeutic Dosage: 100 mg

Water Soluble

Depleted By	Fried foods; excess consumption of fat
VATA	Sesame Seeds and butter (tahini), Wheat, Brown Rice, Quince
PITTA	Rye, Spelt, Sunflower Seeds, Apricot Kernel
KAPHA	Pumpkin Seeds, Brewer's Yeast, Spelt, Almonds, Basmati Rice

VITAMIN B-17 — LAETRILE (NITROSIDES)
Cancer Prevention

Utilized in the Body	Cell regeneration, hair, skin, endocrine (particularly the thyroid)
Deficiencies	Cancer, immune disorders, viruses, autoimmune disorders
Functions	Controls cancer growth, prevention properties, reverses aging process, prevents cancer, strengthens organs, assists metabolism, balances endocrine system, protein assimilation, assists reproductive organs, cell regeneration
Synthetic	Not available
Toxicity	Over 1.0 gr. may be toxic.
R.D.A.	Unknown. Therapeutic Dosage: .25 - 1.0 gr. with meal

Water Soluble

Depleted By	Stress, anxiety, fear
VATA	Pork, Cheese, Lamb, Banana, Comfrey, Catnip, Concord Grapes, Cheese, Eggs, Seaweeds (Kelp, Dulse), Wheatgrass, Apricot, Peach, Almonds, Cranberries, Raspberries, Flaxseed, Plums

PITTA	Freshwater Fish, Milk, Banana, Alfalfa, Catnip, Miso, Sunflower seeds, Garbanzo Beans, Mung Beans, Lima Beans, Wheatgrass, Raspberries
KAPHA	Kelp, Peanuts, Alfalfa, Miso, Millet, Flax, Blackberries, Cranberries, Mung Beans, Almonds

PABA — PARA AMINO BENZOIC ACID (B-COMPLEX)

Utilized in the Body	Red blood cells
Deficiencies	Tooth decay, muscle wasting, constipation, low/high thyroid function, premature gray hair, aging, extreme tiredness, depression, miscarriage, intestinal disorders
Functions	Sunscreen, hair pigmentation, healthy skin, intestinal functions, protein utilization, production of folic acid
Synthetic	
Toxicity	High doses over time can be toxic to the liver
R.D.A.	None established. Therapeutic Dosage: 30 mg.
Water Soluble	
Depleted By	Sulfur drugs; depression; constipation
VATA	Organ Meats, Wheatgerm Oil, Yogurt, Molasses, Rice Bran, Wheat
PITTA	Green Leafy Vegetables, Rice Bran, Legumes, Peanuts
KAPHA	Green Leafy Vegetables, Legumes, Yeast

VITAMIN C — ACEROLA, CITRUS, ASCORBATE ACID, SAGO PALM, AMLA

Strong Bones, Circulation, Night Sweats, Infections, Immune Builder, Adrenal Builder, Menopause

Utilized in the Body	Brain, heart, circulation, endocrine system, bones, ligaments, blood vessels
Deficiencies	Weak bones, mouth sores, anemia, weight loss, frequent infections, colds, flu, bleeding gums, thyroid disorders, poor digestion, bruising
Functions	Gum and teeth formation, smooth skin, collagen production, clear complexion, assists digestion and assimilation, strengthens immune system, prevents diarrhea
Synthetic	Ascorbic acid, ascorbate
Toxicity	
R.D.A.	60 mg. Therapeutic Dosage: Up to 10,000 mg.
Water Soluble	
Depleted By	Aspirins, pain relievers, coffee, stress, smoking, baking soda, fevers, pain killers
VATA	Acerola, Tamarind, Lemon, Saffron, Strawberries, Rosehips, Comfrey, Primrose Oil, Tomatoes, Guavas, Sweet Potatoes
PITTA	Yellow Dock, Dandelion, Raspberries, Red Clover, Alfalfa, Rosehips, Green Pepper, Saffron, Kale, Sago Palm, Cabbage, Primrose Oil, Cauliflower, Green Leafy Vegetables
KAPHA	Red Clover, Alfalfa, Yellow Dock, Raspberries, Rosehips, Spinach, Beet

Greens, Parsley, Strawberries, Cayenne, Cabbage, Primrose Oil, Guava, Bell Peppers, Green Leafy Vegetables

Note: Ascorbic acid is best for Vata and Kapha. The ascorbate form is best for Pitta because it is alkaline.

VITAMIN D — ERGOSTEROL
Strong Bones, Cancer Prevention, Balances Glucose

Utilized in the Body	Bones, nerves, skin, teeth, thyroid
Deficiencies	Anemia, constipation, diarrhea, myopia, muscle weakness, poor absorption, tooth decay, soft bones (rickets)
Functions	Assimilation of vitamin E and calcium in the intestinal tract; normal blood clotting
Synthetic	Calciferol or irradiated Ergosterol
Toxicity	25,000 IU may be toxic
R.D.A.	400 IU. Therapeutic Dosage: Up to 1,500 IU
Fat Soluble	
Depleted By	Mineral oil
Best Source	Sunshine on the skin produces it in the body
VATA	Ghee, Eggs, Cod, Liver, Shrimp, Tuna, Mackerel, Sardines, Sunflower Seeds, Butter, Salmon, Fish Oils
PITTA	Trout, Egg White, Ghee, Butter, Sunflower Seeds, Alfalfa, Nettles, Raspberry Leaves, Red Clover, Fresh Water Tuna, Sprouted Seeds
KAPHA	Ghee, Trout, Sunlight, Alfalfa, Nettles, Raspberry Leaves, Red Clover, Sprouted Seeds

VITAMIN E — D-ALPHATOCOPHEROL; TOCOPHEROL ACETATE

Night Sweats, Cancer, Wrinkles, Arthritic Joints, Aging Process

Utilized in the Body	Heart, liver, lungs, adrenals, pituitary, all fatty tissue
Deficiencies	Baldness, prostate disorders, heart disorders, dry skin, premature aging, miscarriage
Functions	Blood vessel dilator, reduces cholesterol, circulation, red blood cell production
Synthetic	D-Alpha tocopherol, Alpha tocopherol acetate
Toxicity	When taken for long periods of time in large amounts may produce toxicity.
R.D.A.	10 IU. Therapeutic Dosage: Up to 1,000 IU
Fat Soluble	
Depleted By	Stress, alcohol
VATA	Brown Rice, Oats, Shatavari, Cold Pressed Oils-(diet/dosha specific), Organ Meats, Black Strap Molasses, Sweet Potato, Watercress, Rosehips, Nuts-(diet/dosha specific)
PITTA	Alfalfa, Rosehips, Buckwheat, Sunflower Oil, Sweet Potato, Dandelion, Cold Pressed Oils-(diet/dosha specific), Soybean
KAPHA	Wheat, Corn, Rye, Almond Oil, Cold Pressed Oils-(diet/dosha specific), Watercress, Dandelion, Soybeans, Greens

VITAMIN F — LINOLEIC, LINOLENIC, AVACHIDONIC SEED, VEGETABLE & NUT OILS

Utilized in the Body	Adrenal, thyroid, cell production, skin, heart, arteries
Deficiencies	Allergies, dry skin, eczema, baldness, kidney disorders, cancer, nail problems, varicose veins
Functions	Normalizes blood pressure, blood coagulation, all glandular activity, healthy hair
Synthetic	None
Toxicity	None established.
R.D.A.	10% of total calories. Men can take 5 times more than women
Fat Soluble Depleted By	Radiation treatments,
VATA	Ghee, Sunflower Seeds, Vegetable Oils-(diet/dosha specific), Avocados, Flaxseed Oil
PITTA	Butter, Ghee, Sunflower Seeds, Vegetable Oils-(diet/dosha specific), Peanuts, Castor oil
KAPHA	Ghee, Vegetable Oils-(diet/dosha specific), Flaxseed Oil; Pumpkin Oils

VITAMIN K — ALFALFA

Utilized in the Body	Blood, circulation, liver
Deficiencies	Jaundice, bleeding ulcers, miscarriage, fatigue, cramps, menstrual problems, colitis, bruising, aging, varicose veins, miscarriage
Functions	Blood clotting, healthy liver, intestinal tract

Synthetic	Menadoine
Toxicity	1,000 mcg.
R.D.A.	70 mcg. Therapeu
Fat Soluble	e: 250 mcg.
Depleted By	Frozen foods, rancid fats, sulfate drugs & sulfates in ion,
VATA	Safflower Oil, Black Strap Molas, Kelp, Green Leafy Vegetables-(diet, specific), Fish Oil, Cherries, Pickles, Blackberries, Yogurt, Molasses, Fermented Vegetables
PITTA	Safflower Oil, Cauliflower, Alfalfa, Nettles, Green Leafy Vegetables-(diet/dosha specific), All Berries
KAPHA	Cauliflower, Alfalfa, Nettles, Kelp, Green Leafy Vegetables-(diet/dosha specific), Safflower Oil

VITAMIN P — CITRIN, RUTIN, BIOFLAVONOIDS, HESPERIDIN

Varicose Veins, Circulation

Utilized in the Body	Bones, blood, gums, teeth, ligaments, skin, stomach
Deficiencies	Asthma, bleeding gums, gum infections, liver disorders, hardening of the arteries, fevers, miscarriage, varicose veins, influenza, tremors, Alzheimer's, Rheumatic Fever
Functions	Prevents bruising; strengthens immune system; blood vessel strengthening, habitual miscarriage, strengthens nervous system; memory enhancement, ulcer prevention
Synthetic	None
Toxicity	None known

R.D.A.	None established. Therapeutic Dosage: Up to 400 mg.
Water S Deple	Excessive bleeding, poor diet, lack of exercise, pregnancy, gaining & losing weight, antibiotics, aspirin & pain relievers, sulfa, stress, inhalation of petroleum fumes, genetics
VATA	Apricots, Black Strap Molasses, Citrus, Amla or Amalaki, Plum, Rosehips, Tomatoes, Black Currant, Grapefruit, Cherries
PITTA	Buckwheat, Greens, Bulgar, Broccoli, Papaya, Algae, Shepherd's Purse, Chervil, Elder Berries, Horsetail, Apricot, Sweet Pepper, Violet Leaf, Grapes
KAPHA	Buckwheat, Greens, Blue Green Algae, Rosehips, Pepper, Prune, Pippali, Lemon, Parsley, Violet Leaf, Tamarind, Horsetail, Citrus-(diet/dosha specific)

VITAMIN T —SESAME SEED FACTOR

Utilized in the Body	Blood, skin, hair, bones, nails
Deficiencies	Senility, dry skin, bleeding, constipation, anemia
Functions	Circulation, skin moisturizer, hair growth, calcium, healthy skin, memory enhancement, blood platelet formation
Synthetic	None
Toxicity	None known
R.D.A.	None established. Therapeutic Dosage: Achieved by including foods in diet

Fat Soluble

Depleted By	Deficient Diet
<u>VATA</u>	Sesame Seeds, Egg Yolk, Raw Seeds-(diet/dosha specific), All Seeds
<u>PITTA</u>	Butter, Raw Seeds-(diet/dosha specific), Sunflower Seeds
<u>KAPHA</u>	Raw Seeds-(diet/dosha specific), Pumpkin Seeds, Almonds

VITAMIN U

Utilized in the Body	Stomach, intestines
Deficiencies	Ulcers, colitis, underweight
Functions	Assists digestion and assimilation, protects stomach lining
Synthetic	
Toxicity	Not known
R.D.A.	None established.
	Therapeutic Dosage: Achieved by including foods in diet

Fat Soluble

Depleted By	Stress, anger
<u>VATA</u>	Fermented Vegetables, *Rejuvelac, Sauerkraut
<u>PITTA</u>	Raw Cabbage, Leafy Green Vegetables
<u>KAPHA</u>	Raw Cabbage, Sauerkraut, Leafy Green Vegetables

* Rejuvelac is the water poured off of wheat berries which have been soaked overnight in preparation for sprouting.

AYURVEDIC MINERAL CHART

CALCIUM

Utilized in the Body	Bones, teeth, hair, nails, circulation, blood, skin
Deficiencies	Heart palpitation, menstrual cramps, nervousness, numbness, tooth problems, tremors, muscles
Functions	Repairs bones, regulates heartbeat, calms nerves, relieves muscle spasms
Synthetic	Calcium lactate, calcium gluconate, dolomite, pantothnate, bone meal, dolomite, egg shell calcium, oyster calcium
Toxicity	No known toxicity
R.D.A.	100 mg. Therapeutic Dosage: 400 - 1,500 mg. In addition to what is in diet
Depleted By	Enemas, lack of exercise, coffee, sugar, alcohol, cortisone
VATA	Raw Egg Yolk, Shellfish, Cheese, Apricots, Figs, Bran, Comfrey, Chamomile, Borage, Chicory, Kelp, Dulse, Sardines, Salmon, Walnuts, Sesame Seeds, Almonds, Well Cooked Greens, Raisins (best soaked)
PITTA	Milk, Apricots, Figs, Cabbage, Alfalfa, Red Clover, Nettles, Shepherd's Purse, Horsetail, Plantain, Chamomile, Borage, Chicory, Dandelion, Kelp, Kale, Sun Flower Seeds, Oats, Navy Beans, Raisins (best soaked), Greens
KAPHA	Greens, Apricots, Cabbage, Bran, Alfalfa, Red Clover, Comfrey, Nettles, Shepherd's Purse, Horsetail, Coltsfoot, Plantain, Chamomile, Borage, Chicory,

Dulse, Leafy Vegetables, Kale, Chard, Legumes, Almonds, Corn, Raisins (best soaked), Sesame Seeds

CHLORINE

Utilized in the Body	Arterial walls, stomach, liver, gallbladder
Deficiencies	Low agni (digestion), hair loss, edema
Functions	Production of hydrochloric acid; production of enzymes; electrolyte balance, muscle contraction
Toxicity	14-28 gr. is considered to be in excess
R.D.A.	500 mg.
Depleted By	Drinking too many liquids with meals, salt free diet, excessive sweating
VATA	Salt, Fish, Cheese, Coconut, Beets, Radishes, Avocado, Kelp, Saltwater Fish, Olives, Watercress, Celery, Turnips
PITTA	Goat & Cow Milk, Cream Cheese, Coconut, Radishes, Asparagus, Celery
KAPHA	Celery, Asparagus, Turnips, Fish, Beets, Radishes, Avocado

CHROMIUM

Utilized in the Body	Blood, arteries
Deficiencies	Diabetes, low blood sugar, pancreatic disorders
Functions	Regulates sugar levels, increases vitality
Toxicity	No known toxicity
R.D.A.	50 mcg. Therapeutic Dosage: Up to 300 mcg.

Depleted By	Excess sugar; too much dairy; too much meat
VATA	Corn Oil, Clams, Whole Grain Cereals, Catnip, Sarsaparilla, Sugar Cane Juice, Shellfish
PITTA	Whole Grain Cereals, Barley Grass, Bee Pollen, Red Clover, Catnip, Sarsaparilla, Freshwater Fish
KAPHA	Corn Oil, Clams, Brewer's Yeast, Barley Grass, Bee Pollen, Red Clover, Catnip, Meat, Corn

COBALT

Utilized in the Body	Blood, circulatory system
Deficiencies	Anemia, low blood pressure
Functions	Production of red blood cells and enzymes
Toxicity	Excess may produce side effects
R.D.A.	6 mcg. Therapeutic Dosage: 5-8 mcg.
Depleted By	Long fasting, enemas
VATA	Organ Meats, Oysters, Clams, Green Leafy Vegetables, Fruits-(diet/dosha specific), Ginseng, Comfrey, Watercress, Ashwagandha
PITTA	Organ Meats, Poultry, Green Leafy Vegetables, Fruits (diet/dosha specific), Comfrey, Ginseng, Watercress, Blue-Green Algae, Ashwagandha
KAPHA	Oysters, Green Leafy Vegetables, Fruits-(diet/dosha specific), Garlic, Spirulina, Blue-Green Algae, Chlorella, Ashwagandha

COPPER

Utilized in the Body	Circulatory system, nervous system, brain
Deficiencies	Respiratory problems, canker sores, fatigue, weak blood
Functions	Mental clarity, coordination of thoughts, bone development, connective tissue, formation of red blood cells
Synthetic	Copper sulfate
Toxicity	20 times the RDA over time may be toxic
R.D.A.	2 mg. Therapeutic Dosage: 2-10 mg.
Depleted By	Hallucinogenic drugs, antibiotics
VATA	Organ Meats, Seafood, Nuts, Molasses, Watercress, Spinach, Chard, Almonds
PITTA	Legumes, Raisins (best soaked), Spinach, Kale, Cabbage, Chickweed, Chard, Whole Grains
KAPHA	Legumes, Watercress, Garlic, Kale, Cabbage, Chickweed, Prunes

FLUORINE

Utilized in the Body	Bone, teeth, hair
Deficiencies	Split nails, hair loss, weak bones, tooth decay
Functions	Increases growth of hair, strengthens nails and bones
Toxicity	Fluoride is toxic (rat poison)
R.D.A.	1 mg. Therapeutic Dosage: 1.5 - 4 mg
Depleted By	Excess sugar; carbonated sodas

VATA	Cheese, Egg Yolk, Carrots, Black Tea, Shellfish, Watercress
PITTA	Cauliflower, Cabbage, Raw Goat Milk, Brussel Sprouts, Sunflower Seeds
KAPHA	Cauliflower, Cabbage, Brussel Sprouts, Seafood, Watercress, Spinach, Garlic, Carrots

GERMANIUM

Utilized in the Body	Cell regenerator, endocrine system
Deficiencies	Autoimmune diseases
Functions	Builds immune system, rejuvenator, life extension
Toxicity	None known
R.D.A.	None established. Therapeutic Dosage: None known
Depleted By	Processed foods; smoking; alcohol
VATA	Aloe Vera, Comfrey, Watercress, Ashwagandha
PITTA	Aloe Vera, Comfrey, Chlorella, Ginseng
KAPHA	Garlic, Chlorella

IODINE

Utilized in the body	Hair, nails, endocrine (thyroid), brain, bones
Deficiencies	Cold hands and feet, anger, manic-depression, obesity, thyroid disorders
Functions	Mental development, enhances digestion, stabilizes fat metabolism, improves circulation
Synthetic	Potassium oxide (added to table salt). Natural source is seaweeds

Toxicity	Over 1,800 mcg. can cause problems
R.D.A.	150 mcg.
	Therapeutic Dosage: Up to 1,000 mcg.
Depleted By	Too much protein
VATA	Seaweeds, Kelp, Seafood, Carrots, Tomatoes, Pineapple, Dulse, Mushrooms, Irish Moss, Citrus Fruit, Artichokes, Turnips, Watercress, Sea Salt
PITTA	Seaweeds (soaked), Pears, Onions, Parsley, Sarsaparilla, Dulse, Mushrooms, Artichokes, Turnips, Greens
KAPHA	Carrots, Pears, Onions, Pineapple, Parsley, Sarsaparilla, Turnips

IRON

Utilized in the Body	Circulation, bones, skin
Deficiencies	Anemia, fatigue, pale skin, constipation, poor assimilation
Functions	Improves immune system, clear complexion, red blood cell formation & hemoglobin
Synthetic	Ferrous fumarate (best - gluconate, worst - sulfate)
Toxicity	1,000 mg.
R.D.A.	10 mg. (Men) - 18 mg. (Women)
	Therapeutic Dosage: 10-50 mg.
Depleted By	Black tea, high protein diet, bleeding (ulcers, etc.)
VATA	Organ Meats, Eggs, Shellfish, Poultry, Prunes, Blackstrap Molasses, Apricots, Comfrey, Sorrel, Watercress, Fennel, Bananas, Dulse

<u>PITTA</u>	Lentils, Shellfish, Organ Meats, Poultry, Apricots, Potato Peelings, Nettles, Dandelion, Alfalfa, Yellow Dock, Comfrey, Chickweed, Mullein, Fennel
<u>KAPHA</u>	Lentils, Shellfish, Poultry, Potato Peelings, Nettles, Dandelion, Alfalfa, Yellow Dock, Chickweed, Mullein, Sorrel, Watercress, Fennel, Prunes

LITHIUM

Utilized in the Body	Brain, muscular system, nervous system
Deficiencies	Manic-depression, nervousness, anxiety
Functions	Balances and transports sodium metabolism to nerves, brain and muscles
Toxicity	None
R.D.A.	None available
Depleted By	Alcohol; hallucinogenic drugs, bi-polar disorder
<u>VATA</u>	Cream, Yogurt, Milk, Kelp, Dulse, Seafood
<u>PITTA</u>	Kelp, Dulse, Seafood
<u>KAPHA</u>	Buttermilk, Kelp, Dulse, Seafood

MAGNESIUM

Utilized in the Body	Brain, endocrine system, arteries, nervous system, stomach
Deficiencies	Weak bones, infections, confusion, irritability, excessive anger, trembling
Functions	Balances acid/alkaline, regulates blood sugar, metabolism of calcium and vitamin C.
Synthetic	Magnesium palmatate, Magnesium sulfate

Toxicity	Large doses over a period of time
R.D.A.	400 mg.
	Therapeutic Dosage: 300 - 1,800 mg.
Depleted By	Chemical drugs, alcohol
VATA	Lemons, Peaches, Beet Tops, Nuts, Figs, Seafood, Molasses, Yellow Corn, Watercress, Oatstraw, Carrots, Almonds, Raspberries, Brown Rice, Sesame Seeds
PITTA	Peaches, Beet Tops, Sunflower Seeds, Apples, Alfalfa, Green Vegetables, Nettles, Burdock, Horsetail, Sage, Raspberries, Clover
KAPHA	Lemons, Beet Tops, Apples, Almonds, Green Vegetables, Coconut, Apples, Watercress, Alfalfa, Oatstraw, Nettles, Burdock, Carrots, Horsetail, Almonds, Sage, Clover

MANGANESE

Utilized in the Body	Circulation, blood, brain, endocrine system (especially the pituitary and thyroid)
Deficiencies	Stomach disorders, hot flashes, dizziness, loss of hearing
Functions	Production of enzymes, hormonal functions, muscular system, nervous system
Synthetic	Manganese gluconate
Toxicity	5 - 7.5 mg.
R.D.A.	4 - 6 mg. Therapeutic Dosage: 2-50 mg.
Depleted By	Too much fat; constipation
VATA	Egg Yolks, Beets, Citrus, Rice Bran, Kelp, All Nuts, All Seeds, Pineapple, Wheat Germ

PITTA	Peas, Rice Bran, Green Vegetables, Sunflower Seeds, Blueberries
KAPHA	Peas, Citrus, Green Vegetables, Almonds, Kelp

MOLYBDENUM

Utilized in the Body	Circulation, blood, stomach
Deficiencies	Poor digestion and assimilation
Functions	Important for oxidation
Toxicity	In large amounts
R.D.A.	None established. Therapeutic Dosage:150 mcg - 500 mcg.
Depleted By	Alcohol; carbonated drinks
VATA	Whole Grain Cereals-(diet/dosha specific), Liver
PITTA	Legumes, Milk, Liver, Dark Green Vegetables
KAPHA	Legumes, Whole Grain Cereals-(diet/dosha specific), Brewer's Yeast, Millet

PHOSPHORUS

Utilized in the body	Circulation, blood, heart, urinary tract, nerves, teeth
Deficiencies	Loss of appetite, breathing disorders, sudden weight loss or gain, low blood sugar
Functions	Cell regeneration, vitality, assists heart and muscle contractions, calcium metabolism, assists nerve activity, assists muscular activity, assimilation of vitamins
Synthetic	Calcium phosphate

Toxicity	None known
R.D.A.	1000 mg. Therapeutic Dosage: 1500 mg.
Depleted By	Sugar, mental stress, high fat diet
VATA	Cheese, Meat, Whole Grains-(diet/dosha specific), Egg Yolk, Lentils-(well cooked), Caraway Seeds, Parsley, Comfrey, Watercress, Licorice, dried fruit-(well soaked), All Nuts
PITTA	Dried Fruits-(well soaked), Milk, Fish, Poultry, Whole Grains-(diet/dosha specific), Legumes-(diet/dosha specific), Peas, Comfrey, Nettles, Chickweed, Alfalfa, Marigold, Dandelion, Licorice
KAPHA	Almonds, Whole Grains-(diet/dosha specific), Legumes-(diet/dosha specific), Peas, Caraway Seeds, Parsley, Watercress, Nettles, Chickweed, Alfalfa, Marigold, Dandelion

POTASSIUM

Utilized in the Body	Blood, heart, urinary tract, muscle tissue, nerves, skin
Deficiencies	Fatigue, constipation, insomnia, weak reflexes
Functions	Balances sodium, assists all body activities, nerve functions and tissue growth
Synthetic	Potassium gluconate, Potassium chloride
Toxicity	None known
R.D.A.	2,500 mg. Therapeutic Dosage: Up to 6,000 mg.
Depleted by	Excessive urination, excessive perspiration, salt
VATA	Sweet Potatoes, Tomatoes, Watercress, Dried Soaked Fruits, Vegetables, Whole

	Grain Cereals-(diet/dosha specific), All Nuts, All Seeds, Comfrey, Coltsfoot, Parsley, Kelp, Dulse
PITTA	Potatoes, Sweet Potatoes, Sunflower Seeds, Lean Meats, Dried Soaked Fruits, Legumes-Well Soaked-(diet/dosha specific), Vegetables, Whole Grain Cereals-(diet/dosha specific), Alfalfa, Comfrey, Coltsfoot, Borage, Chicory, Eyebright, Mint, Plantain
KAPHA	Potatoes, Lean Meats, Dried Fruits, Vegetables, Whole Grain Cereals-(dosha/diet specific), Alfalfa, Coltsfoot, Water Cress, Borage, Chicory, Eyebright, Mint, Plantain, Parsley

SELENIUM

Utilized in the Body	Male reproductive system, blood, circulation
Deficiencies	Premature aging, hair loss, brittle nails, fatigue
Functions	Slows the aging process, antioxidant, blood oxidation
Synthetic	Natural sources only
Toxicity	Nausea occurs with excessive dosage
R.D.A.	50 mcg. Therapeutic Dosage: Up to 150 mcg.
Depleted By	Stress; smoking; lack of B-vitamins
VATA	Tuna Fish, Herring, Brewer's Yeast, Wheat Germ & Bran, Whole Grains-(diet/dosha specific), Eggs, Wheat Germ, Kelp
PITTA	Milk, Herring, Broccoli, Whole Grains-(diet/dosha specific), Kelp

KAPHA	Brewer's Yeast, Broccoli, Whole Grains-(diet/dosha specific), Kelp

SILICON

Utilized in the Body	Bones, nails, hair, teeth, endocrine system, reproductive system
Deficiencies	Premature aging (early wrinkles, hair loss), weak bones
Functions	Promotes hair growth; strengthens bone tissue and nails, complexion, enhances immune system
Toxicity	None known
R.D.A.	None known
Depleted By	Stress, smoking, alcohol, fear, lack of B vitamins
VATA	Steel Cut Oats, Beets, Kelp, Grapes, Sweet Onions-(well cooked), Almonds, All Seeds, Parsnips, Whole Grains-(diet/dosha specific), Tomatoes, Horsetail, Leeks, Strawberries, Flaxseed
PITTA	Peanuts, Strawberries, Apples, Sweet Onions, Grapes, Parsnips, Whole Grains-(diet/dosha specific), Spinach, Horsetail, Dandelion, Nettles, Leeks
KAPHA	Peanuts, Strawberries, Apples, Almonds, Parsnips, Whole Grains-(dosha/diet specific), Spinach, Horsetail, Dandelion, Nettles, Leeks, Strawberries, Flaxseed

SODIUM

Utilized in the Body	Lymph movement, muscular, arterial balance, all glandular activities, blood
Deficiencies	Chronic pain, diarrhea, sugar imbalance, gallbladder problems

Functions	Lymphatic system, production of bile, adrenaline production, pancreatic enzymes, perspiration
Synthetic	Sodium chloride (table salt)
Toxicity	Excess causes loss of potassium; high blood pressure
R.D.A.	500 mg. Therapeutic Dosage: 2,000 mg.
Depleted By	Too much sugar, meat and dairy
VATA	Watermelon, Celery, Kelp, Sea Salt, Asparagus, Okra, Pork, Carrots, Beets, Organ Meats
PITTA	Romaine Lettuce, Celery, Asparagus, Okra, Coconut, Pork, Beet Greens
KAPHA	Romaine Lettuce, Celery, Asparagus, Carrots, Coconut, Irish Moss, Beet Greens

SULPHUR

Utilized in the Body	Bone tissue (hair, nails, skeletal), nervous system
Deficiencies	Early aging
Functions	All body tissue formation, collagen production
Toxicity	Possible with inorganic sources
R.D.A.	None established. Therapeutic Dosage: 500-1,000 mg. Considered adequate when protein needs are met
Depleted By	Not known
VATA	Lean Meats-(diet/dosha specific), Eggs, Ocean Fish, Horseradish, Shrimp, Parsley, Sage, Celery, Watercress, Coltsfoot
PITTA	Celery, Legumes-(diet/dosha specific), Freshwater Fish, Cabbage, Brussel

	Sprouts, Chestnuts, Nettles, Plantain, Kale, Coltsfoot, Mullein, Shepherd's Purse, Cabbage Family
KAPHA	Legumes-(diet/dosha specific), Celery, Meat-(diet/dosha specific), Freshwater Fish, Cabbage, Brussel Sprouts, Horse Radish, Shrimp, Parsley, Kale, Coltsfoot, Mullein, Shepherd's Purse, Cabbage Family, Sage

VANADIUM

Utilized in the Body	Circulatory system, blood
Deficiencies	High blood pressure, heart disorders
Functions	Breaks down cholesterol
R.D.A.	None established
Depleted By	Not known
VATA	Herring, Sardines
PITTA	Sea vegetables
KAPHA	Sea vegetables

ZINC

Utilized in the Body	Blood, brain, prostate, reproductive system, skin
Deficiencies	Late blooming, low appetite, loss of taste, poor circulation, liver disorders, prostate disorders, reproductive disorders, infertility, insulin insufficient
Functions	Heals cuts & burns; assists breakdown of pancreatic enzyme production, prostate functions, maturity and development of all organs
Toxicity	None

R.D.A.	15 mg.
	Therapeutic Dosage: Up to 50 mg.
Depleted By	Air pollution, alcohol, pregnancy
VATA	Sunflower Seeds, Seafood, Organ Meats, Mushrooms, Watercress, Pumpkin Seeds
PITTA	Sunflower Seeds, Mushrooms, Soybeans
KAPHA	Soybeans, Brewer's Yeast, Watercress, PumpkinSeeds

TRACE MINERALS

ARSENIC

VATA	Asparagus, Celery, Salmon
PITTA	Celery
KAPHA	Asparagus, Celery

BORON

VATA	All Sweet and Sour Fruit, Purslane
PITTA	Dandelion, Yellow Dock, Chickweed, Astringent Fruit
KAPHA	Chickweed, Bitter Herbs

BORIUM

VATA	Organic Fruit, Vegetables, Nuts, Purslane, Dandelion Root
PITTA	Organic Fruit, Vegetables, Chickweed, Purslane, Nettles, Dandelion Leaf, Yellow Dock
KAPHA	Organic Fruit, Vegetables, Chickweed, Nettles, Dandelion Leaf, Yellow Dock

BROMINE

Utilized in the Body	Heart, circulation

Deficiencies	Heart disorders, kidney/bladder disorders, and edema
Functions	Circulation and water balance
Depleted By	Excess alcohol and sugar
VATA	Melons, Cucumber, Seafood
PITTA	Melons, Cucumber, Alfalfa
KAPHA	Alfalfa, Turnips, Seafood

NICKEL

Utilized in the Body	Tissue repair, bones, heart, and circulation
Deficiencies	
Functions	Builds strong bones, healthy tissue
Depleted By	Not known
VATA	All vegetables (diet/dosha specific), All Herbs (diet/dosha specific), Fenugreek
PITTA	All Vegetables (diet/dosha specific), All Herbs (diet/dosha specific), Alfalfa, Red Clover, Oat Straw
KAPHA	All Vegetables (diet/dosha specific), All Herbs (diet/dosha specific), Alfalfa, Red Clover, Oat Straw, Fenugreek

CHAPTER 10

HERBS & THEIR USES

PRIMITIVE MAN LIVED CLOSE to the earth learning and experimenting as they used the different plants around them. They made observations of their properties by watching the animals and noticing what they ate when they were sick. They used only what they needed, having respect and reverence for this earth. They became aware of the herbs as the gift from the Divine to heal their wounds and give them strength in their bodies. They harvested these precious plants with care and gratitude. We are the beneficiaries of 10,000 years of herbal study. Herbs and herbal derivatives were the main medicines used by doctors into the 1900's.

Early in this century, medical schools began receiving endowments from the fledgling pharmaceutical industry and soon "modern science" had abandoned the old herbal remedies for the new, fashionable, scientific drugs. Mercury, now known to be a deadly toxin, was an early favorite for purging the intestines. Later they gave us thalidomide, which caused thousands of birth defects. Now they have chemotherapy drugs so toxic that your hair falls out (the oncologists won't take them). One author has dubbed our country, "the 200 million guinea pigs" because we are constantly being tested upon with new and improved drugs and therapies. Americans over 70 are often on ten or more different prescriptions to handle symptoms that could be prevented or treated naturally without side effects by using herbs. Why should we take dangerous chemicals we don't understand?

Once again our Mother Earth is calling us to partake of her gifts. It's time to listen and return and learn from her. Even though we have forgotten nature, nature has not forgotten us. The herbs have survived, and are pushing up through the cement of our city sidewalks. They are waiting for us. Plants still cover the earth, decorating it with green splendor and many colors. The aroma from flowers can bring us joy.

Seaweed's in the oceans give us their minerals. Their oxygen production sustains the life of all beings. In this natural, vast laboratory the vegetable kingdom maintains a constant balance that allows for the evolution for all creatures - by this gift we are able to nourish and heal ourselves. Let us not continue to destroy and pollute our bodies and the earth.

Herbs contain active therapeutic ingredients that aid in the prevention of dis-ease and produce the healing of many illnesses. These wonderful plants contain alkaloids, minerals, vitamins, enzymes, proteins, tannins, and sapponins. They help us with circulation, respiration, elimination and assist with creating balance in our whole body. Nature is a pharmacy.

We can begin to understand how to use these herbs by reading this and other self-help books. Look in your health food store for classes and herbal walks. Begin harvesting and gathering herbs for your own use. Many fresh herbs can be found in the grocery store or grown right in your home under lighted windows, even in the winter. In the summer grow herbs outside such as cilantro (from coriander seeds), parsley, basil, mint, rosemary, marjoram, dill, fennel, borage, violets, lambs quarters, echinacea, nasturtium, comfrey leaves and flowers, dandelion, ginger, turmeric, and nettles. These make excellent additions to salads, steamed vegetables, soups, or stews. They can also be dried for the winter months. Herbs are easy to grow, needing very little care and most are resistant to insects.

HERBAL CONSTITUENTS*

Herbs contain many active therapeutic ingredients such as enzymes, tannins, alkaloids, glycosides, saponins, bitter compounds, and starches. Following is a brief description of each.

Enzymes

They are organic catalysts, which are produced by living organisms (pepsin, pancreatin, rennin, papain, and bromelain), and nitrogenous organic substances composed of amino acid units.

Tannins

They are widely distributed, especially in barks and leaves, and have a faint odor and an astringent taste. Tannins occur as an amorphous powder, glistening scales, or spongy masses that are light brown to yellowish white.

Alkaloids

Organic substances, which are derived chiefly from plants, are basic substances containing carbon, hydrogen, and nitrogen. Most alkaloids are bitter and slightly alkaline. All the important alkaloids produce profound physiological and pharmacological effects. Many of them are the most poisonous of known substances.

Glycosides

Their distinguishing property is that of splitting into glucose's, or into glucose yielding sugars and some other bodies, when heated in the presence of acids or alkalines. Glycosides are also considered sugar ethers.

Saponins

Plant constituents belonging to the glycosidal group (breaking up in the presence of acids or ferments into glucose - grape sugar, and inactive and unknown bodies). They possess the characteristic quality of foaming when shaken with water. Many of them are innocuous, some extremely poisonous (sapotoxins).

Bitter Compounds

Bitters are compounds that stimulate glandular function, particularly digestive.

Starches

Released in granular form from plant cells. Starches are used as tablet fillers, binders, and disintegrants. They swell in boiling water to form mucilaginous pastes such as cornstarch.

* Information excerpted from "Herbal Preparations and Natural Therapies", by Debra Nuzzi, M.H.

HERBAL THERAPEUTIC PROPERTIES

Adaptogenic	Helps the body adapt to stress and creates balance.
Alterative	Tending to restore normal health, cleans and purifies the blood, alters existing nutritive and excretory processes, gradually restoring normal body function.
Analgesic	Eliminates pain.
Antibiotic	Destroys unwanted organisms in the body.
Anticoagulant	Stops blood clotting.
Anti-inflammatory	Reduces inflammation.
Antifungal	Kills fungal infections.
Antioxidant	Prevents oxidation in the tissues.
Antipyretic	Dispels heat, fire and fever (from the Greek word pyre - fire).
Antiseptic	Cleans blood and inhibits organisms that cause infections.

Antispasmodic	Relieves spasms of voluntary and involuntary muscles.
Aphrodisiac	Invigorates the body by nourishing the sexual organs.
Astringent	Firms tissue and organs; reduces discharges and secretions.
Bitter Tonic	Bitter herbs which, in small amounts, stimulate digestion and otherwise help regulate fire in the body.
Cardiotonic	Improves heart condition.
Carminative	Relieves intestinal gas pain and distension; promotes peristalsis.
Cathartic	An intestinal purgator.
Demulcent	Protects and nourishes mucous membranes.
Diaphoretic	Causes perspiration and increased elimination through the skin.
Diuretic	Promotes activity of kidney and bladder and increases urination.
Emetic	Induces vomiting.
Emmenagogue	Helps promote and regulate menstruation. Special female herbs to build and support female organs.
Emollient	Smoothes, softens, and protects the skin.
Estrogenic	Phyto estrogenic plants; stimulates female estrogen or mimics it molecularly on cell receptor sites.
Expectorant	Promotes discharge of phlegm and mucous from the lungs and throat.
Febrifuge	Reduces fever and takes heat from the organs.
Hemostatic	Stops the flow of blood. An astringent that stops internal bleeding or hemorrhaging.

Hepatic	Assists liver function.
Laxative	Promotes bowel movements.
Nervine	Strengthens the functional activity of the nervous system; may be stimulants and sedatives.
Rejuvenative	Prevents decay, postpones aging, revitalizes organs.
Sedative	Calms and tranquilizes by lowering the functional activity of the organ or body part.
Stimulant	Increases internal heat, dispels internal chill, and strengthens metabolism and circulation.
Styptic	Stops bleeding when topically applied.
Tonic (nutritive)	Increases weight and density and nourishes the body.
Tonify	Firms the tissues of the body.
Vasodilator	Opens the blood vessels.
Vermifuge	Assists in expelling worms.
Vulnerary	Assists in healing of wounds by protecting against infection and stimulating cell growth.

WAYS TO USE HERBS

Storing Herbs

Do not store herbs in plastic.

Canning jars are excellent for storing herbs or good glass jars with tight fitting lid. In the summer, or in tropical climates, add a few bay leaves for bug prevention. When working with herbs, it is very important not to use plastic, aluminum, or Teflon containers or utensils. Use enamel, stainless steel, clay or glass.

Herbs can be smoked like cigarettes or used to make douches, enemas, compresses, bath, gargles, syrup, medicated ghee, jellies, creams, suppositories and oils.

Liquid Preparations - (Teas)

These have been given many names such as herbal blends, herbal brews, herbal mixtures, and the most common one, tea. This is one of my favorite ways to take medicine, yet it is a commitment to prepare. We live in a society that wants fast and quick, easy "fix-it" results. Ayurveda teaches that when the individual is involved with the preparation and their own healing, it speeds up the process toward better health. Drinking herbal mixtures instead of water gives the body added nourishment and is one of the best ways to assimilate and absorb the herbal medicine into the body. Drinking tea adds vitamins and minerals that the body may use to build the immune system.

In practice I find herbal brews to be one of the most effective ways to take herbs. Combine all herbs for the condition and, rather than walking around with a bottle of water, carry a bottle of herbal brew and drink the mixture throughout the day.

This book has a variety of herbal blends for specific dis-eases that taste quite good. For most people, when things do not taste good, they don't like taking it, and won't.

Dry Herb Tea

Cut and Sifted.

I find this to be one of the best ways to make a tea. Dry herbs for tea are best in the cut and sifted form. The herb has not been ground and still carries all the volatile components. Anytime fresh herbs are available, use them. When making a tea, the roots and bark are best boiled for 10-15 minutes. Leaf and flower teas are made by bringing water to a boil, then adding the herb. Let it steep for 15 minutes. Strain into container; refrigerate for future use. Make up to one gallon at a time. Pitta may drink cool. Vatas should heat before consuming.

Sun Tea

This is done by placing the herb into a jar, adding water, and putting the jar in the sun for 2-3 hours. This method works well with leaves and flowers. For 1 gallon of water, use 2 oz. herb, or in smaller amounts use 1 teaspoon per cup of water. For variety, or for better flavor, add 1 quart of fruit juice, such as apple, peach, orange, or mango to the gallon of the sun brewed tea. Refrigerate and use.

Juice Tea

Make any tea of your choice. Strain. Add your favorite fruit juice. This works well for children with a ratio of 30-50% fruit juice and 50-70% herb tea.

Infusions - Tea

This is done to keep the volatile components of the herb. Often in the boiling process they are lost. The vitamins and minerals are preserved.

For leaves and flowers (they do best in this form):

- Boil water and pour over the dry herbs.
- Steep for 15-20 minutes. Strain.
- Do not use plastic or aluminum.

Decoctions

These are strong herb preparations where you boil the mixture down until it is very concentrated with the extracted herbs. Chopped roots, barks and seeds are best used for this method. More of the nutritive value is retained. Take 1-3 teaspoons per day with water.

Digestion

One ounce of herbs to 16 oz. water. Boil down and reduce to 1 cup. Strain and store in refrigerator.

Use one of the following herbs: Fennel, Ginger, Pippali, Cyperus, Peruvian Bark, or Red Root.

Lymphatic Cleanser

One or 2oz. herb to 16 ounces water. Boil down to one-eighth the original amount. For burning fat.

Use Poke Root, Lyceum, Burdock Root.

Weight Reduction

One oz. herbs to 16 oz. water. Boil down to 1.3 ounces. For burning fat in the body.

Use Ephedra, Ginger, Guggul, Yarrow, Myrrh, Motherwort.

Pacifying Doshas

One oz. herbs to 16 oz. water. Boil down to 2 ounces.

Use Cinnamon, Cardamon, Ginger.

Tonic - Stimulating - Nutritive

One oz. herbs to 16 oz. water. Boil down to 5 ounces.

Use Ashwagandha, Shatavari, Angelica, Katuka.

Very Dry Condition

One oz. herbs to 16 ounces water. Boil down to 1 oz. It will be like glue. Add honey.

Use Slippery Elm, Shatavari.

Muscle & Bone Problems

One oz. of herbs to 16 oz. of water. Boil down until half volume.

Use Sesame, Nettles, Comfrey.

Dryness in the Body

To 1 ounce water add 3 tsp. powdered herb and 1 tsp. ghee, add honey and 1/4 cup sucanat. Mix well.

Use Jatamasi, Ginger (fresh).

Milk Decoction

One oz. herbs to 8 oz. milk on low heat for two hours. Boil down to 14 oz. Excellent for Pittas.

One oz. herbs to 16 oz. milk. Boil down to 14 oz.

Use Cardamon, Ginger, Cinnamon.

Tinctures

Tinctures and extracts are where the active ingredients of the plant have been extracted by means of a solvent. If you choose to make a standardized potency, use a ratio of l: 4 (1-part herb to 4 parts alcohol). If you choose to make a tincture stronger than the standardized potency, fill the jar with the herbs. When using fresh herbs, take into consideration the water content of the herb and leave space for it. When using a dry herb, use a jar equivalent to the exact size needed after filling with the alcohol. When using fresh herbs, make sure they are clean, especially any roots. Make sure the bottle is sterilized.

To soak, place 4 oz. of dried herbs in 16 oz. (an example of the 1:4 ratio) of alcohol, Ever Clear brandy, rum or vodka may be used. It is preferable to use a dark bottle when available, or to keep in a dark area. After soaking for 30 days, discard the pressed herbs, and rebottle the tincture. Use a dropper full 3-4 times a day.

Tinctures have a shelf life of two or three years. Never use isopropyl alcohol or rubbing alcohol (menthol). Do not use alcoholic tinctures when pregnant or in a high Pitta condition, such as ulcers, inflammation, or high fevers.

Non-alcoholic tinctures can be made with glycerine or vinegar in the same way as alcohol tinctures, although some prefer to use one-half glycerine and one-half distilled water in place of the alcohol, mixed with the herbs.

Fresh Herb Juice

This can be made by putting the fresh herb right into the juicer, juice press, or a wheatgrass juicer. When a juicer is unavailable, chop the herb, and put it into a blender. Add 1-ounce herb to 2 cups of water. Then strain all liquid out. A great electrical juicer is "The Green Machine".

Cold Water Extract

Prepared by immersing the fresh or dry plant for 8-12 hours in cold water. This particular method only extracts small amounts of the bitter part of the herb and the mineral salts. Good as a daily beverage.

Use 2 Tablespoons of the chosen herb and 1 cup of distilled water. Cover. Steep for 8 hours. Refrigerate.

Herbal Vinegar

Infuse herbal vinegar with culinary herbs such as rosemary, basil, tarragon, savory, garlic, onion or cilantro. Soak herbs in the vinegar for 30 days. Keep in a cool place. Strain and rebottle to use on salads, dressings, and for cooking.

Herbal Wine

To make herbal wine, purchase wine ready-made and add fresh herbs. Similar to making herbal vinegar. Let the herbs set in the wine for thirty days and strain. To ensure freshness, keep bottle very tightly closed.

Another Method

Make a strong decoction, then add 1/2-tsp. yeast, 1-tsp. honey or sucanat. Put in a dark bottle and place in a warm place (at least 70 degrees). Leave for three months. This alters the medicinal value of the herb. Use cork to close bottle.

Medicated Ghee

Place fresh powdered herb in a pan, add ghee, mix and cook at low heat for 15 minutes. If you use cut and sifted herbs, you must strain before use. You can add honey to medicated ghee for use on crackers (children will love it).

Medicated or Infused Oils

There are many ways to make or infuse oils. One of the ways is to use a double boiler, add water in the bottom of the double boiler and bring to a boil. In the top of the double boiler, add the oil. Use 1 pint of oil to two ounces of herb. Add the herbs. Steep on very low flame for 24 hours. Strain and press the oil into a glass jar.

Another more potent way of producing this oil is to add the oil and herbs in a large- mouthed jar and keep in a dark place for 30-60 days. Strain and use.

Cold Infusion - Medicated Oil

Vegetable oil infusion. In a quart of vegetable oil (my preference is coconut oil that has been melted), add the petals and leaves into the oil leaving space for the petals to expand. Wait for 2-3 days. Remove the petals. Strain. Add fresh petals. Repeat this for 30 days or until strong. Often made with jasmine or rose petals.

Poultice

Preparation of a fresh poultice can be made by crushing herbs or leaves in a mortar and pestle. Then simmer the herb for 1-2 minutes on low heat, strain, place into a washcloth, and place over the area of injury. You may use a Band-Aid or surgical sleeve to hold the poultice in place. When in nature and there is an injury, take the herb, chew it up, mix with saliva and make a poultice. Place on the injury (example: dandelion or plantain). Herbs may be juiced in a juice press as well. When using a powdered herb, use 1 teaspoon of powdered herb to 1 tablespoon of water. Mix and apply. Ginger poultice is made from powdered ginger and is good for backaches.

Capsuled Herbal Blends

Herbs are medicine and many have a bitter taste and are best taken in capsule form, especially the pungent and bitter tasting herbs such as golden seal, chaparral, bayberry, and gentian. There is a small hand machine called, "Cap'em Quick" which costs $6.95. Gelatin or rice capsules can be purchased for use in this machine.

Herbal Tablets

Herbs are ground into a fine powder and blended together into a very concentrated mixture with compounds and binders to create a hard tablet. They are harder to assimilate due to the concentration of the mixture, especially when there is low Agni. When taking tablets, take them with hot tea or warm milk for easier assimilation, or take them with meals.

Roasted Herbs

These are used for cooking. The herb is roasted in a pan, then added to food. This method is done with digestive herbs such as coriander, cumin, fennel, anise, garlic, onion, and cardamon. Particularly good for Kapha.

Powder or Churnas

When the herbs have been freshly ground, such as cooking spices, they are good for digestion. They can be used in tea or put into capsules. They can be mixed with honey or added to milk. Powders are particularly good for the blood assimilation and are best added to food as you make it or sprinkled as a seasoning at the table.

Pills can be made by mixing the powder with ghee and warm water. Allow to dry. (Ghee 25% - Herbs 75%)

Jelly can be made by using the powder, the pulp or the fresh herb. Sweeten with honey, stevia, raw sugar, or fructose.

Oatmeal Gruel

Drink	Soak 1 cup of steel cut oats overnight in 4 cups of water. Add 1-ounce raisins. Strain the water and add ground herbs - fennel and coriander to taste. Excellent drink for Pitta digestive system and for diarrhea.
Eat	The oatmeal and raisins can be heated and served to eat.

Slippery Elm Breakfast Delight

Soak dry fruit overnight. In the morning, cook slowly. Then add slippery elm powdered herb until thick like porridge.

Immune Broth

Herbalist Brigitte Mars of UniTea Herbs, Colorado, provided this recipe

Pitta & Kapha

1 onion
4 Cloves of garlic
1 tbs. olive oil
1 cup sliced carrots
1 cup cabbage

1 cup broccoli
1/2-cup shitaki mushrooms
3" of wakame seaweed
4 pieces of astralagus
4 dan shen roots
1/2" fresh ginger, well chopped (not for Pitta+)
1/2 bunch cilantro
1/2 bunch parsley
6 cups water

Vata

1 onion
4 cloves of garlic
1 tbs. seasame oil
1 cup sliced carrots
1 cup sweet potatoes
1 cup broccoli
1/2 cup shitaki mushrooms
3" wakame seaweed
4 pieces of astralagus
4 dan shen roots
1/2" fresh ginger, well chopped
1/2 bunch cilantro
1/2 bunch parsley
6 cups water

Directions

- Chop onion and garlic. Sauté in olive or sesame oil.
- Add all ingredients to water and simmer for 1 hour.
- Take out 1 cup broth.
- Mix 6 tsp. of miso into 1 cup broth.
- Mix well and add to the soup pot just before serving. Do not boil again or the enzymes will be destroyed.
- Do not eat astralagus root, but leave it in the soup for flavor.

Rice Water Herbs

Digestion, Ulcers, Heartburn

Add 1 cup of rice to 4 cups water.

Bring to a boil, then remove from stove.

Strain 2 cups of water out.

Place remainder back on the stove, turn to low, and finish cooking the rice.

To the rice water, add spices to taste:

Indigestion: cardamon, ginger, black pepper, saffron, fennel, coriander.

Ulcers & Heartburn: peppermint, fennel, coriander, aloe vera.

Drink before meals.

For Good Digestion

For digestion, herbs taken ten to fifteen minutes before meals help a Vata condition by stimulating the appetite. When herbs are taken with food, it assists with digestion and assimilation of the herbs. When taken after food, it helps Kapha and assists the lungs. (Best taken in tablets or jelly form.) Tinctures, taken after meals with water, can slow down digestion. When taken between meals it is easily assimilated and particularly helps the small intestines.

Specific herbs taken at night are good for insomnia and a peaceful sleep, especially when taken one-half hour before bedtime. Do not take stimulating herbs before bedtime. Warm herbal teas in the early morning help with cleansing, elimination, and get the gastrointestinal tract ready for food.

Suggestions

Whenever possible, make a habit to study herbs. Try to purchase them from your local merchants, or even grow and harvest them yourself. Local herbs are always best for the people living in that area. Many herbs can also be grown on balconies, especially culinary herbs. In the winter, you can bring them indoors.

Drying herbs is an art. It is best to harvest from unpolluted areas. Often, public parks use sprays. Always harvest from plants that are healthy and abundant. Do not yank the plant when harvesting or cutting. First say a prayer, ask permission, and give thanks for the gifts. Do not over harvest wild areas. Taking one plant in ten insures continuation of the herb. Therefore, look for cut stems as a sign that someone has already harvested an area, then find another area for your gathering.

CULINARY HERBS

Best used in cooking, teas, and as churnas (seasonings)

+ increase   - decrease   o neutral or mixed   = balancing

Allspice	VK-P+	Digestive stimulant
Anise Seed	VK-P+	Flatulence, painful period, dry cough
Basil	VK-P+	Sinus, muscle spasms, nervous disorders, headaches
Bay	VK-P+	Circulation, antiseptic, colds, nervousness, hair, nails
Black Pepper	VK-P+	Stimulating circulation, food poisoning, head cold
Caraway	VK-P+	Digestive, flatulence, respiratory
Cardamon	VK-P+	Spleen, heart, clarity, joy, mental fatigue, nervousness, nausea
Cloves	VK-P+	Toothache, Lupus, sinusitis, lymphatic, insect repellent
Cinnamon	VK-P+	Painful joints, tension, fear, antispasm
Coriander	VPK=	Indigestion, rheumatism, assimilation, skin rashes, fevers
Cumin	VPK=	Immune builder, aphrodisiac
Dill	PK-Vo	Antispasmodic, flatulence, suppressed sexual energy, hiccups, frigidity
Fennel	VPK=	Blood purifier, detoxifier

Ginger	VK-P+	Obesity, sluggish digestion, fevers, colds, flu, morning sickness
Juniper Berries	VK-P+	Swelling, congestion
Lemon	PV-Ko	Diabetes, vomiting, kidneys, arthritis, asthma, cataracts
Lemongrass	PK-Vo	Headaches, indigestion, uplifter
Lime	PV-K+	Depression, exhaustion, antiseptic
Marjoram	VK-P+	Anxiety attacks, grief, sorrow, insomnia, low blood pressure, blood dilator, do not use when pregnant
Nutmeg	VK-P+	Bad breath, rheumatism, enhances dream activity, menstrual regulator, diarrhea
Orange	VK-P+	Heart disorders, circulation, cellulite, weight loss
Oregano	VK-P+	Anti-viral for all kinds of infections, appetite, hiccups, edema, asthma, bronchitis
Parsley	VK-P+	Cleansing, toning, broken capillaries
Peppermint	PK-Vo	Digestive, anti-depressant, refreshing
Rosemary	VK-P+	Constipation, flatulence, gallstones, headaches
Rose Water	VPK=	Circulation, heart, skin
Sage	VK-P+	All rheumatic conditions, diuretic, fluid retention, hot flashes, canker sores
Tarragon	VK-P+	Stimulates appetite, hiccups, irregular menstruation
Thyme	VK-P+	Low blood pressure, flatulence, skin, viruses, courage
Turmeric	VK-Po	Oily skin, circulation, respiratory system, antiseptic

CHAPTER 11

ALTERNATIVE THERAPIES

CHELATION THERAPY

Chelation therapy is one of the most effective treatments for the cardiovascular and circulatory diseases of gangrene, arteriosclerosis, peripheral vascular disease, cerebral vascular disease, and is a safe alternative to vascular surgery. Most patients of chelation IV therapy are treated for vascular diseases. However, due to the many direct and indirect benefits of this treatment, it can also be effective for such related conditions as diabetic retinopathy, macular degeneration, osteoarthritis, and scleroderma.

Chelation therapy has also been proven effective in the removal of heavy toxic metals and other harmful substances that have entered the body through food, water, and environmental pollution. Once these damaging metals are removed, the body has greater access to the vital nutrients obtained through diet and supplements.

The most common form of intravenous chelation therapy is with EDTA, and when properly used, it has been found to be nontoxic. This therapy is administered by intravenous infusion (IV) and is significantly different from the program of oral chelation nutritional therapy used for general preventative measures. When undertaking the IV chelation therapy administered by a physician, proper protocol includes a complete physical exam, laboratory tests, and other studies. A specific, safe protocol for EDTA chelation treatment exists and physicians certified by the American Board of Chelation Therapy (ABCT) follow this protocol.

Ultimately, the benefits of chelation therapy include improved blood flow to the entire body, with special emphasis to the heart, legs, and brain.

COLOR THERAPY

Seek out a good Color Therapist in your area. Chapter 12, "Self Care" provides information on how you may use color therapy at home.

HOMEOPATHY - GENTLE AND EFFECTIVE

Homeopathy was developed 200 years ago in Germany by Dr. Samuel Hahnemann. It's premise is that minute doses of substances that would normally cause the symptoms of a disease or condition cure the condition. What defies generally accepted scientific belief is that the more diluted the remedy, the stronger and deeper-acting it is on the patient.

Homeopathy is widely practiced around the world and is steadily gaining more acceptance due to its absence of side effects and its efficacy. Mahatma Gandhi believed that homeopathy cures a larger percentage of cases than any other method of treatment. He also believed, beyond all doubt, that homeopathy is safer, more economical and the most complete medical science in existence.

The homeopathic remedies are tested or "proven" on human subjects, not animals, and there is extensive documentation to back up each remedy's effects. Medical doctors, naturopathic physicians, dentists, veterinarians and others involved in healing are turning to homeopathy in increasing numbers to obtain positive and lasting results.

Treatment is gentle and non-invasive, thereby eliminating the discomfort suffered by patients in conventional therapies, such as long-term drug therapy (with harmful side effects), chemotherapy, radiation, or surgeries. Occasionally with homeopathic treatment, a healing crisis occurs which results in a temporary aggravation of symptoms. The patient should not be alarmed by this effect, but encouraged, because this is a signal that the remedy is doing its job correctly.

There is no one particular homeopathic remedy that cures any specific disease. For example, if a patient were asthmatic, a homeopathic physician wouldn't automatically prescribe the standard textbook remedy for asthma and be done with it. Instead, the history and nature of the person is carefully determined by a lengthy interview, then the specific remedy is selected to match the core makeup of that individual. The challenge of homeopathy is to select the specific remedy that would then be efficacious against any disease manifestation that the person displayed.

There are instances where remedies are prescribed recipe-book style for certain acute or first-aid situations. For example, Arnica Montana is routinely given for tissue trauma and bruising, Arsenicum Album for some forms of food poisoning, and Apis Mellifica is usually given for bee stings.

However, the constitutional remedy, which is selected based upon careful study of the patient, works at deeper levels. They work on the physical, emotional and mental levels as well. If the remedy is well selected, the patient's well being will improve on all levels.

Although homeopathy alone will improve a patient's condition, it makes sense to support it with good nutrition and lifestyle. Even in chronic or terminal illness where destruction is severe and all hope of cure is gone, homeopathy can be used to palliate. In these cases, the patient progresses into death with clarity and more peacefully than with heroic allopathic treatment.

George Vithoulkas, a renowned contemporary Greek homeopath, presents a structure on how pathology progresses. This understanding helps the homeopath know if the patient is moving towards cure or deteriorating further. This is an area that is not well understood by conventional medical doctors whose treatments very often suppress the disease while alleviating the overt symptoms. The most likely effect of this form of treatment is that the dis-ease then transforms into a more life- threatening pathology. It may relocate to a different area of the body or become some form of emotional or mental illness. Cure of the former dis-ease is then declared and then the process begins again to suppress the "new" illness. Eventually, the patient may succumb unless the patient's own defense system is strong enough to rally and overcome the dis-ease - and the treatment.

Homeopathy is continuing to evolve. New remedies are continually being discovered, developed and proven. Exciting work is being done by a group of homeopathic physicians in Bombay, India, headed by Dr. Rajan Sankaran. George Vithoulkas has recently been given an award, customarily referred to as the "Alternative Nobel Prize" for his work in homeopathy. Practitioners who have studied these homeopath's work are likely well equipped to provide excellent homeopathic treatment.

Homeopathy is a complex science and requires extensive knowledge, experience, and sensitivity on the part of the practitioner. Sometimes even the finest homeopaths do not find the correct remedy for the patient on the first try. Patience is the key here. If given a chance, homeopathy can perform miraculous results.

Grateful acknowledgement to Linda Johnson, Molokai, Hawaii for the homeopathic contribution.

KAYA KALPA - "BODIES TRANSFORMATION"

Ten thousand years ago, a King of India had a problematic, headstrong daughter, who refused to marry any of the eligible princes who were presented to her. In anger and frustration the king decreed that she be blindfolded and placed in the castle courtyard in the midst of all her suitors. The man she touched was to be her husband and their children would continue the royal line.

On that day an elderly holy man wandered into the courtyard to deliver herbs to the King's physician and, by chance, was touched first by the princess. Even though he pled exemption due to his advanced age and holy vows, the King's word was law and they were to marry in three months time. The holy man consulted his teacher about his problem, and the teacher instituted an intensive program to rejuvenate and energize.

For 90 days the holy man ate a special diet, performed breathing techniques, took ritual herbal baths and was anointed with sacred oils. At the end of that time his hair had turned from gray to black, a new set of teeth had grown into his mouth, and his skin and body were youthful and strong. He married the princess. They had many children and lived happily ever after.

This was the beginning of KAYA KALPA (body's transformation), a secret healing technique used in India for thousands of years by religious healers to rejuvenate and give longevity to royal and holy sages. Vigorously suppressed by the British, it was almost lost. There are now only 18 practitioners left in the world. Fortunately, they exist in a form more appropriate to Western life-styles. In addition to its rejuvenating qualities, KAYA KALPA is useful in expanding awareness, consciousness, and can be an aid in making decisions and life changes.

The Treatment

1. Begins with an assessment of the person's Ayurvedic type using pulse diagnosis and questionnaire format. You are one of 10 metabolic types and you will be given appropriate lifestyle, diet, herbs and essential oils to bring you back into balance.

2. When maintaining a tantric, connective breath, an herbal paste made from 108 Indian herbs is applied to the entire body. The paste, which is specifically formulated for your metabolic type, draws out impurities while re-vitalizing the skin. The removal process reveals sites of inflammation and concentrates stimulation to these areas while removing old skin. Skin bruising completes the stimulation and cleansing. A special herbal oil is formulated and applied to nourish the skin and a stream of hot oil is directed onto the area of the third eye creating ecstatic sensations and expanded awareness.

3. A hot bath with herbal extracts and aroma-therapeutics, accompanied by Breath of Fire (Kundalini) and primal sounds, creates a fiery state to release unexpressed emotions and fears, establishing a balanced receptiveness. FORGIVE-NESS RITUALS release you from past projections and create an opening for new ways of perceiving all your relationships. A cooling shower returns the person to the body and initiates divine connectedness.

4. The patient is placed in a cocoon of sheets and blankets, the chakras (energy centers) are anointed with the most powerful and spiritual of essential oils, and a deep meditative breath is maintained. A restful state of bliss is obtained that carries over into the next few days, weeks or even months in everything planned and performed. After the treatment, one is at rest from 2 to 5 hours.

Originally and traditionally this treatment was conducted periodically during 3 months of isolation in which the patient ate a special diet, practiced prescribed meditations and lived in a special hut alone.

Today, transformation is produced by receiving a series of 1 to 10 treatments. The purpose of this treatment is to take you to a place within yourself that you may return to anytime through the use of breath, essential oils, baths and meditation.

This treatment is for those who are prepared for transformation and is best for those who have a spiritual practice or spiritual understanding.

MASSAGE

Massage is the application of soothing hands to the body. Many forms of massage have been practiced by ancient people throughout the world, developing intuitive gestures from inner knowledge of what felt good. Today massage has been proven to have therapeutic effects. The laying of hands is used for health, healing, soothing relaxation, and weight reduction. Today massage is one of the most interesting professions of our time.

How do you go about finding a massage therapist? Ask friends, consult with your doctor, call a chiropractor, or contact the American Massage Association through your phone book. Massage is a very personal experience, so make sure you find someone with whom you feel comfortable.

There are many different kinds and techniques of massage. Some use pressure, others long, soothing touch. Despite the many various modes of massage, all have therapeutic qualities.

When you receive a massage for the fist time you may experience some pain. This is caused by the release of lactic acid from the muscles. Fear not, as this does help to alleviate accumulated stress and subsequent massages will not be painful.

Beneficial Effects of Massage

1. Massage dilates the blood vessels, improves the circulation and relieves congestion throughout the body.

2. Massage increases the number of red blood cells, especially in cases of anemia.

3. Massage acts as a "mechanical cleanser," stimulating lymph circulation and hastening the elimination of wastes and toxic debris.

4. Massage relaxes muscle spasms and relieves tension.

5. Massage increases blood supply and nutrition to muscles without adding to their load of toxic lactic acid, produced through voluntary muscle contraction. Massage thus helps to prevent build-up of harmful "fatigue" products resulting from strenuous exercise or injury.

6. Massage improves muscle tone and helps prevent or delay muscular atrophy resulting from forced inactivity.

7. Massage helps return venous blood to the heart. This eases the strain on this vital organ when forced inactivity occurs due to lack of exercise, muscular contractions in persons who have had injuries, illness, or old age.

8. Massage may have a sedative, stimulating or even exhausting effect on the nervous system, depending on the type and length of massage treatment given.

9. According to some authorities, massage may burst the fat capsules in subcutaneous tissue so that the fat exudes and becomes absorbed. In this way massage, combined with a nutritious but calorie-deficient diet, can be an aid in reducing weight.

10. Massage improves the general circulation, thereby heightening tissue metabolism (interchange of substances between the blood and tissue cells.)

11. Massage increases kidney excretion of fluids, protein metabo-

lism wastes, inorganic phosphorous and salt in normal individuals.

12. Massage encourages the retention of nitrogen, phosphorous and sulfurs necessary for tissue repair in persons convalescing from bone fractures.

13. Massage stretches connective tissues and improves its circulation and nutrition, which in turn breaks down or prevents the formation of adhesions and reduces the danger of fibrosis.

14. Massage helps lessen inflammation and swelling in joints and so alleviates pain. It does this by improving the circulation to the joints, thereby increasing nutrition to the joints and hastening the elimination of harmful deposits away from the joints.

15. Massage helps to reduce edema (or dropsy) of the extremities.

16. Massage disperses the edema following injury to ligaments and tendons, lessens pain and facilitates movement.

17. Massage increases respiration when moderately forceful.

18. Massage over the abdomen increases peristalsis and the elimination of intestinal residues and debris.

19. As a by-product of the increased intestinal elimination massage reduces pain.

20. MASSAGE MAKES YOU FEEL GOOD.

Contraindications to Massage

1. Skin infections and ulcerations
2. Local acute inflammatory processes.
3. Acute deep or visceral inflammations.
4. Phlebitis, thrombosis, emboli, or other vascular diseases.
5. Where there is a tendency to hemorrhage, such as varicosity's or peptic ulcers.
6. Acute osteamyelitis, tubercular joints or any infectious bone or joint disease.
7. Malignant neoplasias.
8. High blood pressure.

9. After recent surgery.

10. Malignant tumors.

Massage Oil Recipes

All recipes are done in 4 ounces of vegetable oil:

Vata Skin - Sesame

Pitta Skin - Sunflower, olive or coconut

Kapha - Canola

All Skin Types - Jojoba is good for.

Vata Blends

Morning Divine

- Sandalwood - 15 drops
- Cyperus - 10 drops
- Rosewood - 10 drops
- Lavender - 15 drops
- 4 ounces of sesame (unroasted)

Grounding Presence

- Jatamasi - 5 drops
- Rosewood - 15 drops
- Vetivert - 5 drops
- Ginger - 10 drops
- Lemon - 10 drops
- 4 ounces of Sesame

Opening - Channeling

- Clary Sage - 10 drops
- Orange - 15 drops
- Cinnamon - 5 drops
- Vanilla - 5 drops
- Angelica - 5 drops
- 4 ounces of Sesame

Eastern Flair

- Cardamon - 5 drops
- Myrtle - 2 drops
- Clove - 2 drops
- Ginger - 10 drops
- Frankincense - 5 drops
- Sandalwood - 10 drops
- Jatamasi - 3 drops
- Trifola - 10 drops
- 4 ounces of Sesame

Pitta Blends

Tuning

- Lavender - 10 drops
- Sandalwood - 15 drops
- Vetivert - 5 drops
- Champa - 10 drops
- Rose Geranium - 5 drops
- 4 ounces of Sunflower oil

Clarity

- Hina - 5 drops
- Brahmi - 10 drops
- Rose Geranium - 15 drops
- Sandalwood - 10 drops
- 4 ounces of Sunflower oil

Blissfulness

- Blue Chamomile - 5 drops
- Lavender - 10 drops
- Jasmine - 10 drops
- Vetivert - 3 drops
- Saffron - 2 drops
- Champa - 5 drops
- Lemon - 2 drops
- 4 ounces of Sunflower oil

Harmony

- Rose - 5 drops
- Roman Chamomile - 5 drops
- Lavender - 10 drops
- Geranium - 15 drops
- Champa - 10 drops
- 4 ounces of Sunflower oil

The Vision

- Clary Sage - 5 drops
- Mint - 5 drops
- Lavender - 10 drops
- Jasmine 10 drops
- Sandalwood - 10 drops
- 4 ounces of Sunflower oil

Serenity

- Blue Chamomile - 5 drops
- Vetivert - 5 drops
- Coriander - 5 drops
- Sandalwood - 10 drops
- Fennel - 5 drops
- Sweet Myrrh - 5 drops
- Benzoin - 5 drops
- 4 ounces of Sunflower oil

Kapha Blends

Movement

- Juniper Berries - 10 drops
- Lavender - 15 drops
- Cypress - 5 drops
- Orange - 5 drops
- Ginger - 5 drops
- 4 ounces of Canola oil

Vision

- Trifola - 5 drops
- Orange - 15 drops
- Champa - 10 drops
- Lavender - 10 drops
- Clary Sage - 10 drops
- 4 ounces of Sunflower oil

Awaken

- Bergamot - 15 drops
- Neroli - 5 drops
- Lemon - 10 drops
- Ginger - 10 drops
- Angelica - 5 drops
- 4 ounces of Almond oil

Aliveness

- Juniper Berries - 5 drops
- Lemon Grass - 3 drops
- Champa - 10 drops
- Sandalwood - 5 drops
- Ginger - 5 drops
- Myrrh - 10 drops
- Frankincense - 5 drops
- 4 ounces of Sunflower oil

Eternity

- Jasmine - 15 drops
- Lemon - 10 drops
- Orange - 5 drops
- Clary Sage - 5 drops
- Dharma - 5 drops
- Lavender - 5 drops
- 4 ounces of Sunflower oil

Joyous

- Cinnamon - 5-10 drops
- Ylang Ylang - 10 drops
- Rosewood - 10-15 drops
- Clove - 2-5 drops
- Ginger - 5-10 drops
- Cardamon - 3-10 drops
- 4 ounces of Sunflower or Canola oil

Medicinal Blend

Circulation

- Cinnamon - 5 drops
- Orange - 10 drops
- Juniper Berries - 5 drops
- Rose Geranium - 10 drops
- Lavender - 10 drops
- 4 ounces Sesame or Canola oil

Breath Free

- Myrtle - 10 drops
- Rosemary - 10 drops
- Eucalyptus - 10 drops
- Mint - 5 drops
- Camphor - 5 drops
- 4 ounces Sesame oil

Pain Free

- Birch - 5 drops
- Eucalyptus - 5 drops
- Juniper Berries - 5 drops
- Ginger - 5 drops
- Lavender - 10 drops
- Rosemary - 10 drops
- 4 ounces of Sunflower oil

Tummy Free
- Chamomile - 5 drops
- Fennel - 10 drops
- Coriander - 5 drops
- Lavender - 15 drops
- Mint - 5 drops
- 4 ounces Sunflower oil

Appetite
- Ginger - 15 drops
- Black Pepper - 5 drops
- Orange - 10 drops
- Basil - 5 drops
- Cinnamon - 5 drops
- Cardamon - 5 drops
- 4 ounces of Sesame oil

Rescue Spray
- Lemon - 5 drops
- Lavender - 10 drops
- Mint - 5 drops
- Myrtle - 10 drops
- Bhrami - 10 drops
- Basil - 5 drops
- 2 ounces water

Itch Free
- Lavender - 10 drops
- Eucalyptus - 5 drops
- Lemon - 5 drops
- Gold Chamomile - 5 drops
- Juniper Berries - 5 drops
- Myrtle - 5 drops
- Tea Tree - 5 drops
- 4 ounces water, alcohol, or pure vegetable oil

Awaken

- Cypress - 5 drops
- Cedarwood - 5 drops
- Cardamon - 5 drops
- Bergamot - 10 drops
- Mandarin - 15 drops
- Pettigrain - 10 drops

Home Fresh Spray

- Pine - 15 drops
- Lemon - 10 drops
- Orange - 15 drops
- Tea Tree - 10 drops
- Mint - 5 drops
- Rosewood - 10 drops
- 8 ounces water or pure vegetable oil

Antiseptic

- Tea Tree - 10 drops
- Cajaput - 10 drops
- Thyme - 5 drops
- Lavender - 15 drops
- Eucalyptus - 10 drops
- Lemon - 10 drops
- Rosewood - 15 drops
- 8 ounces of water or vegetable oil

Liniment

- Eucalyptus - 5 drops
- Bay - 10 drops
- Juniper Berries - 10 drops
- Lavender - 15 drops
- Birch - 5 drops
- Cypress - 5 drops
- 4 ounces rubbing alcohol or vegetable oil

Hot Flash Spray

- Clary Sage - 10 drops
- Geranium - 10 drops
- Lavender - 10 drops
- Sage - 5 drops
- Chamomile - 5 drops
- 4 ounces water, coconut or sunflower oil

OR

- Mint - 5 drops
- Lavender 15 drops
- Jasmine - 10 drops
- Tangerine - 15 drops
- 4 ounces Sunflower oil

Immune

- Cumin - 10 drops
- Lemon - 10 drops
- Myrtle - 10 drops
- Saffron - 5 drops
- Myrrh - 5 drops
- Frankincense - 5 drops
- 4 ounces Sesame oil

Fever Free

- Gold Chamomile - 5 drops
- Lavender - 10 drops
- Mint - 10 drops
- Tea Tree - 5 drops
- Blue Chamomile - 10 drops
- 4 ounces Sunflower or Coconut oil

Weight Loss

- Grapefruit - 10 drops
- Orange - 10 drops
- Juniper Berries - 10 drops

- Birch - 5 drops
- Black Pepper - 5 drops
- Ginger - 10 drops
- 4 ounces Almond or Canola oil

Infection Free

- Thyme - 5 drops
- Oregano - 5 drops
- Lemon - 15 drops
- Tea Tree - 10 drops
- Eucalyptus - 10 drops
- Lavender - 15 drops
- Rosemary - 10 drops
- Cumin - 5 drops
- Turmeric - 5 drops
- 8 ounces Olive oil

Easy Now

- Lavender - 15 drops
- Sandalwood - 10 drops
- Gold Chamomile - 5 drops
- Rose Geranium - 5 drops
- Pettigrain - 10 drops
- Rosewood - 10 drops
- 4 ounces Sunflower oil

Uplifting Spirits Blend

- Lemon Grass - 5 drops
- Angelica - 5 drops
- Bergamot - 10 drops
- Myrtle - 5 drops
- Lemon - 5 drops
- Orange - 5 drops
- 4 ounces Sesame oil

Bruise Juice

- Lavender - 10 drops
- Lemon - 5 drops
- Cardamon - 5 drops
- Bergamot - 10 drops
- Lime - 10 drops
- 4 ounces Almond oil or Canola

Burns

- Blue Chamomile - 10 drops
- Lavender - 10 drops
- Lemon Grass - 10 drops
- Coriander - 15 drops
- 4 ounces coconut oil or a blend including aloe vera gel

OR

- Sandalwood - 10 drops
- Myrtle - 10 drops
- Bhrami - 20 drops
- Saffron - 5 drops
- Cumin - 5 drops
- Lemon - 5 drops
- Rosewood - 10 drops
- 8 ounces Sesame oil

Gout Mixture

- Juniper Berries - 5 drops
- Thyme - 5 drops
- Cypress - 5 drops
- Lemon - 5 drops
- Myrtle - 10 drops
- Basil - 5 drops
- 4 ounces Coconut or Sunflower oil

Liver Flow

- Coriander - 10 drops

- Fennel - 15 drops
- Ginger - 5 drops
- Rosemary - 5 drops
- Patchouli - 5 drops
- 4 ounces Sunflower oil

Fibroids Mixture
- Dhavana - 10 drops
- Frankincense - 5 drops
- Cypress - 10 drops
- Lavender - 15 drops
- Tea Tree - 5 drops
- Bergamot - 10 drops
- 4 ounces Castor or Canola oil

MUSIC AND SOUND THERAPY

Seek out a good therapist in your area. See Chapter 12, "Music and Sound Therapy" for practices which you may do at home.

PANCHA KARMA - SEASONAL HOUSE CLEANING OF THE BODY

Early records reveal that ancient peoples understood the various systems of the body and had developed effective methods of purification and cleansing. Pancha Karma, a technique for rejuvenating and opening up blocked channels of the body, was practiced as early as 300 AD. Based on the belief that the body is the temple or vehicle of the soul, Pancha Karma is used to return the mind to its Sattvic, or harmonious, state. Pancha Karma was traditionally performed to prepare the body for the internal changes that correlate with environmental changes occurring with the change of the seasons.

Today Pancha Karma is performed when chronic disease, brought about by environmental toxins and/or self-indulgent lifestyles, produces symptoms of pain or dysfunction. Dis-ease is often our body's way of demanding change. The techniques of Pancha Karma used to open blocked channels bring an awareness of the connection of the self to others and to all of existence. Rejuvenation opens us to the Healer within and creates within us a desire to serve others and to return to life what has been received.

The five basic purification techniques include Oleation (Sneehana), Purgation (Virechana), Sweats (Swedhana), Enema (Basti), and Nasal Therapy (Nasya). Because each cleansing is specifically adapted for each body type (dosha) and takes into account individual conditions, some purification's might include Emesis (Vomiting), Bloodletting (Rakta Moksha), Shirodhara (Third Eye Balancing), and Tarpana (Relationship Healing).

1) OLEATION (Sneehana):

In this process, oil is ingested to prepare the digestive tract for cleansing and to soften the body's tissues so that toxins (ama) can be freely released. Two to four tablespoons of Castor Oil, Ghee, or medicated oils are consumed for several days. Because medicated oils are not easily available in the United States, adding essential oils to vegetable oils can create an acceptable healing substitute.

For Vata body types add one drop of either Angelica, Dhavana, Ginger, Jatamasi, Sandalwood, or Trifola (Tumru) to one-half (1/2) cup of Castor, Sesame, or Ghee oil.

For Pitta body types use one-half (1/2) cup of either Ghee or Olive oil and add one drop of either Chamomile, Coriander, Lavender, Mint, Sandalwood, or Turmeric. Fresh Aloe or Aloe-Olive medicated oils are also excellent choices for Pittas. Add one tablespoon to the essential oil mixture.

Kapha body types respond to either Almond, Canola, Castor, or Mustard oil. Use one-half (1/2) cup mixed with one drop of either Basil, Ginger, Juniper Berries, Lemon, Orange, or Turmeric.

Oils may also be applied externally to assist in preparing external pores, capillaries, and sebaceous and lymph glands for cleansing through sweating. Use a concentration of thirty to one hundred (30-100) drops of an essential oil appropriate to each body type to four (4) ounces of the base oil and apply onto the surface of the skin and allow to absorb. (NOTE: Kaphas need to use less base oil and a higher concentration of essential oils).

2) PURGATION (Virechana):

This is a technique for cleansing the small intestine and reducing excess fire by using laxative herbs.

Vata types respond well to a mild purgation using Castor oil with Aloe.

Pitta types require the use of stronger purgatives like Aloe, Gentian, and Rhubarb while Kaphas respond to Aloe, Rhubarb, and Senna.

To avoid rapid lowering of the digestive fire and depleting the vital forces, purgation should be practiced for only two (2) days. Also effective in stimulating elimination is an abdominal massage in a clockwise direction using two (2) tablespoons of vegetable oil and thirty (30) drops total of either Angelica, Cedarwood, Chamomile, Fennel, Geranium, Ginger, Lavender, Lemon, Mandarin, Patchouli, Peppermint, Rosemary, Tangerine, or Thyme.

3) SWEATS (Swedhana):

In Swedhana, heat and steam are used to open the outer channels and aid the elimination of toxins through the skin (1/4 of all body waste exits through the skin). Heat is beneficial in raising the metabolic rate, increasing elimination of toxins, and stimulating the immune system.

The best type of steam comes from steam cabinets using cool steam. The head is outside and the genitals and heart are protected by covering them with cool, damp towels. Essential oils can be used with the steam to stimulate and energize the skin and add life force. Some sources recommend using dry heat during early elimination and then switching to moist sauna when the channels have been cleared.

In order to allow the body temperature to return to normal, it is important to wrap in a sheet after the sauna. Shower and scrub with a mild PH balanced soap or shampoos to remove the excess oil and body wastes. Follow by a vigorous toweling and then powder with chana (chickpea flour). After the oil has been absorbed, the powder should be removed.

Vatas should drink extra water to replace the fluid lost and to avoid excessive sweating. Beneficial oils include Cardamon, Cinnamon, Chamomile, Eucalyptus, Ginger, Jatamasi, and Valerian.

Pittas should use lower temperatures and less time than the other doshas. Choose from Anise, Chamomile, Coriander, Cumin, Fennel, Lavender, Lime, Mint, or Yarrow.

Kaphas can most benefit from Swedhana and need higher temperatures and longer times. Beneficial oils include Bay, Black Pepper, Cypress, Eucalyptus, Juniper Berries, Orange, Rosemary, Yarrow.

4) ENEMA (Basti):

Used to cleanse, build, and nourish the eliminative tract. Instead of the plain water enema favored by traditional Western medicine, Ayurveda uses the less drying herbal teas, medicated and vegetable oils, and milk and yogurt.

Since Vata types are often dry in the large intestine, the enema needs to be composed of Flax or Sesame oil, plain yogurt, or nourishing and moisturizing teas such as Mullein, Licorice, Comfrey Root, Flax Seed, Slippery Elm, fresh gel Aloe, and heating herbs such as Cardamon, Cinnamon, and Ginger. Any Vata-reducing essential oil may also be added, ten (10) drops per gallon.

For Pittas use cooling herb teas, such as Guduchi, Katuka, or Bhrami, and milk mixed with ten (10) drops per gallon of Pitta-reducing essential oils.

Since Kapha colons usually have excessive mucus, oil, milk, or other dairy products should be avoided. Use instead teas made with a combination of Ajwan, Aloe, Amalaki, Anise, Bala, Cinnamon, Eucalyptus, Fennel, Ginger, Haritaki, Juniper Berries, Manjishta, Prickly Ash, or Rosemary. Coffee is another beneficial additive mixed with up to ten (10) drops of Ajwan, Anise, Bay, Cardamon, Elecampane, Eucalyptus, Ginger, Lemongrass, Myrrh, Orange, or Sage.

Historically, hollowed out gourds or clay pots attached to a hollow reed were used to administer Basti. Today it is traditional to use an enema bag although the Colema Board system (developed by Dr. Bernard Jensen, D.C.) allows the patient to receive and release up to five gallons of Basti mixture while relaxing over the toilet. It is beneficial to massage the stomach counter-clockwise during administration of the mixture to help move it through the colon. Massaging the abdomen in a clockwise direction helps release the mixture. The mixture should be warm and the treatment should be immediately stopped if the patient experiences spasms, pressure, or other discomfort. The flow may be resumed after abdominal massage and the use of deep breathing to release the spasm.

5) NASAL THERAPY (Nasya):

Nasya is used to stimulate the limbic system and clear the head and sinuses from impurities. The relaxation that accompanies the reduction of pain can beneficially affect our moods, emotions, desires, appetites, and memories. The limbic system can be treated through the use of powders, oils, teas, or smoke and also by applying medicated oils to the ears. (See Melanie Sachs' *Ayurvedic Beauty Care* for a recipe for an effective Ginger Tea Nasya. The *Yoga of Herbs* can be consulted for a list of smoking and inhaling herbs.) The most traditional form of Nasal Therapy is the use of medicated oils or a mixture of one (1) drop of an essential oil to one-quarter (1/4) ounce of vegetable oil.

For Vata, use either Calamus, Jatamasi, or Vetiver oils.

Pittas respond best to the oils of Coriander, Lavender, Mint, Rose, or Yarrow. Kaphas should use Basil, Eucalyptus, Orange, or Rosemary oils, and Sandalwood oil can be used by all three doshas.

It is recommended that Nasya be administered after a full body massage or at least a good neck and face massage. Support the neck with a rolled up four to five inch (4"-5") towel. The oil mixture should be between 102 to 106 degrees F. Gently close one nostril and use an eyedropper to place five (5) drops of the mixture into the open nostril as the patient inhales at least three (3) times. This will send the oil deep into the nasal passageway. Gently massage the forehead, around the eye sockets, and on and around the nose and cheekbones. Then repeat in the other nostril.

To oil the ears, the patient should lie on his or her side while ten to fifteen (10-15) drops of warm oil are applied into the ear canal. The auricle should be massaged and the ear lobe stretched gently in both clockwise and counter-clockwise motions. After ten to twenty (10-20) minutes, repeat in the opposite ear while allowing the initial mixture to drain on a cloth.

Periodic Nasya is said to eliminate eye puffiness and dark circles and improve smell and taste. Patients often experience mild burning, warmth, inner light, increased awareness, emotional release, and peace. Nasya is useful in treating ear itching, pain, ringing, or hearing loss.

6) OTHER RELATED THERAPIES

These include Emesis, BloodLetting, Tarpana, and Shirodhara.

EMESIS or vomiting is often used effectively in Pancha Karma therapy, particularly in cases of Kapha imbalance. Vomiting rids the body of excess stomach mucous resulting from lung and sinus drainage and allows for more efficient digestion and nutrient absorption. Emesis must be supervised by a trained Ayurvedic practitioner to avoid damage to the upper GI tract and nervous system.

BLOODLETTING or Rakta Moksha was used from antiquity until the 1800's to cure various illnesses. Donating blood is a form of modern "bloodletting," and in addition to helping save someone's life, a donation of blood can assist the body in eliminating toxins and in stimulating the circulatory and immune system by the production of fresh blood. Essential oils can be beneficial during blood donation. Add a drop of Angelica to a cup of tea or on the tongue to ward off pre-donation nervousness or try Anise or Fennel to settle a nervous stomach. Afterwards, Lavender and Cajeput oils can be used on a Band-Aid to disinfect the wound and to promote healing. To help build back the blood, try Chamomile, Lemon, and Thyme.

TARPANA (Relationship Healing) is a healing ceremony that is used to release constraining thoughts about our relationships to others and to empower ourselves as an active co-creator of our lives. While Ayurvedic practices embrace foods, herbs, oils, and lifestyles as crucial healing modalities, it also acknowledges that our sense of connectedness to all things may be the most powerful factor in our well being. By freeing us from the power of the negative thoughts that we hold about our relationships to others, Tarpana is a way to experience our true connectedness with all of creation. The ceremony helps us understand that it is possible to change how we view the world and how we feel about ourselves and our connection to others in the universe.

Begin the ceremony alone in a quiet and dimly lit space. Light candles and incense and begin a form of breathing called the "rebirthing" or "connected" breath by breathing in through the nose and out through the mouth. Allow the inhalation and exhalation to be connected and don't control the exhalation, allow it to escape at its own pace like a long sigh. When you are in a relaxed frame of mind, begin the unblocking process by first calling forth your ancestors and then anyone you have ever been in a relationship with.

Begin with your mother or father, then continue through each ancestor and other significant people. Visualize them standing before you looking into your eyes. Remember what they looked like, using your own memory or images from photographs. Remember your experiences with them or stories you have heard about them. Visualize them as being receptive to what you want to say to them. Begin the clearing by saying "What I want you to know is_____." Then tell the ancestor what you have felt about them. Are you grateful for gifts or genetic tendencies that you inherited? Do you feel yourself victimized by them in some way? Discuss with them your role in the co-creation of your relationship. Take this opportunity to forgive yourself and your ancestor. If you truly forgive then you are able to leave the experience behind you and no longer carry it with you. With forgiveness comes the ability to turn adversity into a catalyst for growth and a new sense of gratitude for the gifts they have given you.

Conclude your ceremony by symbolically serving your ancestor their favorite food or drink, something they would have enjoyed. In your mind's eye, visualize them taking your offering, consuming it, and smiling. Then look directly into their eyes and see if you can experience them giving you a blessing. The blessing may be wishing you success in life, blessing you as you find your path, freeing you from obligations to them, or freeing you to pursue your own passion and purpose. Accept their blessing and visualize them walking in the light of their own path. Bless their path as they leave.

Conclude the Tarpana session by being centered and repeating positive affirmations: "I am love, I am one with all things, I am peace, I am joy, I am prosperity, I am forgiveness, I am trust, I am fulfillment." And so it is.

SHIRODHARA (Third Eye Balancing) is the technique of administering a stream of warm oil onto the *Third Eye* area of the forehead. Shirodhara is most effective when it is administered after a massage or a Tarpana ceremony when the patient is relaxed and calm. Shirodhara stimulates the nervous system by releasing neuro-hormones and creating ecstatic feelings of relaxation and pleasure. The patient should be advised to plan only light activity for several hours following the treatment.

Position the patient on their back with the neck supported by a rolled up towel. The head should be tilted back and extended off the table. Cover the patient with a sheet or blanket and place a bolster under the knees. Position a large bowl on the floor under the patient's head to catch the oil as it runs off the forehead. Traditionally sesame oil is used, but it is also effective to use oil and essential oils appropriate to the doshic imbalance. The elaborate equipment used in India can be approximated in the United States by purchasing a separation funnel and stand from a chemistry supply store. The treatment usually takes thirty (30) minutes. A five to ten minute satisfying treatment, however, can be administered by using a one-cup plastic bottle with a squirt top.

Begin by applying a small stream of oil in the center of the forehead. While it is pleasurable to move the stream over the entire forehead and top of the head, the focus of the treatment should be on the *Third Eye*, a position one-inch above and between the eyebrows. Protect the eyes from any accidental splattering. When the treatment is over, remove excess oil from the forehead and head with a small towel. The patient should remain in a state of relaxation for at least the next five to thirty (5-30) minutes.

REFLEXOLOGY

Sometimes called Zone Therapy, it is a form of acupressure that dates back about 4,500 years to Egypt. Reflexology, like acupressure, holds that reflexes link each organ of the body to a certain area of the hands and feet, with the nervous system serving as the connection. Whenever an organ is not functioning properly, the corresponding reflex will be tender and even painful upon applying pressure. Stimulation helps break up the lactic acid that forms small crystals. This short-circuiting of the nervous system results in a surge of energy flow to the directed area.

Organ Balancing Techniques

Hand Reflex Points

Points on the hand can reflexively stimulate organs due to nerve connections. Apply chosen oil to the hand reflex points. Press deeply with thumb or knuckle and apply a circular rocking motion for 30 seconds. Tenderness indicates involvement. May be re-stimulated as needed.

Foot Reflex Points

These points are part of 72,000 nerve endings that correspond to the entire body. Apply appropriate oil and rub with thumb or knuckle in deep rolling motion for 30 seconds. May be re-stimulated.

Lymphatic Points

Energetically releases the blocked flow of associated lymph vessels. Apply one drop of appropriate essential oil to each lymphatic point. Using fingertips in front and thumb pads in back, briskly rub each point in a rotary movement for 15 seconds. Tenderness will indicate severity of blockage. A second stimulation can be applied after a two-minute recovery interval. Do not over-stimulate.

Muscle Stimulating

Each muscle shares an acupuncture meridian with an organ. By stimulating muscles you can reflexively energize organs. Apply a small amount of vegetable oil to a few drops of appropriate essential oil. Apply vigorously with circular fingertip movement from muscle origin to muscle insertion, and back again.

Meridians

Meridians are streams of energy which connect our body together with muscles and organs. Place a few drops of essential oil on the fingertips and trace the meridian lightly several times to stimulate flow in the indicated direction of the meridian.

Grateful appreciation to James Minckler for his loving contribution of the organ balancing technique.

REIKI

Reiki (pronounced ray-key) is a gentle healing practice in which one person places their hands on the body of another (or themselves). Reiki can also be practiced at a distance from the recipient. Healing through touch probably dates back to the origins of the family, when one person first reached out to touch or hold another to ease their pain.

During Reiki, there is a channeling or focusing of energy through the hands of the practitioner. The recipient may feel warmth where the hands are placed, although the identification of sensation is not necessary for Reiki to be effective. These benefits are frequently noticed:

- reduced stress
- release of pain or discomfort
- emotional calming
- deep relaxation
- expanded spiritual awareness
- a meditative state
- increased intuition
- heightened well being.

Reiki means "universal life energy". The "ki" in Reiki is the same as the Chinese qi (or ch'i) and refers to the internal life force that animates all beings. Dr. Mikao Usui, a Japanese minister (1865-1926), discovered the healing methods of ancient spiritual masters, including a sequence for placing hands as well as the use of powerful symbols, and he developed and passed these teachings on as Reiki.

Reiki stimulates the body's own natural healing processes and helps create an internal space for healing. According to Deepak Chopra, "a level of total, deep relaxation is the most important precondition for curing any disorder." Reiki is an excellent modality for achieving that deep relaxation.

Energy follows attention. When the body is touched, ki is awakened and flows more easily. The movement of ki is essential for health and happiness. Reiki is an effortless way to promote and increase the circulation of this unseen energy.

Reiki practitioners are associated with either the traditional system, Usui Shiki Ryoho, or with more recent variations. Different levels of certification are related to the "attunements" received. Attunements are formal practices used by a Reiki teacher, or master, to open a channel to the Reiki energy within the student practitioner. The attunement procedure itself can be a transformative spiritual event. Certain mental symbols are taught and used to increase the potency of a session and for distance healing.

While sessions may vary in style, symbols used, or placement of the hands, healing is always influenced by the subtle interaction of the practitioner, the recipient and the universal energy, which has its own intelligence. Some practitioners combine Reiki with massage or chakra balancing, with spiritual or emotional guidance, or with the use of crystals, sound, essential oils or other healing techniques.

The *intentions* of the healer and the recipient contribute greatly to the power of healing. Adherence to the Reiki Principles promotes mindfulness and gives conscious and ethical direction to both the practice and the living of Reiki.

The Reiki Principles

Just for today, I will give thanks for my many blessings.

Just for today, I will let go of worry.

Just for today, I will let go of anger.

Just for today, I will do my work honestly.

Just for today, I will honor my parents and teachers.

Just for today, I will be kind to my neighbors and
every living thing.

Reiki is healing both to the practitioner and the recipient. If you find resonance with the principles and format of Reiki, you might consider not only experiencing sessions as a client, but also receiving the attunements so that you may be encouraged to practice Reiki on yourself or others.

Grateful acknowledgement to Diana Daffner for the Reiki information.

THERAPEUTIC TOUCH

This is a method of using the hands to direct and transfer the flow of electrical energies to improve circulation and restore balance. It will stimulate a renewed flow of life force throughout the body, allowing the channeling of energy for the well being of another. Prana can be transferred from one individual to another. It flows like a river.

Excerpts were taken from "Energy Balancing For Natural Health". Grateful acknowledgement to the author James Minckler.

CHAPTER 12

SELF CARE

ABYANGHA SELF-MASSAGE

Abyangha is an ancient Ayurvedic technique of daily self-massage. It seals and protects the skin, calms and tones the muscles, centers the mind and provides a barrier to outside influence.

The skin is a very elaborate defense mechanism to protect us from invading bacteria, virus and loss of moisture. Sebaceous glands deep in the skin secrete an acidic, oily mantel called sebum which forms a protective layer. This layer can be stripped off if you use ordinary soap, which is alkaline. Abyangha adds vegetable oils and essential oils to the skin mantel supporting, not disrupting, the protection.

Additionally, this mantel is part of our etheric energy field. Keeping it strong can protect us from being unduly influenced by outside emotions, negativity or control. It strengthens your energy centers and prevents you from being diverted from your purpose.

It is traditional to do Abyangha in the morning before you shower or bathe. It can also be helpful for insomnia or very dry skin to perform it at night. I have found that because I take "hot" baths, it is better for me to do my Abyangha after bathing.

The Blend

It is important to make your own personal blend using a vegetable oil appropriate for your body type and essential oils chosen for your specific health concerns. In 8 oz. of vegetable oil use 100 to 150 drops of various essential oils.

THE TREATMENT

Begin by brushing your skin with a sauna brush or dry loofa for 2-4 minutes. This will remove all the dead skin and surface dirt. Take your bath or shower. After you dry your body, begin by applying your oil blend to your left foot, ankle and leg. Work the oil between the toes, around the foot and ankle, turning up and around the shins and calves, over and around the knee. Apply enough oil so that the skin absorbs most of it, but leaves just a little on the surface. By the time you finish your whole body, this excess will probably be absorbed also.

Work up and around your left thigh and buttocks. Massage in a clockwise direction on your stomach and around your body to your lower back. Your movements should be fluid, rhythmic and deep enough to stimulate the muscles. Work the oil across your chest, over and around the breasts, and up and over the shoulders. Follow the arms down into the forearm and massage the hands and fingers. Coming back up to the neck you may switch to Wrinkle Free blend (Earth Essentials Florida) formulated especially for the face. Use delicate circles on the face, being gentle with the delicate skin below the eyes. Scalp massage without oil is stimulating and invigorating. Move down the right arm, the right chest and shoulders, abdomen and lower back, right buttocks, thigh and finally the right leg and foot. End your self-treatment with long strokes from your feet, up the body to the chest, crossing over and going down the opposite arms, ending with a vigorous shake of the fingers, as if flinging water off the fingertips. This entire procedure should take 5-10 minutes. Use a towel to remove any remaining oil.

BATHING

A favorite way to relax, renew, and rejuvenate is to take an essential oil or herbal decoction bath. Do not use hot water as it tends to dry the skin. While the warm bathwater is running, take a few moments for dry skin brushing to stimulate circulation (described later in this book). Use brisk, circular movements over your entire body to remove dead cells and to unclog pores.

Just before stepping into the tub, add 15-30 drops of essential oils to the bathwater. In this way you can enjoy the full benefits of the oils before they evaporate. Baths can be refreshing, stimulating, fragrant, healing, and sleep inducing. They may be enhanced with soft music, candlelight, crystals, and meditation. Take the time to create the atmosphere you want. Enjoy!

BREATH

Breath is life. Without it there is no human existence. Proper oxygen supply is the essence of the life force called Prana by the Hindu's.

Respiration is the act of inhaling and exhaling which results in an exchange of gases between the blood and the air. With each inhalation the chest expands, and the diaphragm is pulled down, causing the lungs to draw in air. During exhalation the chest contracts and the diaphragm is drawn up, forcing the air out of the lungs. The maximum intake of oxygen and explosion of carbon dioxide is accomplished by both the ribs and the diaphragm.

Each individual has their own mature rate of breathing, according to lung capacity. The normal rate for an adult is between 14-20 breaths per minute. The rate of breathing automatically adjusts to our rate of oxygen consumption and CO_2 build-up. When we are under stress the breath becomes shallow and the body stores tension in its tissues and organs. The process of breathing interfaces the conscious mind with the subconscious. If we begin to focus on our breath we can alter our conscious state and relax our tissues.

Breathing can bring about cell regeneration, vitality, and health. Breath work opens the doors to new experiences. Any blockages and holding patterns begin to disappear.

The science of breath has been used by the yogis, Rishis, and saints to achieve a blissful state of consciousness. Breath reforms our belief systems, patterns, and behaviors. Begin to be aware of your breathing during the day. Use your breath when you find yourself in anger, anxiety, or any exaggerated form of emotion that takes you away from peace. Cancer cannot live in a body full of oxygen.

Ten Good Reasons Why Conscious Breathing is Important!

1. To maintain a good hold on our emotions.
2. Make good changes in our mental patterns.
3. Clear up negative thoughts.
4. Strengthens the whole body.
5. Relaxes the mind.
6. Assists with sleep and tension.
7. Assists circulation.
8. Assists the aging process, maintaining a youthful body.
9. To gain more energy.
10. To take responsibility for your life.

DIFFERENT BREATHING TECHNIQUES

The Connected Breath or Alternate Breathing

Connected Breath: Breathe in through the nose and exhale through the mouth. As you breathe, imagine that you are letting go of any emotion other than love. This breath is used to integrate the body-mind and to create spirit connection. You may breathe in slowly or powerfully, but place no control over the exhale. Donít push it or draw it out. Just let it go.

Alternate Breathing: Place your right index and middle finger on your forehead. Position your right thumb over your right nostril and your right ring finger on your left nostril so that you can alternately open and close the nostrils. Then, using your right thumb, close the right nostril. Take a slow deep breath in through your left nostril. Pause. Open the right nostril, close the left nostril with ring finger, and slowly exhale. Then slowly inhale through the right nostril. Pause. Open the left nostril, close the right nostril and slowly exhale. Continue breathing in this manner of alternating nostrils for five minutes. This breath brings balance to the left and right hemispheres of the brain. Good to do before entering meditation.

Diaphragm Breathing or Breath of Fire

This technique is done by sitting in a cross-legged, lotus position, half lotus, or in a chair, depending on what you are most comfortable with. Place your hands in your lap with palms facing out. Forcibly exhale through your mouth making the sound "SAT" (Great), allow yourself to inhale while producing the sound "NAM" (truth). Do this for 108 breaths. End with a deep inhale, held for as long as possible. This breath will harness and stimulate the Kundalini energy.

The Star Exercise

Stand with legs spread wide apart, arms out straight from the shoulders, left hand up, right hand down. Let the head extend back until you are looking up at the stars. Pick one. Focus on it. Begin to breathe in and out through the nose in a fast diaphragmatic breath. Do this breath 108 times. On the last breath, take a deep breath, tighten the pelvic floor muscles and visualize the energy moving up to the forehead. Let your breath out. This exercise strengthens the nervous system, gives stamina and rebuilds tissue.

Breathing into the Elements

This exercise is best done outdoors.

Earth

Sit on the ground with your legs crossed when possible, spine straight as if a string is pulling you upward. Put your left hand flat on the ground and the right hand facing upward. Breathe and feel the earth's energy coming in through your left hand, into your body. As you exhale, feel earth's energy going out through the right hand. Request this energy to make you grounded and steady. Repeat for 7 breaths.

Air

Breathe through the nose slowly with quiet breaths. Bring your attention to your heart center. Tilt your head back and gaze up to the sky without focusing. Allow yourself to merge with air and ether.

Water

Stand in the ocean or water, sit near a body of water (ocean, lake, river, etc.), or, if available, place a container of water in front of you. Ask for the water element to cleanse you. Breathe in and out. Begin to bring the energy of the water to your whole body. Be aware of your breath.

Fire

Light a candle. Sit with your left hand facing upward, relaxing on your knee. With the right hand, hold the candle. Take a breath in and bring it towards your groin area, circle the candle seven times, clockwise. Exhale. Bring the candle to a level of 3 inches below your navel, breathing in, hold the breath, and rotate the candle seven times clockwise. Exhale. Repeat again at the level of the diaphragm, heart and throat.

Then hold the candle to a level even with the center of your forehead and about 10 inches from your eyes. Take a breath. Look at the flame of the candle, first with the left eye for 3 breaths, then with the right eye for 3 breaths. Finally, look at the flame with both eyes for 3 breaths. Set the candle down. Close your eyes and meditate.

COLOR THERAPY

Light is the mask of the Creator. All life on earth depends on light from the sun, a source of life and energy. Color is the different qualities of light. Light is the masculine or positive force in nature; color is the feminine or negative force.

The soul always lives in color. Color is as necessary to the soul as air is to the body. When we take away the motion of light or color, we have no awareness of the appearance of matter. We receive all knowledge of the universe through this electro-magnetic radiation. White light contains the energies of all elements and chemicals found in the sun. This white light of the sun is absorbed from the atmosphere by the physical body and is split into component color energies, which in turn flow to different parts of the body to vitalize them. Light is a force which stimulates growth; every living thing depends upon it to build and maintain its form. Light brings about chemical changes in nature. By changing the qualities of light we can also bring about chemical changes in the body. Therefore light, whose source is solar energy, is one of nature's greatest healing forces.

In 1665 Isaac Newton focused sunlight through a prism and found the presence of the seven basic colors. The human body is also a prism that reflects this white light. Color therapy is the science of the use of different colors to change or maintain vibrations of the body to the frequency which signifies good health and harmony. Healing by means of color was the first type of therapy used by humans. It is nature's own method of keeping the body in balance with the rhythms of life. Color expresses the way we think. Our emotions and actions affect the electro-magnetic field which surrounds us and is reflected in our aura. Color can help to restore balance when a blockage or imbalance of this energy has resulted in disease. The use of color can help to restore vitality to the etheric body through the projection of specific color rays, which are then absorbed by the chakra centers. The pituitary gland transforms these colors into revitalizing energies to rebuild the centers that are lacking in energy. Color healing shows us how to make light work for us. The use of color is one of the many natural tools available to help us walk in balance with the universe.

Life is color and each organ has a specific color. Each color has intelligence and polarity, knows its functional role, and works selectively. Color is a vibratory energy that can activate a particular organ, gland and system in the body. The application of the correct frequency of the electro-magnetic force field will change the altered function of the body and help return it to its original patterns. It is this energy, which is the result of applying color, that is important in the healing process. This method of healing will create harmony and balance in the mind and in the body. Color therapy is very effective because it helps to maintain this balance.

Color healing is not only a physical but also a spiritual force, and thus forms a link between our physical bodies and the finer forces, or vibrations, of the higher levels of consciousness, or spiritual growth. Color is the bridge between our inner and outer bodies. The vibrations of color are energy of the Life-Force itself and are here to aid us in our growth and progress toward the oneness which is our ultimate purpose. The more intimate our color experiences become, the more attuned we will become with the universe.

We have a quota of ultra-violet light that most of us do not fulfill because so many modern products cut out that portion of the spectrum and because we do not spend enough time out of doors. We can increase our exposure to full spectrum light by simply being out in the sun more. Light automatically replaces darkness.

PRIMARY COLORS	RED, BLUE, YELLOW
Color Opposites	Red - Blue Orange - Indigo Yellow - Violet Green is neutral
Warm Colors	Increases activity and circulation. Will stimulate the function. **Red:** The warmest color and longest wave length in the visible spectrum. **Orange:** The seat of the Soul **Yellow:** Gives a feeling of wellbeing
Cool Colors	Decreases activity and circulation. Will retard the function. **Blue:** Sedates, suppresses and inhibits. **Indigo:** The coolest color and the most difficult to visualize. **Violet:** The shortest wave length in the visible spectrum. The color of transformation.
Toning Color	Helps promote the function. **Green:** Self-regulating. A balancer. When the body feels too cool, the application or visualization of green will bring a warming feeling. When the body feels too warm, the application or visualization of green will bring a cooling feeling.
Color pH	**Acid Rays:** Blue, indigo, violet **Alkaline Rays:** Red, orange, yellow **Neutral Ray:** Green

Projection

The application of color can raise or lower the temperature of the body. Color is a very powerful specific electrical vibration. It must be used with discretion and prudence. Always add color to the body, never decrease it. When lights are used, 25 watts is recommended. The higher the wattage, the shorter time of exposure is required. Use color to unlock in any physical and mental therapy.

Procedure

Everything in nature has a certain frequency of vibration. When a person is subject to a given color, their mental, as well as their muscular activities, change. Muscle monitoring can be used to determine which frequency of color is necessary for balance.

1. Test for "major" color required for balance.
2. Test for the length of time required.

Behavior Modification

Color helps us to see that the universe is not in disorder. Color can be used to help us walk in balance.

Bioluminescence

The body creates its own energy. We produce our own world. The change must come from within.

Balancing Breath

To balance the chakras, visualize breathing a rainbow through the nose. Be strong enough to change the color of the air as it enters into the body. A rainbow displays the quality of absolute spirituality. It transcends the distinction between the physical and non-physical dimensions. It is important to breath rainbows as we are what we think. Proper deep breathing will expand the aura or energy field around the body.

Thought Power

The physical gives life to the etheric body. Without emotions, thoughts are of little value. Activity is the result of emotionally charged thoughts. If actions feel good, inner motivation is satisfied. Direct colored breath to the area required by using creative visualization.

Violet	To become masters of our imaginations and attain control over our thoughts.
Indigo	To have a vision of the future that is so powerful that it becomes reality.
Blue	When devotion transcends thoughts, concepts, and assumptions.
Green	To diminish the drive to possess and to feel secure; to trust the Universe so that we may realize our oneness.
Yellow	To discover the self-sense that includes all other self-senses as well as dissolving the separation between ourselves and others.
Orange	To share ourselves and to be able to relate to others.
Red	Highest expression is to reach our fullest potential.

Food

- Food can be used as a type of color therapy as the body turns food into light. Color is a natural food for the body. Food is a method of introducing color to the body. Physical food is the slowest and least effective. We have the least control over our emotional food. Mental food is the best and most effective. Appetite is an affirmation of being.
- Water is a means of storing sunlight. Charge drinking water in colored glass for 24 hours.
- When food is sun dried, the color turns cooler.

Food and Color

Food is an excellent means of getting color into the body.

Violet	Purple broccoli, grapes, blackberries, beets, wine. Anything that changes color when cooked.
Indigo	Same as violet and blue.
Blue	Plums, blueberries, prunes, grapes, potatoes.

Green	Spinach, peas, string beans, cabbage, wheatgrass juice, lettuce.
Yellow	Grapefruit, mangoes, bananas, lemons, peaches, squash, cantaloupe, beans, nuts.
Orange	Carrots, pumpkin, oranges, apricots, sweet corn, tangerines, sweet potatoes, grains.
Red	Cherries, peppers, radishes, onions, tomatoes, tofu and all protein.

Color and the Systems of the Body

Color represents chemical potencies in higher octaves of vibration. There is a particular color that will stimulate each organ system in the body. By knowing the action of the different colors upon the different organ systems, the application of the correct color will help to balance the actions of any system that has become out of balance in its function or condition.

Violet	Diuretic. Purifies the blood. Promotes bone growth. Stops the growth of tumors. Controls excess hunger. Helps maintain the potassium-sodium balance. Depresses the motor nerves and the lymphatic system. Improves thought. Promotes deeper meditation. **Will aid the following conditions:** Bladder problems, skin conditions, mental disorders, sciatic nerve pain, tumors, cramps.
Indigo	Cooling and astringent. Reduces or even stops bleeding. Depresses the respiration and is good for muscle toning. A purifier that gives relief from swelling. Helps filter out radiation. Also affects the emotional and spiritual levels. Improves smell. **Will aid the following conditions:** Convulsions, tremors, insanity, nasal problems, inflammation of the appendix, eye and ear dysfunctions.
Blue	One of the best antiseptics. Helps heal burns quickly. Suppresses fever. Promotes growth.

Increases metabolism. Good for impatience and overactivity.

Will aid the following conditions: itching, hysteria, burns, overweight, fever, vomiting, throat problems.

Green   Disinfectant. Relieves tension. Dilates the capillaries and produces a sensation of warmth. Master healing color that regulates the etheric body.

Will aid the following conditions: Heart conditions, hay fever, breathing, and stomach problems.

Yellow   Digestant. Activates the motor nerves and generates energy in the muscles. Works favorably on the digestion. Loosens calcium deposits and stimulates the flow of bile.

Will aid the following conditions: Inflammation of the joints, indigestion, skin conditions, blood/fuel problems, constipation, and nervous disorders.

Orange   Antispasmodic. Increases lymphatic movement. Aids calcium intake. Raises the pulse rate, but does not raise the blood pressure. Enlivens the emotions and creates a general feeling of well-being.

Will aid the following conditions: Muscle cramps and spasms, underactive thyroid, "colds", gallstones, lung conditions, and disturbances in the metabolism rate.

Red   Energizer. Stimulates the nerves and the blood systems. Releases adrenaline. Excites the cerebrospinal nerves and the sympathetic nervous system.

Will aid the following conditions: Low red blood cell count, lung congestion, paralysis, and blood poisoning.

The preceding excerpts are from James Minckler's book, "Energy Balancing for Natural Health". Grateful acknowledgement for his generous contribution.

COMPRESS

Compresses are effective and immediate treatment because the warm water opens the pores whereby the essential oils penetrate the skin at a rate of two hundred times faster than water alone. To make a compress, mix 5-10 drops of essential oils in one quart of hot water. Immerse a small towel, squeeze out most of the water, and apply to the required area. You may add a hot water bottle or a heating pad to keep the compress warm for a longer period of time, thereby assisting in the penetration of the essential oils.

Compresses are used for specific conditions, therefore,

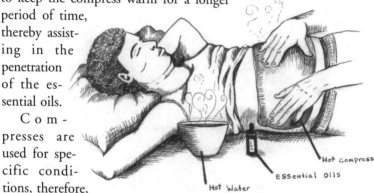

Hot compress

Essential oils

Hot Water

be aware of the body type being treated. Remember that pain is usually an indication of Vata imbalance. Because Vata is cold, you will want to use a warm compress. Pitta conditions are usually characterized by redness, inflammation, and heat. On areas of Pitta imbalance, cool or cold compresses are best. Kapha conditions are characterized by a lack of fluid movement, swelling, and congestion. Here again, warm or hot compresses are best. If placing a compress on an organ use a cool compress for an organ that is overactive, and use a warm or hot compress on an organ that is underactive. Choose the appropriate essential oils for the specific body type being treated.

Contraindications to Cold

1. Whether local or general, cold should not be applied to weakened individuals, such as in old age, infancy, cachexia, advanced cardio-vascular disease, etc.

2. Do not apply when patient is cold and shivering.

General Rules of Application of Local Cold

1. Avoid prolonged application and, therefore, possible chilblains or frost bite.
2. Place cold moist cloth between cold pack and skin - never direct.
3. Apply simultaneous heat to other parts of the body to prevent generalized chilling, or particularly over the heart and head where excess vasoconstriction may be contraindicated.
4. Warm patient after treatment if chilling occurs.

Physiological Effects of Local Heat

A. LOCAL

1. Dilation of blood and lymphatic vessels
2. White blood cell activity
3. Increased perspiration
4. Relieves muscular spasms and thereby pain
5. Sedates nervous system
6. Reflexly dilates blood and lymphatic vessels in deeper tissues, depending upon applied skin site.

B. GENERAL

1. Increases perspiration
2. Increases circulation and heart rate
3. Lowers blood pressure
4. Increases respiration
5. Increases urine formation with loss of water, salts, urea and nitrogenous substances
6. Slight rise in alkalinity

Contraindications to Local Heat

1. Acute inflammatory process particularly when accompanied by fever and/or suppuration.
2. In conditions where there is a tendency to hemorrhage.
3. In malignant tumors.

4. Over the gravid uterus.

5. Over encapsulated swellings where vasodilation may cause dispersion and/or rupture.

6. Where there is a deficiency of thermal nerve reaction.

7. Acute tuberculosis.

8. Diabetic gangrene.

General Rules of Application of Local Heat

1. Test heated object before application to judge temperature.

2. When heat is increased, such as with an infrared lamp or electrical pads, lower or discontinue when excess warmth occurs.

3. In fomentations or other direct contact heat, make certain skin is dry. Enclosed moisture may become steam and cause burning.

4. In direct contact heat, pad bony prominences and/or sensitive areas.

5. When there is cerebral congestion, and in cases of fever, apply cold compress to head.

6. Never apply heat for an extended period of time to avoid prolonged tissue congestion.

DRY SKIN BRUSHING

The gentle friction of dry skin brushing is a highly effective technique for cleansing the lymphatic system and stimulating blood flow. Daily brushing promotes the quick elimination of toxins and helps tone and tighten the skin. A bath-type brush of natural vegetable bristles works best. It must be kept dry and not be used for bathing. Brushing may be performed on any part of the body except the face. The skin must be dry. Use a one-way sweeping motion, directing strokes toward the lower abdomen area. Brush down the neck and trunk. Brush up the arms, legs and buttocks. Perform this highly stimulating and invigorating therapy five minutes at a time. Twice daily is ideal.

FASTING

Fasting is taking a break from food consumption. It allows the vital organs to rest, cleanse, and rebuild. Some people fast for spiritual reasons, some to cleanse the body, and others for mental clarity. Mahatma Gandhi fasted for his country to be free from oppression and to get the Moslems and Hindus to stop fighting each other. Fasting is a way to improve health. Fasting supports the body to cleanse and eliminate excess toxins. It also frees the vast energy used in the digestive process to rebuild itself or to heal any illness. When you observe animals in nature or even your own pets, they will stop eating when they don't feel well. When we become ill with a virus or flu, we often lose all desire to eat.

When Ama (toxicity) has built up in the body, it is a good time to fast. Signs of Ama include tiredness, bad breath, strong body odor, coated tongue, indigestion, and foul gas or stool.

People who find themselves in good health have no need to fast. However, they may wish to fast seasonally, in order to preserve their health and prevent disease. When someone has sunk to a level of severe illness and is too weak or emaciated, fasting is not recommended until some strength has returned.

The best time to fast or do house cleaning in the body is when the energy is high and the individuals mind is ready to take on the discipline of doing without food.

When someone recognizes that they are consuming a junk diet of meat, sugar, refined, processed, and fried foods, it is best to follow a cleansing diet before attempting to fast. After following this diet, then you can more easily do a fast.

ELIMINATION OR CLEANSING DIET

This program can be used to prepare yourself for a water or juice fast, especially if you have been eating a junk food diet.

1. Eliminate all meats from your diet. Eat eggs, dairy, nuts, grains, herbs, beans, vegetables and fruit for 1 week.

2. Then, eliminate all dairy and eggs. Eat grains, herbs, beans, vegetables, nuts, seeds and fruit for 1 week.

3. Then, eliminate all nuts, seeds, beans, and grains. Eat vegetables, herbs, and fruits for 1 week.

4. Then, eliminate all vegetables. Eat only fruits, herbs and herbal teas for 1 week.

Note: Be sure to drink plenty of water.

Now you are ready for a water fast. During this cleansing, choose foods that are best for your body type (organic if possible).

This elimination diet may not be appropriate for some health problems. Consult a physician if in question.

It is ideal to combine fasting with a retreat. Take time off from work, go into nature and focus on yourself. Work, noise, disturbances, unpleasant personalities, people eating or preparing food all make fasting difficult. It is good to be some place warm or be prepared to dress warmly. Allow yourself long hours to sleep and rest. Read inspirational books.

There are many different kinds of fasts such as a juice, fruit, herbal, or water fast.

However you do it, it is most important to create a quiet supportive environment for yourself. Do not attempt to fast while remaining on the job. If you have never fasted, begin with one day, then the following week do two, then three days and work up to fasting for one week. Drink plenty of liquids or water, selecting those juices which are best suited for your body type. For Vata, fasting should be limited, but if it is necessary, fast with juices or spring water.

Skin brushing is important, to stimulate and cleanse the skin. Colon cleansing should be done every day of fasting to eliminate toxins which are being released. Herbal teas are preferable to plain water for colon cleansing. Colonics by a professional, a home Colema board or plain home enemas are all helpful. Light exercise (walking, swimming), sweats, saunas, and breathing all assist in toxin release.

After a few days of fasting you may experience tongue coating, bad breath, headache, or aches and pains. These symptoms will pass. Drink more fluids. In a long fast, it is possible to experience a recurrence of old illnesses which is called a "healing crisis" by natural health practitioners. This will pass also. If you do the cleansing recommended on the preceding page, this is less likely to happen.

When fasting due to an illness, make sure that you are under the supervision of a healthcare practitioner. Pancha Karma programs are specially designed Ayurvedic seasonal cleanses which clean and rebuild all the organs in a systemic, time-tested manner.

BREAKING YOUR FAST

Breaking your fast correctly is as important as how you begin your fast. Fasting and feasting can be dangerous to your health. A gradual transition back to solid foods is necessary . When the fast is only 3 days long, begin to break it with fruit and fruit juices on the fourth day. On the fifth day, drink vegetable juices and eat steamed vegetables. On the sixth day, eat salads, broths, and whole grains. Then on the seventh day, begin to eat a complete diet of good wholesome foods, being careful to eat moderate amounts and observe good food combinations.

Remember, your stomach is only as big as your hands placed wrist to wrist, fingertip to fingertip, and palms separating to make a ball. The stomach is muscular and will stretch more, but it works best when not overfilled.

Fasting may be a very rewarding experience. We may learn that our strength comes not from food, but from our inner connections. If we allow ourselves to let go of our daily concerns and rely on our inner strength and determination, we may experience an internal healing process. A process which, when completed, brings a sense of inner peace and serenity.

ESSENTIAL OIL PATCHES

Essential oil patches are very easy to prepare and to use. The most convenient method is to place essential oil on regular or dot bandaids and place on the body; they are very inconspicuous, especially when worn under clothing. Another method is to place 10 drops of flaxseed oil or primrose oil on gauze or a cotton ball, then add up to three drops each of essential oils of your choice. These are particularly useful when taped over the ovaries, behind the ear, or any other area. Refresh patches with essential oil again during the day, or reapply new ones. (See "Reflexology" section in Chapter 11 for areas in which to use these patches.)

FOOT BATH

A foot bath is very beneficial when the body is under stress or long hours of standing. The bottom of the feet, as well as the hands, have numerous nerve endings corresponding to different organs in the body. It is good to do a foot bath before going to bed, which can be done while reading or watching TV.

It can also be a great aid before meditation by doing a concentration exercise while foot bathing. Raise a candle in front of a picture of your Guru, a mentor, or a beautiful image. Sit comfortably in a chair with your hands out on your lap, palms face-up. Place your feet in a basin or bowl of water. Add 30-40 drops of essential oil (this varies according to what condition you wish to treat), and a handful of sea salt into the water. Sit in meditation with a picture and a candle in alignment with your eyes for 15 minutes. Dry and oil your feet with essential oil. Dispose of water, wash your hands, and meditate for a further 10 minutes. This is an ideal therapy for restless sleep.

INHALATION

Inhalation is a great way to experience immediate benefits of the essential oils which quickly bring relief to any congestion, sinus headache, mood, or various other symptoms. Perhaps the most convenient and effective method is to purchase a small inhalation device expressly for this purpose. Another method is to boil water, pour it into a bowl or into the bathroom sink, and use 3-5 drops of essential oils. Place a towel over your head to make a "tent", bend over the steaming bowl, close your eyes, and take long, deep, relaxed breaths. Avoid getting too close to the steam as it may burn. After three minutes the fragrance will diminish, at which time you may add more essential oils or end the treatment.

MANTRA

"Mantra" is a Sanskrit word which means advise, repetition or suggestion. It is a sound of sacredness that manifests as spiritual power. Mantras are also known as "primordial sounds" because they were the primal cause of the formation of the universe according to the ancient Vedic creation story. Even modern science speaks of the beginning of the universe in terms of sound, "the big bang". When we make the sounds of mantra, we align ourselves with universal forces.

There are many different uses for mantra. The main purpose is to open the energy channels of the body and bring it to a higher vibratory frequency. By resonating sound from the throat you can help to open communication and self expression. Sound waves increase the vibratory rate in the vital organs, bringing the awareness of pure spirit in and taking away negative emotions.

The Transcendental Meditation group (and teachers trained by Dr. Deepak Chopra) give mantras created from "individual" birthdates. Your numerical birthdate contains within it the memory of why you incarnated. It is also possible to simply sit in the space of quietness, and listen to the voice within you. Harmonic sounds will come through you as you connect with the universal currents. The universe is within you.

When I chant a mantra, it brings me into a state of bliss and harmony. If I feel separate or alone or if I create realities which are not conducive to my path or serve my purpose, I can chant a mantra and instantly it calms my mind and brings inner peace. Rather than feeling constricted by negative experiences, the mantra begins to resonate the core of my being, creating expanded feelings and peaceful thoughts. The sounds relax my whole body and a transformational shift occurs in my experience of life. A positive and joyful state awakens within me. At this point I can reconnect with my purpose of service and love.

One does not need to know Sanskrit or be a Hindu, Buddhist, or Sufi to chant. Any sound that vibrates and brings positive emotion and positive invocation will work. Gregorian chants, for example, are beautiful and harmonious. I chant any time I feel my body tense. When I am stopped in traffic, I begin chanting and flow with divine energy. On the days that I pick up my two year old grandson from day care, we chant together so that he begins to resonate with, and take in, the sounds. We bond as he smiles and the ride in the car passes quickly and peacefully.

Until such time as you may receive your own personal mantra, the following wonderful, easy sounds are recommended:

In one breath: **Ahhhh Uuuu-oh MMMM (Aum)**
This is the sound of creation; the background sound in the universal field. I am one with the universal force.

OM SHANTI
Peace, peace in this universe. Peace in me. Divine order.

RAM
The God of light, take away darkness; I am one with the light.

KLIM (Kleem)
Nature spirit, forces of nature, I am in harmony with nature.

SHYAM (Sham)
Ether, space, essence, all creation is mostly space. I am one with the spirit which prevails all space.

HUM (Sham)
Bliss permeates me displacing negative thoughts and energies. I am bliss.

SHREEM
Creativity, prosperity, and abundance is my true nature.

AIM (Aymn)
Concentration, focus, centered I am.

MEDITATION

Meditation offers us an opportunity to reach a higher potential by fine tuning our minds, and places us on the road to discovering our true Self. Meditation creates an opening to live a life free of fears, blame, attachments, judgements, stress, negativity, and illusions. It is a process where we begin to unfold the magic of being, release the beauty from within and experience ourselves as a lotus flower opening its magnificent splendor to the world.

As we begin meditation, it is important to be still and to know that there is nothing to do, but just be. With regular practice, our thoughts will slow down, then cease and we will ultimately go to that space...the void...the initial step to freeing ourselves.

Within this space of self-realization, one can go beyond conventional reality and attachments and establish a connection with the absolute; the only real truth that exists. We become Pure Light.

As meditation practice becomes a daily part of our life, we can accept that we are in this world but not of it and, subsequently, release attachment to the "I", the "ego". Our physical body will continue to function in the world but with more knowledge and awareness of the absolute. We no longer question why or how, we are the flower that becomes the fruit. It is already within us, but through meditation the space is opened to be Divine.

In the west, the word meditation has several applications. Guided imagery and visualization are two of the ways to induce a meditative state. You do not need to renounce all worldly possessions, or sit at the foot of a guru listening for answers. You do not need to look for wisdom on tapes or in music or through controlling thoughts with special techniques such as bio-feedback.

Meditation is the stillness of self; the space where you become the observer, the knower, and the known. Through meditation the Divine awakens within you. The being that is always there, radiating pure joy and eternal bliss, returning time after time through many existences; a physical self wanting to give expression to the God Self in bodily form. The self that we have forgotten in the midst of our crazy thoughts becomes awakened and remembers the sole purpose of this existence. The remembrance of who we are, the discovery of the space we are, and will always be. Through meditation, the ego mind gets glimpses of this space and finally surrenders. With surrender, we become absolute compassion and power. The words, thoughts, and disruptions stop. We become Divine, feeling the oneness with everything that is. When we reach this point, there is no worry if we are alone - there is no need to be around anyone. We are alone, yet connected to all beings simultaneously. Only through this experience do we enjoy the divinity in others.

How To Meditate for Serenity and Bliss

- Sit in a comfortable place in a cross-legged position or, if possible, a half or full lotus posture. If this is not possible, sit in a chair with your feet flat on the ground and your spine erect. Be in whatever position is comfortable for you.

- Close your eyes and allow the eyelids to totally relax. You can focus attention on the area above and between the eyebrows known as "the third eye".

- Begin to observe your breath. Relax your diaphram and breathing muscles. Let your abdomen expand as you breathe in.

- Allow the thoughts to be. Don't try to stop them. Just let them pass like birds flying over your head.

- Relax and pay no attention to your body. Gradually remove awareness from your physical body.

- Feel the experience of the moment - beyond words, thoughts and feelings.

- As you breathe, repeat the words, Amaram Hum Madhuran Hum (I am bliss, I am eternal.) Keep repeating this mantra over and over without thought and allow the sound to transport you. As you repeat the sound, move into that space where nothing can touch you.

- Remain aware of your breathing while repeating the sound and go to that place where nothing can burn you.

- Breath into that space where no wind can dry you.

- The body will begin to call for attention, but keep your attention on the sound.

- Breath into that space where no water can make you wet.

- Repeat the sound, Amaram Hum Madhuran Hum.

- Allow yourself to be aware of the space and continue to slip deeper and deeper into that space. Pay no attention to the seconds, the minutes passing by. Keep repeating, Amaram Hum Madharan Hum and before you realize it, time will

have no meaning.
- You are now in the space of Peace, Love and Truth

In order to master and live in this space, it is recommended that you practice every day for seven to twenty minutes. Everything that we do is learned by practice. When we were small children, we could not read or write. We began by printing each letter of the alphabet numerous times and when that was mastered, we then learned to write. After many years, writing becomes automatic with no thought. The same rule applies when learning to ride a bicycle, driving a car, operating a computer, and meditating.

Many people feel that their life is too busy. "I don't have time for meditation, I have too much to do". My guru/teacher says that if everyone took five minutes of every waking hour and closed their eyes and repeated the mantra, they would be meditating for one hour every day. Try combining your bath time with meditation.

Try meditation and experience yourself feeling more alive, calm and beautiful. Use it to transform your life. It's simple, just close your eyes and join with the divine energy that gave you life. It lives in you and every part of the universe that we have created.

AMARAM HUM MADHARAN HUM

MUST WE SEARCH FOR A GURU?

When the student is ready, the teacher will appear. It is good to find someone to teach us meditation in the beginning since it is probably not something you have done in this lifetime. There may be meditation centers or teachers in your area. Check around and see what your area has to offer, and what form you are drawn to (what feels good to you). Ask for guidance and the path will open. Trust that you will be shown the way. When you listen, you will be guided step-by-step and you will find your guru. He or she may appear in many forms.

Do the work and the teacher will find you. All knowledge is within you already. You have only to remember.

My deepest and most sincere gratitude to my great teacher, Swami Shyam, Kulu, India.

MUSIC AND SOUND THERAPY

Sound is a condensed form of energy. Music is humanity understanding spiritual information clearly. The whole body responds to sound. At a cellular level, this stimulus is understood and assimilated. Sound works directly on the nervous system, radiating energy, which creates specific effects according to frequency and intensity. Every sound emits a certain color. Sound and color are just different rates of vibration. Healing with vibration will help us to fulfill our evolutionary potential.

Existence is full of vibration. It is everywhere. The wind passing through the pines is music, the water descending from the mountains is music, the birds and animals are music. The whole existence is a kind of great orchestra. It is a symphony.

We are born to be a song of bliss. Humanity is hidden music, and the music is trying to explode, but we have created such a hard crust (ego) around ourselves that neither can the music of existence enter into us nor can our music have a meeting with the music of the without. We have created a wall between the without and the within; the wall is the ego. That wall is the idea of separation, that we are separate from the Universe. We are not. We are all One.

The only illusion that humankind has to drop is the illusion of separation. Then suddenly the inner song will burst forth and meet with the outer. They will become one, a pulsation and a rhythm. That experience of the within and the without becoming one is the peak of joy, of ecstasy, of life, and the glorious beauty of it all.

The idea of separation has to be dropped slowly. See and search for moments when you feel more in tune with existence so that the layer of separation becomes thinner and thinner. Listening to music, in meditation, seeing a beautiful sunset, the starry night, or just sitting silently doing nothing, emerging, melting, and disappearing. Allow more and more moments of this rare kind. We are so preoccupied that we never allow those moments to erupt, or if sometimes they do occur, we are in such a hurry we do not take note of them.

Start taking note of those beautiful moments as they are the windows of the Creator.

Keynotes

B	Violet	493.0 Cycles	385 Hertz
A	Indigo	440.0	427
G	Blue	392.0	385
F	Green	349.2	342
E	Yellow	329.1	322
D	Orange	292.0	289
C	Red	261.2	259

Color

Violet	Transcendental, romantic, space music, non-structured jazz
Indigo	Classical
Blue	Country Western
Green	Easy listening
Yellow	Structured jazz
Orange	Folk, reggae
Red	Rock 'n Roll

Instrument	Color	Scale	Color
Wind Instruments	Violet	Ti	Violet
Reed Instruments	Indigo	La	Indigo
Fine String Guitar	Blue	So	Blue
Piano	Green	Fa	Green
Harp	Yellow	Mi	Yellow
Thick Strings	Orange	Re	Orange
Base Tones	Red	Do	Red

Mantra

A sequence of powerful words or sounds used to achieve a result. Sound is vibration that creates matter and form. Chanting changes the frequency of the body. OM (pronounced AUM) is the sound of the Earth.

Chanting

Vibration of tone. Very effective to open the body to receive new information.

Heartfelt appreciation to James Minckler's Sound Therapy information - truly a gift of love.

MUSIC FOR HEALING

Sound is a basis for health and for balancing the energies of the body. Certain selections of music affect responses in the listener far beyond mere "mood setting".

Musical Instruments and Their Vibrations

Drums	Lower back problems; extremely energizing, stimulates the blood and the nervous system. Drums are not the instrument for relaxing unless they are played very slowly.
Violin	Spleen, liver and gall bladder. Stimulates all vital organs, also should be played slowly. Not everyone is ready for this instrument. A person with lots of stress will be aggravated by the sound.
Harp	Works with opening the chakras and taking one to the other dimension of themselves. It opens the psyche and cleanses the mind. (They say that people who play the harp start hearing voices of the angels.) FOR MENTAL STRESS: Opens the doors to new understandings.
Guitar	Classical can be energizing and stimulating to the digestive system and the colon.
Piano	Works with relaxing and enhancing the whole body.
Most string instruments	Work with the nervous system.

The basic theory is that music, as an energy, can work on the energy body of an individual and speak the vibrations language, the mother tongue, to the various organs and systems to help bring the body into physical alignment and attunement with its own perfect pattern of perfection.

Food cannot be digested properly in a tense environment. Tibet, Morocco, Africa and many other cultures used music to drive out evil spirits.

Rhythmic music is necessary for relaxation to allow the body to find its own rhythm. Rock music is much too stimulating to the physical body, and listening to this music at a time of confusion can be very disturbing to the mind. Rock music can be very disturbing at a time of sickness also.

Harp and piano together speaks to the spirit within and provides a direction for those energies. Harps are also good for a healing environment.

NONI — MORINDA CITRIFOLIA

"The Miracle of Paradise"

The noni fruit, due to its medical and nutritional value is considered to be the "queen" of the other 80 species of the Old World Rubiaceae family. Common names: Indian Mulberry (India), Noni (Samoa and Tonga), Nono (Tahiti and Raratonga), Polynesian Bush Fruit, Pain-killer tree (Caribbean Island), Lada (Guam), Mengkudo (Malaysia), Nhau (Southeast Asia), Grand Morinda (Vietnam), Cheese Fruit (Australia), Kuru (Fiji), Bumbo (Africa).[1] It grows on a beautiful tree with large heart shaped leaves that range from a shrub to a large tree in Tahiti that bears 2000 pounds of fruit per month. Where one fruit is picked another grows in its place, ready for picking three months later. The fruit looks kind of like a potato with a lumpy surface ranging in size from small to big, green in color turning yellow then white as it ripens and then to almost black. Because of its strong smell it is not a fruit one would ever come across on a tropical fruit plate! The tree needs volcanic soil rich in calcium and a tropical climate to thrive. The most abundant source of this fruit is on the Tahitian and French Polynesian Islands where whole noni valleys exist as far as your eye can see.

Traditional Polynesian healers (Kahunas) employed every part of the noni plant – root, leaves, flowers, bark, fruit, and seed - to treat health problems ranging from thrush to rheumatism.[2] On a recent trip to one of the Polynesian Islands my trail guide remarked "So you know noni?" I said "Yes, I love noni!" He then shared with me that you don't take noni alone, you take it with a prayer!

Noni is receiving more and more attention from modern herbalists, medical physicians, and high-tech biochemists. Scientific studies within the last few decades lend support to the Polynesian claims of its unusual healing power. These studies have shown the fruit juice to contain several healing attributes including but not limited to, antibacterial, anti-inflammatory, analgesic, anticongestive, hypotensive, and cancer-inhibiting compounds.[3] The seeds have a purgative action, the leaves are used to treat external inflammation and to relieve pain, the bark has strong astringent properties and can treat malaria, root extracts lower blood pressure, flower essence relieves eye inflammation, and the fruit has a number of medical actions.[4]

Dr. Ralph Heiniche, Ph.D. formerly at the University of Hawaii, has pinpointed within the fruit's juice a proenzyme, called proxeronine, that stimulates the human body to produce xeronine, a vital element to the body's protein molecules.[5] A large portion of health related compounds have been isolated from noni; these are Terpene compounds, Morindone, Morindin, Acubin, I. Asperuloside, various Anthroquinones, Alizarin, Caproic acid, Caprylic acid, Scopetin, Damnacanthal, and Alkaloids.[6] It is the ability of the compound proxeronine found abundantly in noni which initiates the increased production of xeronine that Dr. Heinicke believes makes the noni fruit different from all other natural remedies. Xeronine is an alkaloid used by the body to strengthen and revitalize cells.[7]

Dr. Mona Harrison, MD, has had many great results with her patients using noni juice.[8] She credits that to noni's enhancement of the activities of the pineal gland where serotonin is produced, from which melatonin is synthesized. As one gland becomes balanced, it then activates and balances the gland below it. Noni also balances the body's pH levels, which affect one's ability to absorb minerals and vitamins. In balancing the endocrine system, the body can regain its balance. The word dis-ease can be compared to imbalance. Noni juice actually works at the cellular level.

Dr. Neil Solomon, M.D., Ph.D. was first approached to do an article on Morinda Citrifolia by a medical publication. He became fascinated and after two years of researching both the scientific and non-scientific evidence – case studies, reports from doctors and other experts as well as clinical trials involving the Morinda Citrifolia fruit juice – Dr. Solomon wrote a book, "NONI Nature's amazing Healer", published by Woodland Publishing.

In interviewing over forty doctors and over 8,000 people who had used or were using noni, his conclusions indicated that 78%

were helped in some way. One interesting point that he found was that these doctors were also using the noni juice for themselves, their families and friends! He found that it lowers high blood pressure, fights cancer, reduces arthritic symptoms/pain, improves immune function, enhances cellular health, and promotes general health.[9]

Morinda Citrifolia works as an adaptogen and is absorbed in the body as a whole food. It helps the body help itself. Noni is tri-doshic and, therefore, can be taken by all body types. Noni is used extensively in Ayurveda and is taken internally as well as applied as a compress or poultice externally.

Tucked away from most of civilization for thousands of years, this amazing fruit is finally available to us in juice form. The Morinda Citrifolia fruit has been used traditionally in Polynesia, China, and India and has been a staple food in many tropical climates. Thanks to the pristine environment of French Polynesia and those individuals who have given their lives to the production of noni juice and research of Morinda Citrifolia, we are able to experience this juice in its potent, pristine, and original form.

Bibliography on Noni

1. Noni (Morinda Citrifolia) Prize Herb of the South Pacific, by Rita Elkins, M.H. Woodland Publishing, 1996.

2. Alexandra Dittmar, "Morinda Citrifolia L. Use in Indigenous Samoan Medicine", Journal of Herbs, Spices and Medicinal Plants, Vol 1 (3), 1993.

3. Chafique Younos, Alain Rolland, Jacques Fleurentin, Marie-Claire Lanhers, Rene Misslin, and Francois Mortier, "Analgesic and Behavioral Effects of Morinda Citrifolia", Planta Med., Vol. 56, 1990.

4. Noni (Morinda Citrifolia) Prize Herb of the South Pacific, by Rita Elkins, M.H. Woodland Publishing, 1996.

5. R.M. Heinicke, "The Pharmacologically Active Ingredient of Noni," Bulletin of the National Tropical Botanical Garden, 1985.

6. Noni Polynesia's Natural Pharmacy, Pride Publishing, 1997.

7. R.M. Heinicke, "The Pharmacologically Active Ingredient of Noni", Bulletin of the National Tropical Botanical Garden, 1985.

8. Mona Harrison, M.D., received her degree from the University of Maryland, became assistant dean of Boston University School of Medicine, and Chief Medical Officer for D.C. General Hospital. Health News Triple R Publishing, Inc., Vol. 4 Number 2.

9. Dr. Neil Solomon, M.D., Ph.D., New York Times Best Selling Author. Former CNN-TV Health Commentator; former L.A. Times Syndication Health Columnist; Maryland's first Secretary of Health and Mental Hygiene; John Hopkins trained physician.

Gratitude and Blessings to my sister in spirit, Mary Murphy, for the Noni information.

T'AI CHI / CH'I KUNG

T'ai Chi (modern spelling, T'ai Ji) refers to a system of exercise techniques designed to promote and direct the movement of energy in our bodies. There are various forms and styles of T'ai Chi, each presenting a series of soft flowing movements that, when practiced regularly, can reward the practitioner with physical, mental and emotional health.

Originally taught as a self-defence art, to develop mind/body skills for successful combat, T'ai Chi is related to an ancient system of Chinese health-training called Ch'i Kung (modern spelling, Qi Gong). Ch'i means "energy", or "vital force"; kung is the word for "work" or "development". Both T'ai Chi and Ch'i Kung work and develop the energy systems of the body.

T'ai Chi means "supreme ultimate". The movements may be simple and easy-to-learn, as in T'ai Chi Chih (supreme ultimate knowledge) or other short T'ai Chi forms, or they may be more complicated, requiring years of study, as in the long form of T'ai Chi Ch'uan (supreme ultimate fist), a traditional system of 108 movements first formally taught in the thirteenth century. Ch'i Kung is sometimes practiced in a seemingly static, or non-moving, form, at least from an external viewpoint. The healing benefits result from *internal* movement.

According to Chinese medical philosophy, when the circulation of ch'i is open and flowing, we have healthy bodies and stable emotions. If it becomes blocked or stagnant, disease and illness appear.

Ongoing T'ai Chi or Ch'i Kung training can be an effective therapy for digestive, circulatory, muscular and skeletal ailments. Emphasis on conscious breathing can help strengthen and tone the abdominal muscles, as well as increase bronchial activity and oxygen intake. Relaxed, rhythmic motions lessen pressures on the heart and smooth and regulate the circulation of blood. Metabolism and weight can be normalized.

The emphasis on grounding through the feet enhances a sense of balance and improves posture, while directly stimulating reflexology and acupuncture points in the balls of the feet. With continued and disciplined practice, it is said that even the involuntary actions of the internal organs can be controlled and exercised.

When the physical body is bathed with energy, natural feelings of peace and happiness arise. Training to perform each move deliberately and consciously, creates an on-purpose attitude and encourages mental alertness. At the same time, a detachment from results allows the practitioner to enter into a meditative state of mind. This meditation in movement, being centered in the midst of activity, is practical training that can carry over into the workplace, the family, all areas of daily existence.

Thousands of years ago, these systems of moving energy probably began as part of a search for longevity and spiritual wholeness. The ancient Chinese believed that a unifying principle, called "Tao", underlies everything in the universe. They observed that everything other than the Tao (pronounced "dow") is constantly changing. Morning becomes night; wet becomes dry. Born from the Tao are yin and yang, the feminine and masculine principles from which everything else is created. Yin and yang are interdependent, one continuously changing into the other.

The disciplined movements and postures of T'ai Chi and Ch'i Kung, often drawn from an observation of nature itself, were designed to build internal power by bringing into balance the forces of yin and yang, to return the practitioner to the essential harmony of the Tao.

To determine if this type of exercise program is for you, try out or visit available schools and courses. Some systems place great importance on perfection of form, others are more relaxed, and still others offer training within a martial arts structure. Trust your intuition and, once you have found a teaching that appeals to you, continue to practice faithfully. The benefits are accumulative - they increase the more you practice. And remember that in all healing, it is your intention that directs the therapeutic power.

Grateful acknowledgement to another sweet sister in spirit, Diana Daffner, for the T'ai Chi, Ch'i Kung information.

YOGA

The word yoga means "joining, union, or yoke". It is the science of uniting the mind and body. There are many forms of yoga being taught today and each of these forms guides us to become more connected and aware of the physical body as a vehicle to our soul connection. The teacher's knowledge and spiritual legacy can be passed on to the student. Yoga allows the individual to become awakened to self realization and connected with the Divine. Most people think of yoga as a form of exercise providing fitness to the physical body, yet the ancient basis of this system is of a spiritual connection to the knowledge that lies within us. We, in the west, might call this intuition (the art of listening).

The asanas (postures) that are taught in Hatha Yoga bring harmony to the physical body, accelerates healing processes, adds vitality, enhances the life force, brings suppleness and toning to the muscular system, and enhances the function of all the internal organs. Many of the techniques combine mental control and breath awareness.

Be aware that there are many other types of yoga:

Bakti Yoga	Stresses devotion and selflessness.
Karma Yoga	Emphasises work or service, surrender to God.
Raja Yoga	Focuses on achieving enlightenment through the understanding of true knowledge.
Kundalini Yoga	Teaches specialized breathing techniques along with postures and visualizations to stimulate forces of enlightenment residing in the sacrum.
Hatha Yoga	Using the physical body as a means to enlightenment.

Tantra Yoga	Channels our sexual powers for spiritual purpose, using the body as the vehicle of the mind.
Swara Yoga	Provides balance through the use of breath, which creates balance of the mind.

We mention these branches of yoga because each has healing applications and we will refer to some of them later for assisting with overcoming specific conditions.

TANTRA

Diana Daffner and Light Miller

Tantra, a disciplined practice of energy awareness, teaches how to open yourself to the forces of the universe which pulsate through your body. Derived from Hindu and Buddhist traditions, Tantra is an approach to living which joyously links the physical universe to the cosmic whole.

All activities are influenced by the joy you are able to express. Ayurvedic practitioners inquire about the state of your intimate relationships, knowing that your vitality and your state of well being are dependent on the harmony within your family life.

Western research shows that a loving and supportive relationship has measurably positive effects on the body's health.

A family that lives Tantra has healthy values. With openness of mind and heart, the whole family thrives and grows into a maturity of being.

Sexuality, the most physical and intimate of human interactions, is considered by Tantra to be a sacred activity, continuously reenacting the original creation of the universe. The First One, separating from Itself to know Itself, embracing Itself to experience Itself.

Tantra occurs only in the present moment. Yesterday's experience has no relevance. In each moment that we shift from overt physical pleasure to an internal joy, to a focus on the intrinsic movement of energy, the subtle nature of our being is exposed and Tantra takes place. Nor does Tantra exclude experiences that are not overtly pleasurable. This same internal shift of focus can take place as we experience outward pain, even death.

Tantra is about mastery. The study of Tantra not only benefits personal relationships, it creates focus and vision in all aspects of life. Ancient Tantra communities discovered and developed astronomy, mathematics and the chakra system.

Tantra describes a movement of energy, a welling up within you, of joyous excitation. Unlike forms of meditation that cause you to withdraw from the world of senses, Tantra encourages you to start with the senses, building on their ability to focus you in the present moment.

Some spiritual paths teach you to deny, to say "not this, not that". They teach that who you are is not the body, not the mind, not your actions, not your thoughts. Stripped of what you are not, these paths allow you to see the emergence of who you may be. Tantra takes the seemingly opposite approach and teaches you to say "YES! to this, YES! to that".

All experience can be a doorway to who you are, provided you focus on the experience itself, with the intention of energetic awareness. Tantra provides the training for this focus, through practices that includes breathwork, movement, postures, chanting and meditation.

To be focused in the Tantra way means to be fully present, to allow each moment to be the entire experience. In Tantric lovemaking, there is no goal, no race toward release or orgasm. Instead, there is complete attention to each touch, each breath, each movement of energy.

Every moment in your life can be shaped by Tantra, can be lived in fullness and acceptance. Your relationships, your health, your family and your life will benefit from exploring the path of Tantra.

CHAPTER 13

75 HEALTH CONDITIONS & THEIR TREATMENTS

HOW TO USE THE CONDITIONS AND ILLNESSES SECTION

NAME and descriptions of condition.

FEELING AND EMOTIONS - possible thought and feeling patterns which may be causative at the psycho-physical interface (mind-body).

CELL SALTS - simple homeopathic solutions using readily available simple cell salts.

DIET - Eating the Ayurvedic diet which is specific to your constitutional body type is generally beneficial. In certain conditions a specific diet or food is suggested (i.e., you are constitutionally a vata but in menopause extreme bleeding calls for a Pitta reducing diet).

VITAMINS/MINERALS - specific nutrients and amounts which have been beneficial for the conditions are suggested.

ESSENTIAL OILS - a list of helpful essentials oils is given with body type effects. VP- means that these oils decrease (are good for) Vata and Pitta constitutions or conditions. K+ means that these oils increase (are not good for) Kapha symptoms or constitutions.

HERBS - a variety of herbs are suggested for assistance with the condition. You can use them singularly or make a blend. A specific recipe may be suggested but it can be altered due to herb availability and your personal tastes. Herbs are also marked as to effect. When choices are available, choose herbs which agree with your constitution or counter a particular condition's doshic aspect.

CLEANSE - Always consult a health practitioner when doing a cleanse.

ALTERNATIVE THERAPY - Here are suggested alternative or complementary therapies which can be helpful. Understand you need not do any of the therapies and could be overwhelmed if you try to do everything. Go within and let your inner guidance decide what, of all your choices, to do.

AVOID - This category includes those things which might aggravate the condition.

HERBAL BLENDS - This is a suggested blend of herbs to be used for up to three months. You can make your own blend from the list of suggested herbs.

SELF-CARE - This section describes special procedures to do at home.

How to Use the Condition Section

V   Means Vata.

P   Means Pitta.

K   Means Kapha.

(-)   Means decreases.

(+)   Means increases.

(=)   Balancing to all body types.

(o)   Neutral effect.

Example

VP-   Means this herb or essential oil will reduce Vata & Pitta.

K+   Means Kaphas should avoid as it will increase Kapha.

VPK =   Good for all doshas.

o   Neutral effect.

Author's Comments on herb Choices

After reading my herb recommendations for specific conditions, please don't imagine that you have ever made "wrong" choices in the past. All herbs contain nutrients and healing power. Intuition and the power of personal choice are powerful healers. However, our experience has shown that by choosing herbs based on their Ayurvedic properties, you can experience better results.

May your adventure into Ayurveda be an enjoyable one.

ACNE (Excess Sebum Production)

Acne can be caused by a high Pitta condition, especially during the teen years. During times of development, the body goes through hormonal increases. Other factors include medications, allergic reaction, stress, poor diet, and the buildup of Ama (toxicity). Acne can be triggered at various times of the menstrual cycle and during menopause. The first step is to look at the diet and begin to eliminate foods which could be aggravating the condition. The most common offenders are sugar, chocolate, dairy products, meat with hormones, fried foods, potato chips, salty foods, soda pop, and processed foods.

Vata Acne: The boils are dry and scaly with some patches of oil, yet the skin is dry. **Pitta Acne:** Reddish pimples appear with yellowish discharge and inflammation (redness). **Kapha Acne:** There is a fluid buildup with white discharge.

Feelings and Emotions: Not feeling good about the way you look.

Diet	Vitamins & Minerals (Daily)	Essential Oils (Always dilute)	Herbs	Alternative Therapy	Avoid
Ayurvedic diet for body type	A: 50,000 IU before meals E: 400 IU before meals	Juniper: KV-P+ Sandalwood: PV-Ko	Turmeric: KV-Po Sandalwood: PV-Ko	Facials Steam	Sugar Chocolate
Elimination diet	B6-Pyrodoxine: 50 mg. 2x day	Jatamasi: KV-P+ Tea Tree: VPK=	Rose Petals: VPK= Gentian: PK-V+		Dairy Female Hormones
High fibre	Zinc: 90 mg. Multi-Mineral	Lemon: PV-Ko	Oat Straw: VP-K+ Licorice: VP-K+		Iodine Inorganic Iodine
	Flaxseed or Evening Primrose: 4 tablets per day	**Blended Oils:**	Burdock: PK-V+ Red Clover: PK-V+		B-12 Commercial Soaps
	C: 3,000 mg.	*Acne Free: VPK	Peppermint: PK-Vo Lemongrass: PK-Vo		Soft Drinks
			Acnenil Ayurvedic Blend Noni Juice: VPK- Amalaki: VPKo		

* Product of Earth Essentials Florida

Acne Herbal Brew

See directions for preparing herbal brew on page 407

VATA		PITTA		KAPHA	
Turmeric	1 oz	Witch Hazel	1 oz	Echinacea	1 oz
Sandalwood	2 oz	Dandelion	2 oz	Myrrh	1 oz
Rose Petals	1 oz	Burdock	2 oz	Red Clover	2 oz
Amalaki	1 oz	Red Clover	1 oz	Lemongrass	2 oz
Gentian	1 oz	Peppermint	1 oz	Lemon Balm	1 oz
Oat Straw	2 oz	Lemongrass	2 oz	Guggul	1 oz
Licorice	1 oz				

VATA ACNE		VATA-PITTA ACNE	
Sandalwood	2 oz	Use: 1/4 teaspoon of Sandalwood powder	
Turmeric	1 oz	1/4-teaspoon turmeric powder	
Chamomile	2 oz	1/3 of a lemon (juice)	
Ginger	1 oz		

Mix all dry ingredients and lemon juice into a paste.
Apply to your face.
Dry. Wash well.
Apply aloe vera gel.
Wash.

Recipes for Acne

Ayurveda clays, Bentonite clays, fresh clays:

1/2 teaspoon of clay
1 Tablespoon lemon juice
Mix well to create a paste.
Apply and let dry.
Wash.
Note: Do not use apple cider vinegar even though some brands of clay call for it.

In the morning, wash face with chana flour (garbanzo flour):

Mix enough flour to make a watery paste.
1 drop of Sandalwood essential oil.
1 drop of Turmeric essential oil.
(*Note: Tea Tree essential oil may be substituted*)
Apply mixture and rub/scrub lightly
Wash with water.

Do not use soap on the skin.

For Kapha: Use Cajaput, Juniper or Lavender essential oils

Acne Free essential oil blend can then be applied. Use either a dry skin blend that contains carrier oil, or use a blend specifically for oily skin.

Essential oil blends can be made for Vata with equal amounts of:
Sandalwood
Jatamasi
50% sesame oil base

Essential oil blends can be made for Pitta & Kapha with equal amounts of:
Sandalwood
Rose
Lavender
50% jojoba oil base

Be sure to follow your Ayurvedic diet and avoid foods that could aggravate the condition. Keep skin clean; wash often with a pH balanced soap (do not use regular soap). Avoid makeup and clogging of the skin pores while healing the acne.

Self Care

Flaxseed or Evening Primrose oil for hormonal balance
Vitamin C with bioflavonoids: Pittas do best with Sago Palm or Ascorbate C - 3,000 mg.
Facial Sauna

AIDS

This is a disease of the immune system where the body is run down due to stress, poor diet, excessive sexual activities, drugs, alcohol, or through diseased blood transfusions. This is a Vata/Pitta condition with both doshas involved.

Feelings and Emotions: Guilt, shame, confusion about sexuality.

Cell Salts: Silica

Diet	Vitamins & Minerals (Daily)	Essential Oils (Always dilute)	Herbs	Alternative Therapy	Avoid
Ayurvedic diet for body type	A: 50,000 IU E: 600 IU C: 10,000 mg	Sandalwood: PV-Ko Tea Tree: VPK= Saffron: VPK= Jatamasi: VK-P+	Isatis: PKV+ Suma: PK-V+ Saw Palmetto: V-PK+ Ginko Biloba: VPK	Chakra balance Energy work Acupuncture Massage	Masturbation Spices Smoking Alcohol
Yellow vegetables	B-Complex: 200 mg. 3 x per day	Geranium: PK-V+ Egg Lecithin: 20 gms Cumin: VPK-	Shilajit: PKV+ Myrtle: PKV+ Guggul: KV-P+	Counseling	Sodas Red meat Sugar
Shitaki mushrooms	Digestive Enzyme Zinc: 50 mg Acidophilus: 3 times/day	Rose: VPK=	Sandalwood: PV-Ko Red Clover: PK-V+ Gotu Kola: PKV=		Reduce sexual activities
Meat broth	Copper: 3 mg RNA-DNA: 1500 mg.		Sarsaparilla: PV-Ko Coriander: PVK-		
Immune soup	Sustain (Metagenics) Q 10: 100 mg Haelen: Soybean extract - 8 tablets		Ashwagandha: VK-P+ Marshmallow: PV-K+ Diamond Ash: VPK		
Sesame oil	Germanium: 200 mg.		Aloe Vera Gel: VPK= Triphalla: VPK- Immune support+ (Banyan herbs)		

Chayanprash

Lotus seeds
Almonds
Ghee

Medicated Jelly - (Chyavanprash)

Medicated Oil:
Amla: VPKo
*Blends: (Do not dilute)
*Immune Free
Brahmi

**ImmuniTea: VPK+
Trikatu: VK-P+

Vatas: Need to increase digestion. Take Trikatu (2 tablets) before each meal during lunchtime with yogurt and fennel.

Pitta: Use ginger, coriander, cardamon, acidophilus.

*Product of Earth Essentials Florida. **Product of UniTea Herbs.

Aids Herbal Brew

See directions for preparing herbal brew on page 409

VATA		PITTA		KAPHA	
Astralagus	2 oz.	Saffron	1 oz.	Burdock	2 oz.
Ashwagandha	1 oz.	Rheumania	2 oz.	Plantain	3 oz.
Saw Palmetto	1 oz.	Astralagus	3 oz.	Solomon's Seal	1 oz.
Licorice	2 oz.	Gotu Kola	2 oz.	Gokshura	1 oz.
Ligustrum	1 oz.	Sarsaparilla	2 oz.	Saffron	1 oz.
Shatavari	3 oz.	Gokshura	1 oz.	Saw Palmetto	2 oz.
Bala	1 oz.	Plantain	2 oz.		
Ginseng	1 oz.	Sandalwood	3 oz.		
		Solomon's Seal	2 oz.		

DRINK

Turmeric 1 Tbs.
Aloe vera 1 Tbs.

Mix all ingredients together. Use 1 teaspoon per cup of water, and drink 3 times a day.

Self-Massage (Abyangha)

Self-massage is very important. The following recipes are for preparing your own massage oil.

VATA		
	Brahmi	30 drops
	Sandalwood	20 drops
	Cumin	10 drops
	Jatamasi	15 drops
	Himalayan Cedarwood	20 drops
	Sesame oil	4 oz.

PITTA		
	Brahmi	30 drops
	Sandalwood	20 drops
	Cumin	10 drops
	Rose	20 drops
	Lavender	15 drops
	Sunflower oil or Ghee	4 oz.

Self-Care

Breathwork, Meditation, Mantra

ALCOHOLISM

Alcoholism can be associated with repressed feelings and emotions consistent with "holding on" or hiding. A poor diet and a deficiency of nutrients can also result in addiction. Alcohol raises Pitta, blocking the functions of the liver and pancreas.

Feelings and Emotions: Suspicion of self. Lack of self-love.

Diet	Vitamins & Minerals (Daily)	Essential Oils (Always dilute)	Herbs	Alternative Therapy	Avoid
Pitta	A: 2,000 IU	Geranium: PK-V	Aloe Vera: VPK=	Counseling	Sugar
Ayurvedic diet	B-Complex: 300 mg.	Sandalwood: PV-Ko	Gentian: PK-V+	Emotional release	Drugs
	B-12: 30 mcg.	Rose: VPK=	Turmeric: KV-Po	Tarpana massage	Coffee
Wheat germ	E: 150 IU	Jatamasi: KV-P+	Barberry: PK-V+	Therapeutic touch	Fried foods
	C: 2,500 mg.	Bergamot: VK-P+	Gotu Kola: PKV=	Energy work	
	Selenium: 1,000 mg.		Skullcap: PV-Vo	Pancha Karma	
	Magnesium: 500 mg.		Hops: PK-V+		
	Zinc: 50 mg.	For withdrawal symptoms:	Burdock: PK-V+		
	Nicotinic Acid: 500 mg.	-Melissa: PKV-	Milk Thistle: PK-V+		
	B2 - Riboflavin: 200 mg.	-Marjoram: KV-P+	Passion Flower: PK-V+		
	Amino Acid: 100 mg.	-Ylang Ylang: PV-K+	Dandelion: PK-V+		
		-Lavender: PK-Vo	Amla: PV-Ko		
	Catechin: 100 mg.				
	L-Glutathione: 300 mg		**Ayurvedic Formulas:**		
	Pantethine: 300 mg. - 2-3 x per day		-Bhanta Rasayana: VPK-		
			-Saraswati: VPK-		

B6 - Pyrodoxine: 100 mg.
B1 - Thiamine: 100 mg.
Folic Acid: 50 mcg.
A good Multi-Vitamin
Evening primrose: ½ gram
3 x per day

-Chyavanprash: VP-K+
-Amla: PV-Ko

Alcoholism Herbal Brew

VATA

Gotu Kola	1 oz.
Ginger	2 oz.
Coriander	2 oz.
Skullcap	2 oz.
Saraswat	1 tsp.

Drink 4 to 6 cups per day.

PITTA

Dandelion Root	2 oz.
Burdock Root	2 oz.
Gotu Kola	1 oz.
Milk Thistle	2 oz.
Mint	2 oz. (or add 1)
Lobelia	1 oz.
Gentian tablets	2 tablets

KAPHA

Ginger	2 oz.
Burdock Root	2 oz.
Peppermint	1 oz.
Cardamon	1 oz.
Passion Flower	2 oz.
Ginger	1 oz.
Turmeric	1 tablet

See directions for preparing herbal brew on page 409

COMPRESS OVER LIVER

Pour 1 cup of boiling water over a 1/4 cup of Dandelion root.
Let steep for 20 minutes.
Strain. Cool to room temperature.
Take a cloth and soak it for 5 minutes in this liquid. Squeeze out excess.
Place cloth over liver for 15 minutes.
Repeat 2-3 times per week.

LIVER FLUSH

For instructions, see page 349.

ALLERGIES

Caused by low immunity and/or long term use of allopathic drugs (particularly antibiotics). The body is not able to produce antihistamines because of stress, poor diet, overwork, nervousness, environmental pollution, or food allergies. More common in Vata body types because of their weak digestive system and sensitivity. Pitta types often suffer more with skin rash or sweating type allergies. Kaphas usually experience sinus congestion, hay fever, or water retention.

Feelings and Emotions: Something, someone is irritating them. Life is too much. Feeling overwhelmed.

Diet	Vitamins & Minerals (Daily)	Essential Oils (Always dilute)	Herbs	Alternative Therapy	Avoid
Ayurvedic diet for body type	A: 25,000 IU	Myrtle: KP-V+	Bayberry: KV- P+	Tarpana	Foods which are common allergens:
	E: 200 IU	Saffron: VPK=	Calamus: VK- P+	Nasya	-Wheat
Yellow vegetables	C: Ascorbate 2000-3000 mg.	Eucalyptus: KV-P+	Mullein: PK-V+	Pancha	-Dairy
	B-12: 100 mcg. (4 weeks)	Lavender: PK-Vo	Elecampane: VK- P+	Karma	-Beef
Shitaki mushrooms	B-Complex: 100 mg.	Patchouli: VP-K+	**PuriTea: VP- K+		-Corn
	Bioflavonoids: 1000 mg.	Peppermint: PK-Vo	**ImmuniTea: VPK+		-Citrus
Rotation diet	Pantothenic Acid: 2500 mg.	Camphor: VK-P+	Basil: VK- P+		-MSG
Raw foods & juices	Molybdenum: 50 mg.	Cubeb: VK-P+	Nutmeg: VK-P+		-Soy
	Quercetin: 100 mg.	Spruce: VK-P+	Cardamon: VK-P+		-Sugar
Elimination diet	Linoleic Acid: 200 mg.	All Chamomiles: VPK-	Fennel: VPK=		
	Lactobacillus: ¼ tsp. 3 x day	Rosemary: KV-P+	Coltsfoot: PK-Vo		
	Acidophilus: 3 x a day	Angelica: VPK=	Cloves: VK- P+		
Immune building diet	Bifido bacteria: 3 x a day	Lemon Balm: KP-Vo	Eucalyptus: KV-P+		
	Catechine: 100 mg.	Basil: VK-P+	Aloe Vera: VPK=		
		Echinacea: PK- V+	Immune support (Banyan Herbs)		
		Rose: VPK=			

Blended Oils:
*Immune Free: VPK-
*Magnolia: VPK-

Lobelia: K-PV+
Ephedra: K-VP+
Angelica: VPK=,P+(in excess)
Vasa: PK-V+
Kola: VPK-
Trikatu: VK-P+
Triphalla: VPK-
Guduchi: VPK+
Gotu Kola: PKV=

*Product of Earth Essentials **Product of UniTea Herbs*

Allergy herbal Brew

VATA		PITTA		KAPHA	
Eucalyptus	1 oz.	Elecampane	2 oz.	Ephedra	2 oz.
Elecampane	1 oz.	Coriander	1 oz.	Elecampane	1 oz.
Ginger	2 oz.	Vasa	2 oz.	Peppermint	1 oz.
Cardamon	1 oz.	Peppermint	1 oz.	Horehound	1 oz.
Cloves	1 oz.	Mullein	2 oz.	Mullein	2 oz.
Licorice	2 oz.	Gotu Kola	1 oz.		

See directions for preparing herbal brew on page 409

Drink 4 cups in-between meals. Add warm milk at night. Avoid milk if there are dairy allergies; substitute rice or soymilk.

VATA & KAPHA
Warm compress over the chest with equal amounts of:

Eucalyptus 5 drops
Camphor 5 drops
Rosemary 5 drops
Myrtle 5 drops

Mix with 2 Tbs. of mustard or canola oil
Warm the oil and apply to chest. Cover the chest with wool cloth for 15 minutes.
Repeat 2-3 times per week.

PITTA

Compress should be at room temperature.
Cilantro juice - 3 times per day

DRINK — VKP

Mix:

Lemon Balm	5 drops	Take essential oil blend and use
Rose	3 drops	2 drops in 8 oz. of water once per day.
Chamomile	3 drops	

MORE ON HERBS

Vata & Kapha: Take 2 tablets of Trikatu before every meal. 1 tsp. coriander before each meal.

Vata-Pitta-Kapha: Take 500 mg. of Triphalla at bedtime.

EYEWASH TO REDUCE REDNESS IN EYES

Make infusion of 1 oz. Chrysanthemum herb in 2-oz. water - or use Eyebright.

Strain well. It is best to use cotton cloth on strainer.

Keep formula refrigerated. Wash eye 3 times per day.

Self Care

Essential oil inhalation every 2 hours	Compresses over the area
Colon cleanse	Vaporizer at night in the bedroom with essential oils

ALOPECIA (Hair Loss)

At first, the hair begins to thin slowly in patches eventually being followed by baldness. It can result from old age, radiation, endocrine disorders, hormone imbalance, sudden weight loss, stress, overwork, pregnancy, or heredity factors. When the condition is due to heredity, one needs to begin to work on it at at an early age. Vitamin and mineral deficiency can also be consistent with alopecia.

Feelings and Emotions: Anger, irritability. Thinking too much. Having to do the right thing. Compulsiveness

Diet	Vitamins & Minerals (Daily)	Essential Oils (always dilute)	Herbs	Alternative Therapy	Avoid
Ayurvedic diet for body type	B-Complex: 200 mg.	Ginger: VK-P+	Bhringaraj: VPK=	Shirodhara	White sugars
	F: 100 mg.	Brahmi: VPK-	Alfalfa: PK-V+	Head massage	Over eating fruit
Protein foods	Inositol: 100 mg.	Coriander: VPK-	Gotu Kola: VPK=		Fried foods
	Folic Acid: 150 mcg.	Gold Chamomile: KP-V+	(Brahmi)		Coffee
	C: 3000 mg.	Birch: PK-V+	Ginger: VK-P+		Tobacco
Foods high in sulfur	E: 150 IU	Sandalwood: VP-Ko	Rose Petals: VPK=		Hot spicy foods
	Lecithin: 2 tablets before meals	Aloe Vera: VKP-	Sage: KV-P+		Stress
Eggs	Choline: 100 mg.		Rosemary: KV-P+		Hormone therapy
	Zinc: 50 mg.	**Medicated oils:**	Aloe Vera: VPK-		
Legumes	Multi-vitamin	- Bhringaraj: VPK=	Nettles: PK-V+		
	Multi-mineral	- Amla: PV-Ko	Burdock: PK-V+		
Cabbage	Flax oil: 2 tsp.	- Brahmi: VPK=	Yarrow: PK-V+		
Sunflower seeds	Evening Primrose: 3-6 capsules		Yucca: VPK-		
Juice therapy	Amino Acids Complex	**Vegetable oils:**			
	Copper: 100 mg.	- Coconut: P-K+Vo			
	Acidophilus: 2 tablets 3 x day	- Sesame: V-PK+			
	Iodine: 100 mg.				

Hair Oil Formulas

VATA		PITTA		KAPHA	
Sesame Oil	1 oz.	Coconut or Jojoba oil	1 oz.	Almond oil	1 oz.
Rosemary	10 drops	Brahmi (gotu kola)	10 drops	Sage	10 drops
Brahmi	5 drops	Sandalwood	5 drops	Rosemary	10 drops
Sandalwood	5 drops	Coriander	10 drops	Coriander	10 drops
Coriander	5 drops	Birch	5 drops	Brahmi (gotu kola)	10 drops
Chamomile	5 drops	Chamomile	5 drops		

Mix all ingredients. Apply on scalp for 20 minutes before shampooing.

Herbal Brew

VATA		PITTA		KAPHA	
Gotu Kola	2 oz.	Gotu Kola	2 oz.	Yarrow	1 oz.
Rosemary	1 oz.	Rose Petals	1 oz.	Gotu Kola	2 oz.
Sage	1/2 oz.	Coriander	1 oz.	Coriander	2 oz.
Ginger	2 oz.	Chrysanthemum	2 oz.	Ginger	2 oz.
Coriander	1 oz.	Mint	1 oz.		
Bhringaraj	1 oz.	Chamomile	1/2 oz.		

See directions for preparing herbal brew on page 409

Self-Care

Yoga: headstand (inversion therapy)

Head massage/scalp massage

Stress reduction tapes

Add herbs and essential oils to shampoo and conditioner

Oil treatments for the hair

ALZHEIMERS

Another name for Pre-senile Dementia. It begins with personality changes, difficult communication, and mood swings. Vata types can become "spacey" and leave out words when speaking. Pitta types can become irritable and on edge about life. Kapha types shut down communication and become disoriented. Causes are hereditary, with some controversy about other possible causes, namely; excess amounts of aluminum, silicon, sulfur, and calcium. Hair analysis can be used as a diagnostic tool for monitoring any heavy metals within the body. Chelation can remove them and increase arterial blood flow.

Feelings and Emotions: Life is becoming too much. Life is overwhelming, not worth dealing with.

Cell Salts: Silica; Kalphos; Potassium phosphate

Diet	Vitamin & Minerals (Daily)	Essential Oils (always dilute)	Herbs	Alternative Therapy	Avoid
Ayurvedic diet for body type	B-Complex: 200 mg.	Brahmi: VPK-	Gotu Kola: VPK=	Head massage	Aspirin
	B-12: 200 mcg.	Ginger: VK-P+	Ginko Biloba: VPK-	Chelation	Antacids
Foods high in minerals	A: 100,000 IU	Ashwagandha: VK-P+	Basil: VK-P+	Shirodhara	All products with aluminum:
	Beta-Carotene: 1500 IU	Amla: VPK	Rosemary: KV-P+	Nasya	- Makeup
	C: 2500-3000 gm.	Cyperus: PKV-	Dandelion: PK-V+	Hair analysis	- Baking powder
Fiber (oat bran)	E: 150 IU	Basil: VK- P+	Myrrh: KV- P+	Pancha Karma in the early stages	- Shampoo
Foods rich in sulfur (legumes)	Selenium: 200 mcg.	Cardamon: VK- P+	St. John's Wort: PK-V+		- Cookware
	Boron: 100 IU	Hyssop: VK-P+	Calamus: VK-P+		- Deodorant
Oats	Zinc: 50 mg.	Mint: PK-Vo	Irish Moss: V-PK+		- Beer cans
	Co Q-10: (2) 50 mg.: 2 x day	Lemongrass: PK-Vo	Lotus Seed: PV-K+		
		Camphor: KV-P+	Jasmine Flowers: PK-V+		
			Mental clarity (Banyan Herbs)		

Lots of yellow & orange vegetables
Kidney beans
Lots of seaweed
Potassium broth
Juice fasting
Ghee
Salmon /Sardines

Lecithin: 200 mg.
L-lysine: 4 tablets daily
L-phenylalanine: 100 mg.
Amino Acid Complex: 700-900 mg. 2 x day
Germanium: 75 mg.
DHEA: 150 mg.

Angelica: VPK=
Bergamot: VK-P+

Blended Oils:
(do not dilute)
*Mental Clarity: VPK-

Burdock: PK-V+
White Musal: VPK-
Cardamom: KV-P+
Chrysanthemum: PK-V+
Ghee: PV-K+
Chicory Root: PK-V+
**Mental ClariTea: VP-K+

Fried foods
Fast foods

Ayurvedic Herbal Formulas:
-Triphalla: VPK
-Trifolia: VK- P+

* Product of Earth Essentials Florida   ** Product of UniTea Herbs, Colorado

See directions for preparing herbal brew on page 409

Alzheimers Herbal Brew

VATA		PITTA		KAPHA	
Basil	1 oz.	Gotu Kola	2 oz.	Chicory Root	2 oz.
Gotu Kola	2 oz.	Ginko Biloba	1 oz.	Cardamon	1 oz.
Rosemary	1 oz.	Dandelion	1 oz.	Spearmint	1 oz.
Cardamon	1 oz.	Chrysanthemum	2 oz.	Irish Moss	1 oz.
Calamus	1 oz.	Burdock	1 oz.	Burdock	1 oz.
Ginko Biloba	2 oz.	Jasmine	1 oz.	Ginko Biloba	2 oz.
		Peppermint	1 oz.		

Potassium Broth

Cut all ingredients. Add to two quarts of water and bring to a boil. Cover. Simmer for two hours.

VATA		PITTA		KAPHA	
Potatoes & peelings	5	Peelings of sweet potatoes	5	Potatoes & peelings	5
Carrots	4	Parsley	1/2 bunch	Parsley	1 bunch
Ginger, fresh	2"	Cilantro	1 bunch	Ginger	3"
Celery	1/2 stalk	Mint	1/2 bunch	Juniper berries	1 handful
Cilantro	1 bunch	Yellow squash	2	Cilantro	1 bunch
Spinach	1/2 bunch	Coriander seeds	1/2 oz.	Spinach	1/2 bunch
Watercress	1/2 bunch	Borage	1/2 oz.	Borage	1/8 oz.
Tomatoes	2	Water	2 quarts	Carrots	4
Water	2 quarts	Add Bragg's Liquid Aminos to taste		Water	2 quarts
Add Bragg's Liquid Aminos to taste				Add Bragg's Liquid Aminos to taste	

Alzheimer Prevention Formula for Massage

Basil	5 drops	Lemongrass	3 drops
Camphor	3 drops	Angelica	2 drops
Bergamot	3 drops	Base Oil	4 oz.

Self-Care

Use essential oils in an aromatherapy lamp when studying or during activities that require concentration and memory. Inhalations: Three times per day - especially with essential oils of Rosemary, Basil, Mint, and/or Lemon. Early prevention. Alzheimer's can be prevented when symptoms begin to appear. Abyangha (self massage)

AMENORRHIA

Amenorrhia is the absence of menstruation. It can be due to low caloric intake or excessive exercise that lowers the body weight and body fat. It is also consistent with low protein or low mineral levels. Long term incidence may cause bone loss.

Feelings and Emotions: I don't enjoy being a woman. Fear of the unknown.

Cell Salts: Nat Sulph; Calci-Phos

Diet	Vitamins & Minerals (Daily)	Essential Oils (always dilute)	Herbs	Alternative Therapy	Avoid
Ayurvedic diet for body type	B-6: 200 mg.	Cyperus: VPK-	Saffron: VPK=	Acupuncture	Exercise
	Folic Acid: 50 mcg.	Valerian: VK- P+	Ignatia: PK-V+	Rolfing	Weight loss
	E: 150 IU	Angelica: VPK-, P+ (in excess)	Nettle Leaf: PK-V+	Ayurvedic consultation	Excess protein
Spices	Calcium: 1200 mg.		Dong Quai: VK-Po		Stress
	Magnesium 100 mg.	Basil: VK-P+	Rose: VPK=	Therapeutic touch	Birth control pills - "post pill syndrome"
Sesame seeds	Evening Primrose: 200 mg.	Sage: VK- P+	Ginger: VK-P+	Woman's support group	
	FlaxSeed Oil: 200 mg.	Clary Sage: VPK-	Cyperus: VPK		
Saffron rice		Geranium: PK-Vo	Squaw Vine: PK-V+		
			Angelica: VP-P+ (in excess)		
			Aloe Vera: VPK=		
			Fennel: VPK=		
			Black Cohosh: PK-V+		
			Vitex: VPK-		
			Yarrow: PK-V+		
			Cotton Root: V-KP+		
			Cinnamon: VK- P+		
			Woman's Treasure***		

*** Product of Planetary Herbs

Amenorrhia Herbal Brew

See directions for preparing herbal brew on page 409

VATA		PITTA		KAPHA	
Ginger	2 oz.	Nettles	2 oz.	Vitex	2 oz.
Catnip	2 oz.	Shatavari	1 oz.	Ginger	1 oz.
Angelica	2 oz.	Mint	1 oz.	Angelica	2 oz.
Rose Petals	2 oz.	Fennel	1 oz.	St. John's Wort	1 oz.
Vitex	1 oz.	Black Cohosh	1 oz.	Yarrow	2 oz.
Shatavari	1 oz.	Chamomile	1 oz.	Cyperus	1 oz.
		Rose Petals	1 oz.		

Drink 4 times per day.

All Doshas:

Two weeks before periods, drink 1 cup daily

Vata: Aloe Vera Gel with Basil or Ginger added.

Pitta: Aloe Vera Gel with 1/2 tsp. Fennel or Mint added.

Kapha: Aloe Vera Gel with Turmeric added.

VATA		PITTA		KAPHA	
Vitex	1 oz.	Chamomile	2 oz.	Angelica	1 oz.
Rose Petals	2 oz.	Yarrow	2 oz.	Motherwort	1 oz.
Angelica	2 oz.	Blessed Thistle	1 oz.	Ginger	2 oz.
Cinnamon	1 oz.	Motherwort	1 oz.	Cinnamon	1 oz.
Ginger	1 oz.	Rose Petals	1 oz.	Yarrow	2 oz.
Cotton Root	1 oz.	Hibiscus	1 oz.	Hibiscus	1 oz.

Drink 4 times per day

Self-Care

Supportive counseling

Abdominal massage

Aromatherapy (especially in the morning)

Dance movement

ANEMIA

A blood disorder caused by a deficiency of iron and minerals. The blood becomes thin and weak. There are many kinds of anemia: Micro Cystic - VK; Sickle Cell - VK; Side Roblastic - VK; Metablastic - PK. Vatas may experience copper skin, insomnia, dizziness, constipation, or dehydration. Pittas will have fevers, inflammation, thirst, and yellow on the eyes and skin. Kaphas will often have water retention, fatigue, tiredness or pale, almost white skin.

Feelings and Emotions: Feeling tired of life. I don't deserve.

Diet	Vitamins & Minerals (Daily)	Essential Oils (always dilute)	Herbs	Alternative Therapy	Avoid
Ayurvedic diet for body type	B-Complex: 200 mg. A-E: 450 IU (easier) Folic Acid: 200 mcg. B2 - Riboflavonoids: 25-30 mg.	Chamomile: VPK Lemon Thyme: PK-Vo	Aloe Vera: VPK= Bibhitaki: PK-Vo. Amalaki: PV-Ko Saffron: VPK=	Naturopath Ayurvedic consultation	Blood cleansers Excessive exercise Iron Ferrus Sulfate
Bone soup	B1 - Thiamin: 100 mg.		Shatavari: PV-K+ Manjishta: PK-V+		
Sesame seed	Folate: 300 mcg. -especially during pregnancy (for anemia)		Punarnava: PK-V+ Agrimony: PK-V+		
Pomegranate juice	Copper: 50 mg. Iron: 100 mg. Zinc: 40 mg.		Yellow Dock: PK-V+ Shata Root: best taken in tablet form		
Spinach	Hydrochloric Acid: 2 before protein meals		Fo Ti: PV-K+		
Carrots					

Molasses
Beets
Organic
  whole milk
Red organic meats

Iron (Ferrus Fumerate): 80 mg.
-(helps with constipation)

Ayurvedic Formulas:
- Chyavanprash: VP-K+
- Triphalla: VPK-
- Iron Ash: VPK
- Women's Treasure: VPK-

See directions for preparing herbal brew on page 409

Anemia Herbal Brew

VATA

Amalaki	1 oz.
Shatavari	2 oz.
Ashwagandha	1 oz.
Lotus	1 oz.
Fo Ti	1 oz.
Ginger	1 oz.
Raspberry Leaves	½ oz.
Comfrey	1 oz.

PITTA & KAPHA

Yellow Dock	2 oz.
Bibhitaki	1 oz.
Peppermint	1 oz.
Nettles	1 oz.
Barberry	1 oz.
Agrimony	1 oz.
Dandelion Root	2 oz.

Recipes

Saffron	½ gram
Milk or Yogurt	1 cup
Molasses	1 tsp.

Take 3 times per day with 1 teaspoon of ghee.

ANOREXIA - BULIMIA

Anorexia and bulimia involves suppression of the digestive fire due to eating and vomiting or skipping meals. People with this condition usually have the tendency to make poor food choices. Vatas will tend to fast and feast. Pittas will often have burning in the stomach. Kaphas force themselves to throw up.

Feelings and Emotions: I am not good enough the way I am. Low self esteem. Fear of gaining weight. Distorted view of self. Sees self as overweight, even when emaciated.

Diet	Vitamins & Minerals (Daily)	Essential Oils (always dilute)	Herbs	Alternative Therapy	Avoid
Ayurvedic diet for body type	B Complex: 200 mg.	Ginger: VK-P+	Comfrey: PV-K+	Counseling	All sugars - until the condition is under control
Lots of digestive spices (especially carminative)	Good Multi-Vitamin	Cardamon: VK-P+	Ashwagandha: VK-P+	Massage	Depressing situations
	Zinc: 50 mg. w/every meal	Bergamot: VK-P+	Slippery Elm: PV-K+	Breathwork	
	Pancreatic Enzymes: 2 with each meal	Orange: VK-P+	Cardamon: VK-P+	Therapeutic touch	
	Comfrey: 2 with each meal	All Citrus: VK-P+	Ginger: VK-P+	Polarity therapy	
	Pectin: 2 with each meal	Rose Geranium: PK-V+	Fennel: VPK=		
	Papaya Enzymes: 2 tablets before meals	Clary Sage: VPK	Hing: VK-P+		
Lots of green leafy vegetables	Trikatu: 2-3 before meals	Sandalwood: PV-Ko	Valerian: VK-P+		
		Lemongrass: PK-Vo	Nutmeg: VK-P+		
		Bay: VPK+	Lemongrass: PK-Vo		
Meat broth or chicken broth		Angelica: VPK= P+(in excess)	Angelica: VK-P+		
Lots of yellow (Vata) vegetables			Chitrack: VPK		
Hing with all beans			Shatavari: PV-K+		
Kicharee			Hingatash: VK-P+		
			Chyavanprash: VP-K+		
			Ashwagandha Compound: VK-P+		

Anorexia & Bulimia Herbal Brew

See directions for preparing herbal brew on page 409

KAPHA		VATA		PITTA	
Ginger	2 oz.	Ashwagandha	2 oz.	Fennel	1 oz.
Orange Peel	1 oz.	Angelica	2 oz.	Mint	2 oz.
Cardamon	2 oz.	Slippery Elm	2 oz.	Coriander	2 oz.
Basil	1 oz.	Comfrey	1 oz.	Comfrey	1 oz.
Lemongrass	2 oz.	Licorice	2 oz.	Licorice	1 oz.
Cinnamon	1 oz.	Ginger	2 oz.	Slippery Elm	1 oz.
Fennel	1 oz.	Coriander	1 oz.		
Mint	1 oz.	Shatavari	1 oz.		

MORNING BREAKFAST

Oats or any other grain	
Slippery Elm powder	2 Tbs.
Ginger	½ tsp.
Cardamon	½ tsp.
Coriander	¼ tsp.
Cinnamon	½ tsp.
Kicharee	equal amount of rice, mung dahl, and spices

Cook oatmeal. Add slippery elm, all spices, and kicharee

TAKE

Vata & Kapha: Trikatu - 3 tablets before each meal for 2 weeks, then 2 tablets before meals for 1 month, then 1 tablet before meals for 3 months.

ANXIETY

Anxiety can be associated with excitement, panic, apprehension, or feeling unsure. Anxiety is often elevated by too much coffee, drug usage, excess sugar in the diet, feeling troubled, or not trusting the process of life. Vata types may experience anxiety more often than the other body types.

Feelings and Emotions: No trust of self. Mistrust in general.

Diet	Vitamins & Minerals (Daily)	Essential Oils (always dilute)	Herbs	Alternative Therapy	Avoid
Ayurvedic diet for body type	B-Complex: 200 mg. B6 Pyridoxine: 100 mg. B1 Thiamine: 100 mg. B3 Niacinamide: 500 mg.	Jatamasi: KV-P+ Sandalwood: VP-Ko Lavender: PK-Vo Vetiver: V-KP+	Chamomile: PK-Vo Chrysanthemum: PK-V+ Skullcap: PK-Vo Valerian: VK-P+	Massage Therapeutic touch Tarpana Reiki	Sugar Coffee Cigarettes Processed foods
Lots of yellow vegetables	2 x day Calcium: 300-750 mg. (in extreme cases)	Ylang Ylang: PV-K+ Chamomile: VPK-	Kava Kava: PV-K+ Passion Flower: PK-V+ Bala: PV-Ko	Counseling Shirodhara	Alcohol
Lots of root vegetables	L-tryptophan: 100 mg.		Bhringaraj: VPK= Jasmine Flower: PK-V+ Alum Root: PK-V+ Catechu: KP-V+ Myrrh: KV-P+ Katuka: PK-V+ (Tranquil Mind)		

See directions for preparing herbal brew on page 409

Anxiety Herbal Brew

VATA TEA

Kava Kava	2 oz.
Valerian	1 oz.
Licorice	1 oz.
Fennel	2 oz.

PITTA & KAPHA TEA

Chamomile	2 oz.
Gotu Kola	1 oz.
Skullcap	2 oz.
Passion Flower	2 oz.
Jasmine Flower	1 oz.

At night, drink tea with warm milk.

Self-Care

Abyangha massage: every morning with relaxing formula.

Massage head at night with essential oil formula.

Inhalation: every 2 hours with essential oil of your choice.

Put drops of essential oil on your desk, work area, or pillow; can also use a diffuser.

Meditation: add drop or two of essential oil on your third eye area (on forehead, in between the eyes).

Tai Chi.

Breathwork.

ARTERIOSCLEROSIS

This is a degenerative condition of the arteries caused by an accumulation of lipids or plaque on the arterial wall. It begins at an early age. Often, one-year-old babies show lesions in the aorta. This buildup of mineral deposits and fats on the arterial walls causes blockages, which result in thickening or solidifying of blood, high cholesterol, and circulatory problems. This cardiovascular disease is the great killer of Americans. The presence of a diagonal crease on the earlobe correlates very well with the degree of arteriosclerosis. The earlobe is richly vascularized, and a decrease in blood flow over time is believed to indicate a collapse of the vascular bed, which is indicated by a specific crease on the earlobe.

Feelings and Emotions: Feeling constricted and trapped in the body.

Diet	Vitamin & Minerals (Daily)	Essential Oils (always dilute)	Herbs	Alternative Therapy	Avoid
Ayurvedic diet for body type	B-6: 300 mg.	Sandalwood: PV-Ko	Cayenne: KV-P+	Massage	Carbon monoxide
	Omega 3 oils:	Lemon: PV-Ko	Comfrey: PV-K+	Hypnosis	Barium
Fish (cold water type)	-Cod liver oil	Juniper: KV-P+ (in excess)	Goldenseal: PK-V+	Chelation	Organophosphates
	-Flaxseed oil (2 Tbs. @ night)	Cardamon: VK- P+	Rosehips: V-KP+	Shirodhara	Glues in solvents
-Salmon	Multi-vitamin	Myrrh: VK-P+	Burdock: PK-V+	Pancha Karma	Heat
-Mackerel	Multi-mineral	Rose: VPK=	Arjuna: PK-V+	Biofeedback	Cold
-Herring	E: 200 IU	Orange: VK-P+	1-3 gms day		Carbon disulfide
Raw carrots	C: 1,500 mg.		Guggal: KV-P+		Cigarettes
Lots of fiber	B3 - Niacin: 200 mg.		Saffron: VPK=		The pill; estrogen
Psyllium seed	Magnesium/Calcium:		Salvia danshen: KV-P+		Second-hand smoke
Guar gum	500 mg.		Hawthorn Berries: V-KoP+		Sedentary lifestyle
			Ginger: VK-P+		Red meat

Pectin
Oat bran (not wheat bran)
Pantethine: 900 mg.
Mesoglycan: 100 mg.
Evening primrose: VPK
200 mg. 2 x per day

Cardamon: VK-P+
Cinnamon: VK-P+
Gotu Kola: VPK=
Garlic: VK-P+
Ashwagandha: VK-P+
Aloe Vera: VPK=
Horsetail: PK-V+

Saturated fats
Sugar
Milk
Coffee
Alcohol
Stress
Suppressing emotions
Salt

Recipe

Kapha & Vata:

Arjuna powder	1 Tbs.
Guggul powder	1 Tbs.

Take 2 tsp. twice a day w/lunch and dinner.

Pitta:

Arjuna powder	1 Tbs.
Gotu Kola powder	1 Tbs.

Take 2 tsp. (or 1,000 mg) w/lunch & dinner.

Arteriosclerosis Herbal Brew

See directions for preparing herbal brew on page 409

VATA		PITTA		KAPHA	
Comfrey Root	2 oz.	Gotu Kola	2 oz.	Guggul	2 oz.
Ginger	1 oz.	Burdock	2 oz.	Ginger	2 oz.
Rosehips	2 oz.	Red Clover	1 oz.	Cinnamon	1 oz.
Ashwagandha	2 oz.	Mint	1 oz.	Cardamon	1 oz.
Cinnamon	1 oz.	Cinnamon	1/2 oz.	Burdock	1 oz.
Cardamon	1 oz.	Cardamon	1/2 oz.		

Self-Care

Imagery
Lifestyle modification
Exercise
Stress management
Yoga
Meditation

A degenerative dis-ease that is very common. An autoimmune disorder often consistent with extreme pain and swelling of the joints, degeneration of the cartilage, and/or weakening of the bones. Pittas often suffer with inflammation (heat makes it worse). Vatas generally have aching and dryness (cold increases pain). Kaphas usually experience swelling. Arthritis can be caused by poor diet, poor digestion, and/or a low immune system. Rheumatism is a more advanced condition often affecting all joints; it is more easily diagnosed with blood work.

Feelings and Emotions: Holding on to anger and resentment. Something is eating you. Stuck, not moving forward.

Diet	Vitamins & Minerals (Daily)	Essential Oils (always dilute)	Herbs	Alternative Therapy	Avoid
Elimination diet	B-Complex: 100 mg. -(esp. B-15)	Brahmi: VPK-	**PuriTea	Light massage	Sugar
Ayurvedic diet for body type	C: Ascorbate, 2000-3000 mg.	Oregano: VK-P+	Guggul: VK-P+	Sauna	Dairy
	E: 400 IU	Cyperus: PKV-	Sandalwood: PV-Ko	Steam	Night shades***
Food combining	F: 200 mg.	Sandalwood: PV-Ko	Dashmool: VK-P+		- Peppers
	D: 500 IU	Peppermint: PK-Vo	Galangal: VK-P+		- Tomatoes
Potassium broth	K: 200 IU	Chamomile: VPK	Guduchi: PK-V+		- Potatoes
	B3 - Niacin: 100 mg.	Cypress: VKP+	Aloe Vera: VPK=		- Egg Plant
Nuts (soaked)	B 5 - Pantothenic Acid: 1000-1500 mg.	Eucalyptus: KV-P+	Neem: PK-V+		Meat
	Magnesium: 200 mg.	Sweet Marjoram: KV-P+	Ginger: VK-P+		Acid foods
	Glucosamine Sulfate: 200 mg.	Rosemary: KV-P+	Cyperus: PKV-		White flour
	Bio Flex: 2 tablets	Lavender: PK-Vo	Chaparral: PK-V+		Cayenne
		Juniper: KV-P+	Turmeric: KV-Po		
			Angelica: VK-P+		
			(do not use if tumor or fibroid)		
			Kaishore Guggulu (Banyan herbs)		
			Purnana Vadi Auggulu		

Evening Primrose: 2 tablets
A good Multi-Mineral
Linoleic Acid (Vitamin F):
Calcium: 1500 mg.

Medicated Oils:
-Maharayan: VPK
- Narayan: VPK
- Saharshardi: VP-K+
- Brahmi oil (or mustard oil): VPK

*Blended Oils:
*Joint Free: VPK
-Yogaraj Guggul

Gentian: PK-V+
Buckhorn: PK-V+
Black Cohosh: PK-V+
Myrrh: KV-P+

Ayurvedic Formulas:
-Trikatu, 2 tablets before meals.

-Triphalla, 4-6 tablets at bedtime.

HERBAL BREWS   *See directions for preparing herbal brew on page 409*

VATA

Ashwagandha 2 oz.
Valerian 1 oz.
Ginger 1 oz.
Angelica 1 oz.
Dashmoola 2 oz.
Chamomile 1 oz.
Rosemary ½ oz.

* Product of Earth Essentials-Florida
** Product of UniTea Herbs, Colorado

Arthritis Herbal Recipes

HERBAL PASTE

Mix all ingredients together, apply them on joint, let dry.

VATA

Juice of ½ lemon
1 tsp. Bentonite clay
½ tsp. Ginger powder
1 tsp. Sandalwood
¼ tsp. Mustard oil

PITTA

Burdock	2 oz.
Skullcap	1 oz.
Guduchi	2 oz.
Chamomile	2 oz.
Licorice	1 oz.

Aloe Vera gel 3 x day (best fresh)

KAPHA

Cinnamon	
Ginger	2 oz.
Cyperus	2 oz.
Yucca	2 oz.
Lingusticun	2 oz.

Turmeric powder ½ tsp. (this can be added if desired)

MASSAGE FORMULA

Cypress	10 drops	Juniper	10 drops
Eucalyptus	5 drops	Rosemary	5 drops
Peppermint	5 drops	Vegetable oil	2 oz.

Hot Baths   1 to 3 day fast

Castor oil compresses

PITTA

2 Tbs. Sandalwood powder
10 drops Cyperus essential oil
5 drops Peppermint oil
¼ tsp. Coconut oil or Brahmi*
1 tsp. Bentonite clay
* *Product of Earth Essentials Florida*

KAPHA

1 tsp. Calamus powder
1 tsp. Bentonite clay
½ tsp. Ginger powder
1 tbs. rubbing alcohol
¼ tsp. Cayenne
¼ tsp. Mustard oil

TAKE

Kapha: Triphalla at night; Guggul in the morning
(2 tsp. or 200 mg)

Pitta: Castor oil - 1 Tablespoon at night

Kapha: 1 tsp. Ginger & 1 cup water 2 times per
day before meals.

Self Care   Ice packs for Pitta   Exercise
                Basti oil enemas   Colon Cleanse

ATHLETE'S FOOT

Athlete's foot involves susceptibility to infection by mold-like bacteria, yeast, fungi, parasites, and viruses. Fungus results from "creatures of darkness", moisture, and heat. It is necessary to strengthen the immune system. Athlete's foot can be exacerbated by poor food combining, too much starch, sugar, fried foods, and direct contact in public showers (wear sandals). Vatas may experience dryness, cracking, and itchiness. Pittas and Kaphas experience discomfort between the toes, foul odor, redness, defoliation of skin, cracking, and puss.

Feelings and Emotions: Stagnation. Afraid to move forward. Confusion.

Diet	Vitamins & Minerals (Daily)	Essential Oils (always dilute)	Herbs	Alternative Therapy	Avoid
Ayurvedic diet for body type	E: 250 IU	Tea Tree: VPK=	Echinacea: PK-V+	Acupuncture	Sugars
Eat a well balanced diet	C: 1,500 mg.	Clove Oil: VK-P+	Licorice: VP- K+		Wine
Lots of raw vegetables	Selenium: 100 mcg.	Anise: VK-P+	European Mistletoe: VK- P+		Sodas
Green juice	Zinc: 100 mg.	Basil: VK-P+	Black Walnut: PKVo		Fried foods
Food combining	Beta-Carotene: 2000 IU (critical)	Tarragon: VK-P+	Korean Ginseng: V-KPo		Alcohol
	A: 10,000 IU (until clear)	Marigold (Tagetes): PK-V+	Siberian Ginseng: V-KPo		Grains
	B-6: 200 mg.	Lemongrass: PK-Vo	Barberry: PK-V+		Fruit
	Thymus Extract: 2 tablets	Cajaput: KV-P+	Aloe Vera: VPK=		Fermented food
	Chlorophyll: 2 Tsp., 2 x per day.	Trifolia: VK-P+	Turmeric: VK-Po		
	Q-10: 100 mg.	Turmeric: VK-Po	Marigold: PK-V+		
	(Capryllic acid as per bottle)	Yarrow: VPK-	Burdock: PK-V+		
		Thyme: VK-P+	Dandelion: PK- V+		
		Chamomiles: VKP-	Red Clover: PK-V+		
			Peppermint: PK-Vo		

Cave man diet: (no sugars, low fruit, no grains, some starches, lots of green proteins, oils)

Rotation diet (for allergies)

Iron: 100 mg.   Colloidal Silver

Niaouli: VPK-

Ginger: VK-P+
Goldenseal: PK-V+
Pau d'Arco: PK-V+

Formula:
Caprinex: VPK

Athlete's Foot Herbal Brew

VATA

Ginger	2 oz.
Prickly Ash	1 oz.
Coriander	2 oz.
Lavender	1 oz.
Astragalus	1 oz.

PITTA

Echinacea	2 oz.
Mint	1 oz.
Burdock	2 oz.
Red Clover	1 oz.
Dandelion	1 oz.

KAPHA

Mint	1 oz.
Burdock	2 oz.
Echinacea	2 oz.
Ginger	1 oz.
Dandelion	2 oz.

See directions for preparing herbal brew on page 409

ANTI-FUNGAL POWDER

Arrowroot	4 Tbs.
Goldenseal powder	1 Tbs.
Marshmallow	2 Tbs.
Black Walnut powder	2 Tbs.
Turmeric powder	1 Tsp.

Mix all ingredients together. If the powder is grainy, put it in a coffee or nut grinder. Mix well. Store this powder in a sealed container. Apply to feet as needed. This same mixture can be used as a footbath. Steep herbs in water. Strain. Soak feet.

OINTMENT #1

Turmeric	1 tsp.
Tea Tree oil	20 drops
Basil essential oil	20 drops
Vegetable oil or salve	1/2 ounce

Apply to feet at night. Cover with socks.

See directions for making salve at end of chapter.

OINTMENT #2

Beeswax	1 part
Olive oil	4-6 parts
Tea Tree	20 drops
Cajeput	20 drops

(Total - 1/2 ounce)

Self-Care

Foot baths

Walk barefoot when possible (except public baths)

Spray essential oils in shoes

BACK PROBLEMS

Back problems can result from old injuries, heredity, accidents, poor posture, organ weaknesses, malfunctioning vertebrae, birth defects, and/or long periods of sitting. Vatas are prone to extreme back pain. Pittas may experience inflammation or burning. Kaphas tend to experience swelling.

Feelings and Emotions: Not feeling supported.

Diet	Vitamins & Minerals	Essential Oils (Daily)	Herbs (Always dilute)	Alternative Therapy	Avoid
Ayurvedic diet for body type	B-Complex: 2 tablets	Lavender: VK-Vo	Kava Kava: PV-Ko	Chiropractic treatments	Unsupervised exercise
	B5 - Pantothenic Acid: 2,500 mg.	Ylang Ylang: PV-K+	Passion Flower: PK-V+	Raindrop therapy	Over eating
Foods rich in calcium & Mag-nesium	Magnesium: 800 mg.	Rosemary: VK- P+	Skullcap: PK-V+	Acupuncture	Over stretching
	Calcium: 800 mg.	Brahmi: VPK-	Valerian: VK-P+	Physical therapy	Over bending
	C: 3000 mg.	Eucalyptus: KV-P+	Chamomile: PK-Vo	Massage	Jumping
Green, leafy vegetables		Juniper: KV-P+	Guggul: KV-P+	When caused by digestive & assimilation problems:	Running
		Cypress: VKP+	Cyperus: VPK	- Colonics	
		Valerian: VK-P+	Jatamasi: KV-P+		
		Geranium: PK- V+	Nutmeg: VK-P+		
		Chamomile: VPK-	Oat Straw: VP-K+		
			St. John's Wort: PK-V+		
		Blended Oils: (do not dilute)	Jasmine Flower: PK-V+		
		Relaxing Blend: VPK	Lotus seed: PV- K+		
			Dashmoola: VK-P+		

Product of Earth Essentials Florida

Back Problems Herbal Brew

See directions for preparing herbal brew on page 409

VATA			PITTA			KAPHA	
Gotu Kola	2 oz.		Gotu Kola	2 oz.		Gotu Kola	1 oz.
Valerian	1 oz.		Chrysanthemum	2 oz.		Valerian	1 oz.
Ginger	1 oz.		Chamomile	1 oz.		Guggul	2 oz.
Oatstraw	1 oz.		Skullcap	1 oz.		Passion Flower	2 oz.
Lotus Seed	1 oz.		Jasmine Flowers	1 oz.		Skullcap	1 oz.
Jatamasi	2 oz.		St. John's Wort	1 oz.		Mint	1 oz.
			Mint	1 oz.			

Bedtime: Drink 1/2-cup tea with 1/2-cup warm milk. Add 1-Tbs. ghee. Mix well.

Compresses with Essential Oils

VATA & KAPHA	
Ginger Powder	2 Tbs.
Water	4 Tbs.
Lavender essential oil	5 drops
Eucalyptus oil	5 drops (or any oils of your choice)

Paste will get hot. Take it off after 5-10 minutes, or when it begins to burn.

Self Help

Basti oil enema
Magnetic Blend
Compresses
Yoga

BAD BREATH

Bad breath can be caused by a number of reasons or conditions, including tooth decay, poor digestion, liver trouble, catarrh, poor food combining, lack of chlorophyll in the diet, or a congested colon. This often inflicts Pitta with the feeling of sourness in the mouth.

Feelings and Emotions: I am not important. I don't care.

Diet	Vitamins & Minerals (Daily)	Essential Oils (always dilute)	Herbs	Alternative Therapy	Avoid
Ayurvedic diet for body type or anti-Pitta diet	Acidophilus: 2 caps 3 x day	Peppermint: PK-Vo	Peppermint: PK-Vo	Ayurvedic consultation	Poor food combinations
	Chlorophyll: 2 tsp. 2 x day	Thyme: VK-P+	Rosemary: KV-P+	Colonics	Mucous forming foods
Pungent herbs	B-Complex: 200 mg.	Bergamot: VK-P+	Myrrh: VK- P+	Dental visits	Constipation
Fried foods	Digestive enzymes	Fennel: VPK=	Goldenseal: PK-V+	Pancha Karma treatments	Negative emotions
Fruits	C: 1,500 mg.	Eucalyptus: KV-P+	Ginger: VK-P+		Tongue scraping
Proper food combining	PABA: 100 mg.	Clove: VK-P+	Fennel: VPK=		
Lots of greens	Magnesium: 200 mg.	Tea Tree: VPK=	Mint: PK-V+		
Lots of vegetables	Zinc: 50 mg.		Trikatu: VK- P+		
	Triphala: 3-6 tablets at night with tea				

Bad Breath Herbal Brew

See directions for preparing herbal brew on page 409

VATA		PITTA		KAPHA	
Ginger	2 oz.	Mint	1 oz.	Ginger	2 oz.
Cardamon	1 oz.	Coriander	2 oz.	Angelica	1 oz.
Coriander	2 oz.	Chamomile	2 oz.	Cardamon	2 oz.
Fennel	1 oz.	Fennel	2 oz.	Basil	1 oz.
Angelica	1 oz.			Rosemary	1 oz.

MOUTHWASH #1

10 drops Eucalyptus essential oil
8 oz. hydrogen peroxide (food grade)
Gargle, morning & evening

10 drops Peppermint essential oil in 8 oz. of water.
Mix well. Rinse mouth after meals.

MOUTHWASH #2

4 oz. Prickly ash
2 oz. water
Boil water. Add herbs. Let steep for 45 minutes. Cool
Add 10 drops essential oil of your choice
Add 2-oz. saline solution
Add 1 drop of liquid Stevia
Mix well. Store in bottle

Self-Care

Fennel or Anise essential oil on the tongue
Mouthwash
Flossing
Fasting
Tongue Cleaning

BI-POLAR - (Manic-Depressive)

This is a chemical imbalance in the brain where the person changes from low depressive states to very high energetic states. It can be caused by hereditary factors, severe birth trauma, stress, environmental pollutants, over-exposure to chemicals, or a B-vitamin deficiency. Vatas will experience bouts of anxiety, fear, or nervousness, and their moods will swing both high and low. Pittas often struggle with anger and irritability. Kaphas become depressed, along with problems of phobia and paranoia.

Feelings and Emotions: Unsure of life. I don't know where I belong. General insecurity.

Diet	Vitamins & Minerals	Essential Oils (Daily)	Herbs (always dilute)	Alternative Therapy	Avoid
Ayurvedic diet for body type	B-Complex: 2 tablets; 3 x day C: 3,500 mg. B-12: 500 mcg./or shots	Brahmi (Gotu Kola): VPK- **Mental Clarity: VPK- Basil: VK-P+	Basil: VK-P+ Brahmi: VPK- Rosemary: KV- P+ Skullcap: PK-Vo	Counseling Shirodhara Tarpana B-12 shots:	Foods high in vanadium Herring Sardines
Lots of green, leafy vegetables	B6 - Pyridoxine: 100-200 mg. L-Phenylalanine: 300 mg. (for 2 months)	Rosemary: VK-P+ Myrtle: PK-V+ Lavender: PK-Vo Chamomile: VPK-	Passion Flower: PK-V+ Chrysanthemum: PK-V+ Peppermint: PK-Vo Calamus: VK- P+	(2-3 times per week)	White sugar Alcohol Hallucinogenic drugs
Carbo-hydrates	Blue-green algae: 2-tsp. 3-x day Primrose: 500-mg. 1-3 x day	Myrrh: KV-P+ Frankincense: KV-P+ *Mental Clarity: VPK+	**SereniTea: (manic) **LeviTea: (depression)		
Seaweeds	Amino Acid Complex: 2-x day Natural Lithium: 300-400 mg. Spirulina: 2-tsp. 3-x day Folic Acid: 500-600 mcg.				

*Product of Earth Essentials Florida   **Product of UniTea Herbs

Bi-Polar Herbal Brew

See directions for preparing herbal brew on page 409

VATA

Calamus	1 oz.
Gotu Kola	2 oz.
Ginger	1 oz.
Basil	2 oz.

PITTA

Chrysanthemum	2 oz.
Skullcap	1 oz.
Gotu Kola	2 oz.
Mint	1 oz.

KAPHA

Skullcap	1 oz.
Calamus	1 oz.
Chrysanthemum	2 oz.
Basil	1 oz.

PREPARED TEAS (1 teaspoon per cup of water):

**SereniTea (Vata)

**Mental ClariTea (Pitta)

**LeviTea (Kapha)

Self-Care

Breathing exercises	Yoga
Meditation	Tai Chi
Chi Qong	

*** Product of UniTea Herbs*

BLACK EYE

This is an effusion of blood under the loose skin over and around the eyes. Can be caused by an injury or weak kidneys. With Vatas the eye becomes yellow, Pittas experience a black eye, and Kapha's eye may turn dark brown. Dark circles under the eyes.

Feelings and Emotions: Angry.

Cell Salts: Calcium Fluoride

Diet	Vitamin & Minerals (Daily)	Essential Oils (always dilute)	Herbs	Alternative Therapy	Avoid
Ayurvedic diet for body type	C: 25,000 mg.	+Hydrosols:	Arnica: KV-P+	Reiki	Fried foods
Foods high in bioflavonoids	K: 200 mcg.	Lavender: PK-Vo	Comfrey: PV-K+	Therapeutic Touch	Congesting foods
Cooling foods	B Complex: 100 mg.	Rose: VPK=	Aloe Vera: KPV	Homeopathics	Watching TV
	P: 200 mg.		Chamomile: PK-Vo	Shirodhara	
			Cinnamon: VK-P+		
			Ginger: VK-P+		

+ Hydrosols are composed of the water remaining after the distillation of essential oils. This water is suitable for eye washing.

Self-Care

Comfrey ointment
Cool compresses with rose or neroli essential oil
Ice compresses
Inhalations

Black Eye Herbal Brew   *See directions for preparing herbal brew on page 409*

VATA	PITTA	KAPHA
Comfrey - equal amounts	Mint - equal amounts	Ginger - equal amounts
Ginger	Chamomile	Mint
Cinnamon		

Mix in equal parts and drink until eye has cleared.

BLEEDING

Bleeding can be caused from a injury or an accident. Nosebleeds are common for Vatas; Pittas and Kaphas experience more head injuries. Women, especially Pitta types, have excessive bleeding during menstruation or menopause. Hemorrhoids are common with constipation and straining which cause Frank "Red" blood with stool. Bleeding ulcers are a Pitta condition and cause a black tarry stool.

Feelings and Emotions: Not feeling harmonious. Scattered.

Cell Salts: Ferr Phos, Iron phosphate

Diet	Vitamin & Minerals	Essential Oils (Daily)	Herbs (always dilute)	Alternative Therapy	Avoid
Anti-Pitta Diet	A: 5,000 IU	Cajaput: KV-P+	Comfrey: VP-K+	Therapeutic touch	Dairy
Astringent foods	K: 500 mcg.	Tea Tree: VPK=	Plantain: PK-V+	Reiki	Hot spices
Green vegetables	B17: 2 grams with meals	Cypress: VPK+	Yarrow: PK-V+		Meat
Wheatgrass juice	Calcium: 800 mg.	Lavender: PK-Vo	Horsetail: PK-V+		Excess salt
Liquid chlorophyll	Magnesium: 500 mg.	Chamomile: VPK-	Calendula: PK-V+		
Egg yolk		Tagetes: VK-P+	Shepherd's Purse: PK-V+		
Seaweeds		Sandalwood: PV-Ko	Cayenne: VK-P+		
			Aloe Vera Gel: VPK=		
			Witch Hazel: PK-V+		
			AlumRoot: PK-V+		

Bleeding Herbal Brew

See directions for preparing herbal brew on page 409

HERBAL BLEND FOR ALL BODY TYPES

Drink for two weeks:

Horsetail	1 oz.
Plantain	2 oz.
Calendula	1 oz.
Shepherd's Purse	1 oz.
Witch Hazel	2 oz.
Fennel	2 oz.

Self-Care

Direct pressure can be applied onto the cut to stop the blood flow.

When in the wild, Plantain can be used as a natural Band-Aid.

Nosebleeds: Put head back. Place a copper penny on forehead. Hold the head back for 15 minutes.

Salves

Cold baths

Cold compresses

Ice

BRUISES

Bruises are more or less extensive injuries of the deeper part of the skin and underlying tissues, accompanied by an outpouring of blood from damaged vessels. The simplest type of bruise is one in which the deeper layers of the skin are damaged, causing a slight bluish discoloration. When a severe blow occurs, the muscles may be bruised and torn without an opening in the skin. The resulting effusion of blood may cause a large swelling which sometimes results in the formation of an abscess. If the bruise is close to a bone, it can become calcified.

Feelings and Emotions: Guilt. Self-punishment.

Cell Salts: Calcium Fluoride

Diet	Vitamins & Minerals (Daily)	Essential Oils (always dilute)	Herbs	Alternative Therapy	Avoid
Ayurvedic diet for body type	C: 2,000 mg. 3 x day	Pine: KV-P+	Arnica: KV-P+	Reiki	Dairy
Berries	D: 200 IU	Amber: VPK-	Triphala: VPK-	Therapeutic touch	Clogging foods
Cherries	Bioflavonoids: 500 mg.	Orange: VK-P+	Guggel: KV-P+	Aura balancing	
Proteins	B-Complex: twice a day	Bergamot: VK-P+	Camphor: KV-P+	Chakra balancing	
Green vegetables	Folic Acid: 300 mcg.	Lavender: PK-Vo	Salvia: KV-P+		
Cooling foods	Iron: 40 mg.	Cardamon: VK-P+	Turmeric: VK-Po		
	F: 200 IU	Lemon: PV-Ko	Comfrey: PV-K+		
	P: 200 mg.	Lime: PK-V+	St. John's Wort: PK- V+		
	K: 200 mg.	Yarrow: VPK+	Red Clover: PK-V+		
			Burdock: PK-V+		
			Noni Juice: PKV-		

Bruise Herbal Brew

See directions for preparing herbal brew on page 409

VATA		PITTA		KAPHA	
Skullcap	1 oz.	Marshmallow	1 oz.	Ginger	2 oz.
Ginger	1 oz.	Mints	2 oz.	Mint	1 oz.
Rosehips	2 oz.	Comfrey	2 oz.	Lemongrass	2 oz.
Comfrey	1 oz.				

TO MAKE A SALVE *See directions on page 409*

1 part beeswax	Arnica tincture	30 drops	Lavender essential oil	20 drops
3-5 parts vegetable oil	Comfrey tincture	30 drops		

Place beeswax in pan. Melt.

Add oil, tincture, and essential oils - check hardening with a cold spoon. Add more oil if too hard; more wax if too soft.

Place in refrigerator for 20 minutes to harden.

Apply to area when cool.

AS AN ANTI-COAGULANT

Sesame oil 1/4 cup

1 Tbs. Black mustard seeds, ground with 2 oz. water.

Make a paste and apply to area around the bruise.

Self-Care

Castor Oil Pack   Ice Compresses

Cold Water Baths

BURNS

Burns are injuries caused by dry heat or scalds caused by moist heat. Burn injuries can also occur through contact with electric wires or with acids or other chemicals. Simple sunburn produces redness and disappears quickly. More severe burns produce blisters, tissue damage (scars), severe deformations, and sometimes—even death.

Feelings and Emotions: Feeling aggravated with life. Tired of life. Burnout.

Cell Salts: Calcium Fluoride

Diet	Vitamins & Minerals (Daily)	Essential Oils (always dilute)	Herbs	Alternative Therapy	Avoid
Pitta reducing diet	C: 1,000 mg, every hour	Sandalwood: PV-Ko	Aloe Vera Gel: VPK-	Chakra Balance	Heat
High caloric diet	B Complex: 200 mg.	Vetiver: V-KP+	Chickweed: PK-V+	Energy Work	Warm water
High protein diet	Potassium: 200 mg.	Lemongrass: PK-Vo	Comfrey: PV-K+	Cranial Sacral	Ointment
Lots of fluids	A: 75,000 IU	Lavender: PK-Vo	Ghrita: PK-V+	Color Therapy	Butter
Fresh fruits	E: 200 IU after each meal	Blue Chamomile: PV-K+	Coriander: VPK-		
Fresh vegetables	PABA: 200 mcg.	Coriander: VPK-	Plantain: PK-V+		
Rosehips	D: 600 IU	Tea Tree: VPK=	Slippery Elm: VP-K+		
Cherries	F: 300 mg.		Shepherd's Purse: PK-V+		
Green peppers	Zinc: 40 mg.		Turmeric: VK-Po		
Citrus			Rescue Remedy		
Cooling foods			Noni Juice: PKV-		

Burn Recipes

RECIPE

Fresh leaf of aloe vera - cut off spiny edges.
Lay leaf flat on a table and cut open with knife.
Scoop the gel out with a spoon.
Put in blender.
Spread over the burned area or use cut open leaves to rub on the burned area.

MAKE A SALVE *See directions on page 409*

1 part beeswax   3-5 parts vegetable oil
30 drops essential oils: Chamomile & Lavender
(Total volume liquid should equal 1 ounce.)
Melt vegetable oil in pan
Add beeswax
Add essential oils

Self-Care

Immediately immerse the burned area in cool or ice water for 5-10 minutes (within a 20-minute period)
Cold compresses   Liquid honey
Comfrey poultice   Apple cider vinegar
Saline water   Ghee or coconut oil with lavender. Apply to area.
Salve - with cooling oils of coconut or sunflower

CANCER

Cancer is a process of the cells reproducing out of control and attacking other tissues of the body. Rebelling against the central authority of the body/mind. It can be caused by chronic constipation, poor digestion, food sensitivity, poor diet, suppressed emotions, lack of spiritual connection, exposure to chemicals, and environmental hazards. Vatas are more prone to colon, bone, stomach cancers and dry tumors; Pittas are more prone to liver, stomach, pancreas, skin, brain, and lymph cancer. Kaphas are more prone to melanoma, tumors, lung, and breast cancer.

Feelings and Emotions: Self hate, criticism, judgements, and belief in suffering and separation.

Diet	Vitamin & Minerals (Daily)	Essential Oils (always dilute)	Herbs	Alternative Therapy	Avoid
Ayurvedic diet for body type	A: 100,000 IU	Ginger: VK-P+	Chaparral: PK-V+	Ayurvedic consultation	Canned foods
Cleansing	C: 10,000 mg.	Rose: VPK=	Essiac Blend: PR-V+	Biofeedback	Processed foods
Short period of fasting	E: 75,000 IU	Lavender: PK-Vo	Burdock: PK-V+	Sound therapy	Sugars
Foods which support the immune system	F: 200 mg.	Yarrow: PK-V+	Astralagus: VP-K+	Pancha Karma	High protein
Shitaki mushrooms	Calcium: 800 mg.	Rose Geranium: PK-V+	Pippali: VK-P+	Tarpana	Refined grains
Yellow & orange vegetables	Potassium: 800 mg.	Sandalwood: PV-Ko	Ashwagandha: VK-P+	Wholistic medical doctor	Junk foods
	Chromium: 100 mcg.	Saffron: VPK=	Guduchi: PK-V+		Sour foods
	Digestive Aids: 2 before meals		Solomon's Seal: PV-K+		Dairy
	B complex: 200 mg.		Yarrow: PK-V+		Meat
	B17 (laetrile): 200 mg.		Goldenseal: PK-V+		Fried foods
	B12: 400 mcg.		Turmeric: VK-Po		Iron supplements
	Niacin: 160 mg.		Manjishta: PK-V+		All chemicals
	Haelan soybean extract: 1 bottle once day for 2 months then		Ginger: VK-P+		Household cleansers
	1/2 bottle once day until remission		Saffron: VPK=		
			Haritaki: VK-Po		

Raw foods Sustein: (by Metagenics): 1-cup 3-x day Guggul: KV-P+
Wheatgrass Q-10: 100 mg.   Myrrh: KV-P+
Alfalfa   Gotu Kola: VPK-
Barleygrass   Calamus: VK-P+
Green juices
Dandelion greens

See directions for preparing herbal brew on page 409

Cancer Herbal Brew

VATA		PITTA & KAPHA
Astralagus	1 oz.	Essiac Blend
Ginger	1 oz.	10 drops Chaparral
Burdock Root	1 oz.	
Slippery Elm	1 oz.	

Vata: Need tonics, colon cleansers, and digestive aids

Pitta: Need blood purifiers

Kapha: Need strong expectorants

CANDIDIASIS

A yeast type fungus infection which is able to live in many parts of the body where there is moisture and wetness, such as; intestines, mouth, sinuses, lungs, urinary tract, and the vagina. Candida easily multiply with poor diet (sugar and yeast), weakening the immune system and digestive tract causing many problems in them. This condition can be triggered by antibiotics and birth control pills. In Vata body types it creates allergies, dryness, constipation, muscle pain, and adrenal insufficiency. In Pitta types, there can be rashes, athlete's foot, jock itch, and heartburn. In Kapha body types, it may cause water retention, congestion, depression, diabetes, and kidney problems.

Feelings and Emotions: Not trusting the flow of life.

Diet	Vitamin & Minerals (Daily)	Essential Oils (always dilute)	Herbs	Alternative Therapy	Avoid
Ayurvedic diet for body type	A: 25,000 IU (until clear)	Trifolia: VK-P+	Prickly Ash: VK-P+	Chiropractic treatments	Antibiotics
	B-Complex: 200 mg.	Tea Tree: VPK=	Hing: VK-P+		Fermented foods
Cleansing diet	Biotin: 300 mcg.	Cloves: VK-P+	Aloe Vera: VPK=	Naturopathic consultation	Nut butters
Proteins	B12 Shots 1 x week	Rosewood: VK-P+	Asafoetida: VKP+		Pickles
	Megadolophilus: 1/4 tsp.	Rosemary: VK-P+	Katuka: PK-P+	Ayurveda consultation	All yeast foods
Colloidal silver	3 x day	Peppermint: PK-Vo	Barberry: PKV+		& breads
	Capryllic Acid:	Tarragon: VK-P+	Goldenseal: PKV+	Pancha Karma	Chemical cleansers
Raw foods, (kapha, pitta)	2 caps 3 x day	Palmarosa: VPK-	Pau d'Arco: PKV+		Acid foods
	Selenium: 200 mcg.	Myrrh: KV-P+	Cardamon: PK-V+		
Rotation diet	***Niastatin (powder/oral form)	Bergamot: KV-P+	Bay: VKP+		
		Bay: VKP+	Ginger: VK-P+		

*** *Doctor's prescription required. This is the only antibiotic that does not kill friendly bacteria within the body.*

Candidiasis Herbal Brew

See directions for preparing herbal brew on page 409

VATA		PITTA		KAPHA	
Prickly Ash	2 oz.	Pau d'Arco	2 oz.	Pau d'Arco	2 oz.
Ginger	1 oz.	Barberry	1 oz.	Katuka	1 oz.
		Mint	1 oz.	Cardamon	1 oz.

Morning: Drink 2 Tbs. Aloe Vera juice in 8-oz water.

SALVE *See directions on page 409*

Beeswax	1 part
Vegetable oil	3-5 parts
Essential oils	40 drops
(of your choice)	

Melt wax. Add vegetable oil. Test consistency with cold spoon.

Add more wax for hardness; oil for softness.

Let cool.

Add essential oils.

Self Care

Use Hing with cooking of all beans and soups

CANKER SORES

Canker sores begin as a swelling in the mouth and progresses into an ulcerated lesion, with much pain and burning. They are caused by stress, poor diet, too much sugar, and/or deficiencies of B-12 and iron. Pittas may experience inflammation with puss. Vatas may experience dryness and pain. Kaphas may experience large sores with swelling (puss).

Feelings and Emotions: Not good enough. I can't do it. Too much stress.

Cell Salts: Calcium Sulph

Diet	Vitamin & Minerals (Daily)	Essential Oils (always dilute)	Herbs	Alternative Therapy	Avoid
Ayurvedic diet for body type	A: 1000 IU B-Complex: 2 tablets 2 x per day Folic Acid: 400 mcg. B-12: 300 mcg.	Tea Tree: VPK= Bergamot: VK-P+ Geranium: PK-V+ Cajaput: KV-P+ Frankincense: VK-P+	Burdock: PK-V+ Golden Seal: PK-V+ Pau d'Arco: PK-V+ Neem: PK-V+ Red Clover: PK-V+	Acupuncture Therapeutic Touch Reiki Chakra Balancing Shirodhara	Wheat Cheese Tomato Lemon Pineapple
Elimination diet	Iron: 100 mg. Copper: 40 mg. Zinc: 50 mg.	Myrrh: VK-P+ Neem: PK-V+ Lavender: PK-Vo Sandalwood: PV-Ko	Guduchi: PK-V+ Comfrey: VP-K+ Red Raspberry: PK-V+ Red Root: PK-V+		Sugar Mustard Vinegar Most citrus
Chlorophyll	B-5: 150-200 mg. L-lysine: 2500 mg. Amino Acid Complex: 2 tablets 2 x day		Slippery Elm: VP-K+ Noni Juice: VPK-			

Canker Sore Herbal Brew

See directions for preparing herbal brew on page 409

VATA TEA

Comfrey	1 oz.
Chitrak	1 oz.
Cardamon	1 oz.

PITTA-KAPHA TEA

Burdock	1 oz.
Red Clover	1 oz.
Pau d'Arco	1 oz.
Mint	2 oz.
Guduchi	2 oz.

SALVE *See directions on page 409*

Beeswax	1 part
Vegetable Oil	3-5 parts

Essential Oils - 30 drops per ounce of beeswax - (of your choice from list)

In a small pan, melt the wax and vegetable oil. Remove from stove.

Add essential oils. Let cool.

APPLY TO CANKER SORE

Vata-Kapha: Mix 2 drops Aloe Vera Gel with 1/2 tsp. Turmeric and 1 drop essential oil.

Pitta: Mix 2 drops Aloe Vera Gel with 1/3 tsp. Sandalwood powder and 1 drop Sandalwood essential oil.

CHICKEN POX

A highly contagious viral disease that is characterized by generalized skin eruptions. It most commonly afflicts children. One attack usually protects one against the disease for life. The rash first shows up across the trunk, arms, and face as red bumps that contain drops of clear fluid eventually breaking out to form a crust. This cycle continues for 3 or 4 days. The patient should be isolated for 10-14 days.

Feelings and Emotions: Sensitive to the opinions of others.

Cell Salts: Aconite, Belladonna and Pulsatila

Diet	Vitamins & Minerals (Daily)	Essential Oils (always dilute)	Herbs	Alternative Therapy	Avoid
Ayurvedic diet for body type	A: 25,000-100,000 IU (until clear)	Peppermint: PK-Vo	Echinacea: PK-V+	Homeopathics	Scratching
	E: 50 IU	Geranium: PK-V+	Cayenne: KV-P+		Heating foods
	Multi-Mineral	Blue chamomile: PV-K+	Chickweed: PK-V+		Massage
Protein	Potassium: 1000 mg.	Lavender: PK-Vo	Cleavers: PK-V+		Hot Baths
	Zinc: 10 mg.	Clary Sage: PVK-	Lobelia: K-VP+		
Light diet	RNA & DNA: 3 x day, until condition clears	Rose: VPK=	Red Clover: PK-V+		
		Sandalwood: PV-Ko	Burdock: PK-V+		
	C: 2,500 mg.				

Note: When I had chicken pox as an adult, I tested very low in vitamin C so I took 10,000-13,000 mg. daily. I also took Vitamin A supplements in doses of 75,000-125,000 IU per day, and RNA tablets in doses of 7-10 capsules per day (300 mg. each). I am happy to say that I've come through quite well with no scarring.

Chicken Pox Herbal Brew

See directions for preparing herbal brew on page 409

VATA			PITTA			KAPHA		
Chamomile	1 oz.		Chickweed	1/2 oz.		Mint	1/2 oz.	
Rosehips	1 oz.		Burdock	1 oz.		Burdock	1 oz.	
Mix with Berry juice	1/2 cup		Chamomile	1 oz.		Mix with Apple juice	8 oz.	
			Mix with Apple juice	8 oz.				

Mix 1/2-cup tea with 1/2 cup juice and drink every 2 hours.

CHILDREN

Echinacea   10 drops every 2 hours - until rash is gone

RECIPE FOR TOPICAL OINTMENT

Aloe vera gel	equal amounts
Sandalwood powder	equal amounts

Make a paste. Apply to area.

Self-Care

Take a cotton ear swab. Apply Blue Chamomile essential oil, dab lightly on all sores.

Chickweed bath	Cool baths with Chamomile
Chickweed ointment	Basti oil enema

CHRONIC FATIGUE

A virus related to Epstein Bar Herpes family, affecting with flu type symptoms, as well as low energy. Vata's experience extreme tiredness, loss of appetite, anxiety, intestinal problems, mood swings, and muscle pain. Pitta's experience fevers, liver problems, irritability, and swollen glands. Kapha's experience respiratory problems, depression, sleepiness, and spasms.

Feelings and Emotions: Tired of not knowing what one's life purpose is all about.

Cell Salts: Silica oxide

Diet	Vitamin & Minerals (Daily)	Essential Oils (always dilute)	Herbs	Alternative Therapy	Avoid
Ayurvedic diet for body type	A: 50,000-100,000 IU	Angelica: VPK-	Astralagus: VK-P+	Color therapy	Frequent flying
	C: 5,000-8,000 mg.	Lavender: PK-Vo	Ashwagandha: VK-P+	Reiki	Radiation
	B-Complex: 100 mg.	Immortelle: VPK-	Shatavari: PV-K+	Tarpana	Chemical cleansers
	Megadolphilus: 3 x day	Saffron: VPK=	Gotu Kola: VPK-	Dance	Processed foods
Yogurt	E: 800 IU	Bergamot: VK-P+	Ginger: VK-P+	Acupuncture	Fried foods
	Calcium: 1200 mg.	Myrtle: PK-V+	Fennel: VPK=	Life purpose counseling	Poor food combining
Juices	Magnesium: 1,000 mg.	*Immune	Saw Palmetto: V-PK+		Yeast
	Bioflavonoids: 300 mg.	Free: VP-K+	**ImmuniTea: VPK+		All chemicals
Broths	Selenium: 200 mcg.		Solomon's Seal: PV-K+		Preservatives
	Zinc: 50 mg.		Chrysanthemum: PK-V+		Fluorescent lights
Sesame seeds	Potassium: 100 mg.		Fo-Ti: PV-K+		Overuse of computers
	DHEA: 50 mg. 2 x day				
Nutmilk					

*Product of Earth Essentials Florida   **Product of UniTea Herbs

Chronic Fatigue Herbal Brew

See directions for preparing herbal brew on page 409

VATA

Astralagus	equal amounts
Saw Palmetto	
Solomon's Seal	
Ashwagandha	
Ginger	
Shatavari	

PITTA

Shatavari	equal amounts
Gotu Kola	
Fo Ti	
Fennel	
Chrysanthemum	

KAPHA

Ashwagandha	2 oz.
Ginger	2 oz.
Guggul	2 oz.

Self Care

Yoga
Meditation
Walking
Dancing
Tai Chi

COLITIS

Irritation and inflammation of the colon, poorly formed stools, and pain due to toxins in colon. Vata's experience food sensitivities and irregular bowel movements; Pitta types may experience severe inflammation; Kapha types may lose weight and have loose stools with mucous.

Feelings and Emotions: Experiencing lack of support, fear, and insecurity.

Diet	Vitamin & Minerals (Daily)	Essential Oils (always dilute)	Herbs	Alternative Therapy	Avoid
Ayurvedic diet for body type	A: 25,000 IU	Helichrysum: PK-V+	Bayberry: PK-V+	Massage	Red meat
Oat bran	B-Complex: 200 mg.	Tea Tree: VPK=	Katuka: KP-V+	Biofeedback	Dairy
Steamed vegetables	C: 4,000 mg.	Geranium: PK-V+	Aloe Vera: VPK=	Reiki	Sulpha drugs
Cabbage juice	Multi-vitamin	Sandalwood: VP-Ko	Cyperus: VPK	Therapeutic touch	Fried foods
Carrot juice	Calcium: 800 mg.	Myrrh: VK-P+	Chamomile: PK-Vo	Gem Therapy	Sugars
Baked foods	Magnesium: 700 mg.	Cypress: VKP+	Dandelion: PK-V+	Color Therapy	Alcohol
Broiled foods	Zinc: 50 mg.	Chamomile: VPK-	Comfrey: VP-K+	Food allergy testing	Spicy foods
Steamed foods	Bioflavonoids: 1,000 mg.		Papaya: PK-Vo		Allergic foods
Rotation diet	Acidolophilus: 3 x day		Alum Root: PK-V+		Yeast foods
Allergy/ avoidance diet			Triphalla: VPK-		
Cave man diet			Marshmallow: PV-K+		
			Fennel: VPK=		
			Coriander: VPK-		
			Nutmeg: VK-P+		
			Mint: PK-Vo		
			Noni Juice: VPK-		

Colitis Herbal Brew

See directions for preparing herbal brew on page 409

VATA		PITTA		KAPHA	
Katuka	1 oz.	Papaya Leaves	1 oz.	Fennel	1 oz.
Cyperus	1 oz.	Chamomile	1 oz.	Mint	1 oz.
Comfrey	1 oz.	Dandelion	1 oz.	Cyperus	1 oz.
Coriander	1 oz.	Alum Root	1 oz.	Katuka	1 oz.
Nutmeg	1/2 oz.	Fennel	1 oz.		

Self Care

Relaxation techniques

Meditation

Yoga

COMMON COLD

Infection due to low immunity describes the common cold. Pittas get fevers and sometime diarrhea. Vatas may experience restlessness, pain in the joints, sneezing, and/or headaches. Kaphas suffer from congestion and excess mucus.

Feelings and Emotions: Not paying attention to one's needs. Confusion. Stressed.

Diet	Vitamins & Minerals (Daily)	Essential Oils (always dilute)	Herbs	Alternative Therapy	Avoid
Kelp	A: 1500 IU	Eucalyptus: VK-P+	Slippery Elm: PV-K+	Homeopathy	All dairy
	Beta-Carotene: 15000 IU	Rosemary: KV-P+	Ginger: VK-P+	Saunas	Sugar
Garlic detox	B-Complex: 3 tablets	Myrtle: PK-V+	Echinacea: PK-V+	Music therapy	
	C: 5000-10000 mg.	Lavender: KP-Vo	Goldenseal: PK-V+	Color therapy	
Fast	Amino acids	Sandalwood: PV-Ko	Astralagus: PV-K+		
		Peppermint: PK-Vo	Mint: PK-Vo		
Colloidal		Camphor: KV-P+	Clove: VK-P+		
Silver		*Immune-Free: VP-K+	Basil: VK-P+		
		Cinnamon: VK-P+	Yarrow: PK-V+		
Ayurvedic diet		Hyssop: KV-P+	Elderberry: KP-Vo		
for body type		Anise: VK-P+	Shatavari: PV-K+		
		Basil: VK-P+	Ajwan: VK-P+		
Plenty of fluids		Angelica: VPK=, P+	Triphalla: KVP		
		Lemon Balm: PK-Vo	Licorice: VP-K+		
Immune broth			Lemongrass: PK-Vo		
			Burdock: KP-V+		
			**PuriTea: VP-K+		
			**ImmuniTea: VP-K+		

Product of Earth Essentials Florida

**Product of UniTea Herbs*

Common Cold Herbal Brew

See directions for preparing herbal brew on page 409

VATA

Basil	1 oz.
Astralagus	2 oz.
Elder berries	1 oz.
Ginger	1 oz.
Cinnamon	1 oz.
Shatavari	1 oz.

PITTA

Elder berries	1 oz.
Echinacea	1 oz.
Shatavari	1 oz.
Mint	1 oz.
Burdock	2 oz.

KAPHA

Burdock	1 oz.
Lemongrass	1 oz.
Clove	1/2 oz.
Cinnamon	1/2 oz.
Elder berries	2 oz.
Mint	1/2 oz.
Ginger	1/2 oz.

Drink herbal blend 3 times a day.

Inhalation Therapy

VATA

Lemon	3 drops
Ginger, fresh	3 inch piece
Eucalyptus	3 drops

PITTA

Mint	3 drops
Lime	2 drops
Myrtle	2 drops

KAPHA

Lemon	3 drops
Ginger	2 inch piece
Camphor	2 drops

COUGH

Myrtle	1 drop
Hyssop	1 drop
Anise	1 drop
Honey	2 Tbs. Take 2 x per day.

COLD REMEDY MASSAGE BLEND

Basil	3 drops
Angelica	2 drops
Eucalyptus	5 drops
Lemon Balm	3 drops
Vegetable Oil	2 oz.

Self-Care

If fever is present: do cold sheet treatment. (See "Fever")

Aromatherapy inhalations

Dry skin brushing

Necessary to increase the digestive fire - use spices for appropriate dosha (body type)

Steam

Hot bath

Rebounder

Foot baths

Colon cleanse

CONSTIPATION

Constipation is retention of waste materials in the body. Some indications of accumulation of toxins in the colon include a coating at the back of the tongue, bloating, gas, and abdominal pain. Cultures consuming high fiber diets (100-170 grams daily) have a transit time of 30 hours and a fecal weight of 500 grams, whereas the typical low fibre diets of most Europeans and Americans (+20 grams daily) have a transit time of 48+ hours and a fecal weight of 100 grams. This condition is more common to a Vata body type. It affects other doshas under extreme circumstances, such as when traveling.

Feelings and Emotions: Holding on. It's hard to let go.

Cell Salts: Mag-Phos (Magnesium Phosphate)

Diet	Vitamin & Minerals (Daily)	Essential Oils (always dilute)	Herbs	Alternative Therapy	Avoid
Ayurvedic diet for body type	Folic Acid: 200 mcg.	Rose: VPK=	Plantago Psyllium: PV-K+	Massage	Anti-depressants
	A: 25,000 IU	Trifolia: VK-P+	Haritaki: VK-Po	Acupuncture	Anticholinergics
Drink plenty of water	B-Complex: 100 mg.	Ginger: VK-P+	Flaxseed: V-KoP+	Pancha Karma	Antacids
	B1: 100 mg,	Anise: VK-P+	Cumin: PKV=		Tobacco
Ground seeds	Choline: 500 mg.	Fennel: VPK=	Garlic: KV-P+		Cocaine
	Inositol: 500 mg.	Cumin: VK-P+	Rose: VPK=		Amphetamines
Lightly cooked whole bran	B3 - Niacin: 300 mg.	Rosemary: VK-P+	Aloe Vera: VPK=		Mineral Oil
	C: 1000 mg.	Calamus: VK-P+	Senna: PK-V+		Laxatives (addictive)
	Calcium: 200 mg.	Cyperus: VPK-	Barberry: PK-V+		Bad food combinations
Soaked nuts	Potassium: 300 mg.	Cypress: VKP+	Yellow Dock: PK-V+		Fried Foods
	E: 150 IU	Lemon: PV-Ko	Cascara Sagrada: PK-V+		Anti-Psychotics
	F: 200 IU	Lavender: PK-Vo	Cayenne : VK-P+		Sugar
			Black Pepper: VK-P+		Beta-Blockers
			Noni Juice: PKV-		
			Triphalla: VK-Po		

Vata:
-Light cooked apple
with cinnamon & ginger

Pitta & Kapha:
-Raw Grated Vegetables

Lemon Peel: PV-Ko
Ginger: VK-P+
Pippali: VK-P+
Punarnava: PK-V+
Bibhitaki: KP-Vo
Triphala: VPK-; 4-6 tablets;
at night with tea or milk
Slippery Elm: PV-K+
Oregon Grape: PK-V+
Rhubarb: PK-V+

Cheese
Muscle Relaxants
Yogurt
Bread
Pastries
Fried foods
Pork/Meats
Dry foods
Inactivity

Constipation Herbal Brew

VATA		PITTA		KAPHA	
Ginger	2 oz.	Mint	1 oz.	Rose Petals	2 oz.
Slippery Elm	2 oz.	Bibhitaki	2 oz.	Pippali	1 oz.
Plantain	2 oz.	Haritake	1 oz.	Ginger	2 oz.
Rose Petals	1 oz.	Cascara Sagrada	1 oz.	Haritaki	1 oz.
Bibhitaki	1 oz.	Rose Petals	1 oz.		
Tamarind	1 oz.				

See directions for preparing herbal brew on page 409

Mix. Use 1 tsp. per cup.
Pitta Bedtime: 1-2 tsp. psyllium powder with 1-tsp. ghee & warm milk.
Vata Bedtime: Take 2 tsp. of flaxseed powder and 1 tsp. ghee with warm milk.
Kapha Bedtime: Cod Liver Oil, 1 Tbs.

INFUSION
Pitta: Rhubarb 1tbs.
Mint 1/2 tbs.
Ginger 1/2 tbs.

Castor Oil Pack Procedure

(Required: Castor oil, 1 piece of flannel, piece of plastic, hot water bottle or moist heating pad, and 1 large towel)

Warm the castor oil. Fold flannel so that it is thick and is approximately 10" x 14". Lay the flannel on a plastic wrap. Pour the warm oil onto the flannel, covering the entire area. Apply the flannel to the abdomen and cover with the plastic wrap. Then place heat on it, as warm as is tolerable. Keep on for 45 minutes to two hours. Remove. Then wash the area with baking soda (1 tsp.) and water (1 pint). *(Edgar Cayce formula)*

Massage Formula

Massage abdomen clockwise with:

Trifolia	10 drops
Constipation Free*	50 drops
Sesame Oil	1 Tablespoon

* Product of Earth Essentials Florida

Self-Care

Exercise daily
Yoga: sun salutation
Meditation
Relaxation
Fasting/Light Diet
Self-massage, esp. the abdomen
Basti (oil enema)
Tai Chi
Castor Oil Pack

CYSTITIS

An inflammation or infection of the bladder. Although the symptom of burning while urinating is quite frightful, it is not usually serious. Urination may be scant and accompanied by blood or puss. Cystitis may disappear without treatment, but if it persists for more than 48 hours and includes symptoms of chills, vomiting, or pain in the kidneys, consult a practitioner. Urination for Vata will be scanty and painful; Pitta may experience some puss; and Kaphas may experience puss and swelling.

Feelings and Emotions: Not wanting to connect. Wanting to be alone. Feeling irritated.

Diet	Vitamins & Minerals (Daily)	Essential Oils (always dilute)	Herbs	Alternative Therapy	Avoid
Ayurveda diet for body type	A: 50,000 IU (until clear)	Juniper: VK-P+	Barberry: PK-V+	Therapeutic touch	Sugar
	B-Complex: 50 mg.	Sandalwood: PV-Ko	Garlic: VK-P+		Refined carbohydrates
Acidophilus after meals	Beta-carotene: 20,000 IU	Cajeput: VK-P+	Goldenseal: PK-V+	Chakra balancing	Full strength fruit juice
Cranberry juice	C: 500 mg. every 2 hours	Bergamot: VK-P+	Uva-Ursi: PK-V+	Reiki	Coffee: decaf and regular
	D: 600 IU	Eucalyptus: KV-P+	Black Pepper: VK-P+	Counseling	Caffeine in all forms
Watermelon	E: 600 IU	Lavender: PK-Vo	Fennel: VPK=		Cigarettes
Propolis	Choline: 100 mg.	Pine Needle: KV-P+	Buchu Leaves: PK-V+		Alcohol
Cranberries	Calcium: 300 mg.	Benzoin: VPK-	Gotu Kola: VPK-		Dehydration
16 oz. of juice daily	Magnesium: 200 mg.	Cedarwood: PK-V+	Mint: PK-Vo		Stress
Restrict calories	Potassium: 200 mg.	Frankincense: VK-P+	Coriander: VPK-		Poor hygiene
	Bioflavonoids: 1 gm.	Niaouli: PK-V+	Cilantro: PK-Vo		Red pepper
	Zinc: 30 mg.	Tea Tree: VPK=	Dandelion: PK-V+		Hot spices
		Trifolia: VK-P+	Ginger: KV-P+		Garlic
			Gokshura: KVP+		Onions
			Chandraprabha: K-VP+		

See directions for preparing herbal brew on page 409

Cystitis Herbal Brew

VATA

Fennel	1 oz.
Coriander	1 oz.
Ginger	2 oz.
Black Pepper	2 oz.

PITTA & KAPHA

Uva Ursi	1 oz.
Buchu Leaves	1 oz.
Dandelion	2 oz.
Fennel	2 oz.
Coriander	2 oz.
Ginger	2 oz. (Kapha only)

Self-Care
DOUCHE

8 oz. of water

3 drops of Tea Tree essential oil

2 drops of Dhavana essential oil

DIABETES

Diabetes appears in two forms: Diabetes Mellitus and Diabetes Insipidus. Diabetes Mellitus involves the inability to assimilate food, and it primarily affects the function of the liver and the pancreas. Diabetes Insipidus is characterized by constant thirst and an excessive flow of urine. This condition can be caused by excess consumption of sugar and Kapha-producing food due to a low pancreatic function. It can also be inherited. Vata urine tends to be like butter or sesame oil in advanced stages with a noticeable loss of bladder control and weak muscles. Pitta urine can be very alkaline, combined with bladder and kidney inflammation. It can also be acidic and bluish or red due to toxicity in the kidneys. Moreover, vision can rapidly weaken. Kaphas may experience very poor digestion, sweet smelling urine containing mucous, excessive urination, or cold hands and feet.

Feelings and Emotions: Not enjoying the sweetness of life. Not being on purpose.

Diet	Vitamin & Minerals (Daily)	Essential Oils (Always dilute)	Herbs	Alternative Therapy	Avoid
Ayurvedic diet for body type	Zinc: 30 mg.	Lavender: PK-Vo	Blueberry Leaf: PK-V+	Sound therapy	Alcohol
	Iron: 50 mg.	Myrtle: PK-V+	Turmeric: KV-Po	Massage	All sugars
Bitter melons	Magnesium: 500 mg.	Eucalyptus: VK- P+	Myrrh: VK-P+	Acupuncture	Restrict starches (carbohydrates)
Complex carbo-hydrates	Amino Acids	Camphor: KV-P+	Aloe Vera: VPK=P-	Pancha Karma treatments	White potatoes
	Calcium: 400 mg.	Juniper Berry: KV-P+	Gentian: PK-V+	Therapeutic vomiting	Rice
	Fish oil: 5000 IU	Hyssop: K-P+	Katuka: VPK		Processed foods
Bone marrow soup	C: 1000-3000 mg.	Geranium: PK-V	Neem: PK-V+		Dairy
	Manganese: 500 mg.		Barberry: PK-V+		Fat
	B Complex: 200 mg.		Goldenseal: PK-V+		Stress
Ghee:	B1: 100 mg.		Black Pepper: VK-P+		
1-2 Tbs.	B2: 10 mg.		Cayenne: VK-P+		
2-3-x day	B6: 100 mg.		Ginger: VK-P+		
	B12: 400 mcg.		Ginseng: V-KPo		

Lots of water
Lots of greens
Licorice ghee
Milk - (10 gm)
Nuts
Protein
Stevia

B3 - Niacin: 100 mg.
Potassium: 300 mg.
Pangamic Acid: 200 mg.
Co Q-10: 80 mg.
D: 400 IU
E: 400-1200 IU
F: 2 Tbs. cold pressed vegetable oil or 6 capsules
Chromium: 200-400 mcg.

Comfrey: PV- K+
Wintergreen: PK-Vo
Dandelion Root: VK-P+
Buchu Leaves: PK-V+
Raspberry Leaves: PK-V+
Eucalyptus: VKP+
Yarrow: PK-V+
Bitter Root: PK-V+
Vanadium: 100 mcg.
Red Root: PK-V+
Marshmallow: PV-K+

Ayurvedic Herbs:
Chandraprabha: VPK-
Shilajit: VPK-
Trikatu: VK-P+
Triphala: VPK
Guggul: PKV+
Gurmar: PK- V+

Diabetes Herbal Brew

VATA

Eucalyptus	1 oz.
Rosemary	1/2 oz.
Yellow Jasmine	1 oz.
Dashmoola	2 oz.
Ginger	2 oz.

Drink tea all day between meals.

PITTA

Mint	1 oz.
Lavender	1 oz.
Burdock	1 oz.
Red Clover	1 oz.
Raspberry Leaves	1 oz.
Dandelion	1 oz.

KAPHA

Eucalyptus	1 oz.
Red Clover	2 oz.
Ginger	1 oz.
Yarrow	1 oz.
Dandelion	1 oz.

See directions for preparing herbal brew on page 409

Trifala: 2,000 mg. at night (all doshas)

Gurmar or Shardunikha: Take 3 tablets 3 x a day before meals with tea.

WHEN BLADDER CONTROL IS LOST

Vacha   300 mg.
Brahmi   200 mg.
Gotu Kola   250 mg.
Jatamasi   200 mg.

Mix and take with tea 2 x per day

MASSAGE FORMULA

Eucalyptus   10 drops   Hyssop   5 drops
Geranium   5 drops   Juniper   10 drops
Vegetable oil 4 oz.

COMPRESS AT NIGHT WITH ESSENTIAL OILS OVER THE PANCREAS

10 drops   Coriander
10 drops   Eucalyptus
1 oz.   base oil

Place 20 drops on pancreas at night
Place 20 drops over kidneys at night

Self-Care

Exercise (walking, swimming, etc.)   Meditation
Inhalation of essential oils: 3-4 times per day   Mantra
Turmeric Rice: Cook rice with 1 Tbs. Turmeric   Yoga

DYSMENORRHIA (Painful Menstruation)

Sometimes accompanied by incapacitating cramps and often nausea and diarrhea. It has been determined that an excess of a certain type of prostaglandin is found in the uterus. Prostaglandin's are chemicals found in the body, one of which causes contractions of the uterine and intestinal muscles. With too much prostaglandin, the rhythmic contractions of the uterus during menstruation become longer and tighter, keeping oxygen from the muscles. It is this lack of oxygen that we perceive as pain. Vata experiences light menstruation, along with severe pain. Pitta may have the opposite effect with heavy bleeding and painful diarrhea. Kapha suffers from clots, water retention, and fatigue.

Feelings and Emotions: Not having good feelings about their feminine energy. Sexual guilt.

Cell Salts: Magnesium Phosphate

Diet	Vitamin & Minerals (Daily)	Essential Oils (always dilute)	Herbs	Alternative Therapy	Avoid
Ayurvedic diet for body type	E: 400 IU, 2 x day	Clary Sage: VPK-	Dong Quai: VK-P+	Massage	Caffeine
	Evening Primrose Oil 1000 mg.	Geranium: PK-V+	Uva-Ursi: PK-V+	Bio-feedback	Sodas
		Lavender: PK-Vo	Crampbark: KV-P+	Acupuncture	Salt
		Yarrow: PK-V+	Blue Cohosh: KV-P+	Tarpana	Sugar
		Fennel: VPK=	Fennel: VPK=	Therapeutic touch	Alcohol
Seaweeds or kelp	Calcium: 1,000 mg.	Cypress: VKP+	Ginger Root: VK-P+	Reiki	IUD
	Magnesium: 600 mg.	Chamomile: VPK-	Valerian: VK-P+		Fasting
Whole grains	Iron: 30 mg.	Jasmine: PK-V+	Cinnamon: VK-P+		Light diet when
	Iodine: 200 mcg.	Peppermint: PK-Vo	Raspberry Leaf: PK-V+		Vata
Legumes	B Complex: 200 mg.	Sage: VK-P+	Vitex: VPK-		
	C: 2000 mg. (ascorbate is best)	Tarragon: VK-P+	Yarrow: PK-V+		
Vegetables & fruits	Pantothenic acid: 200 mg.	Thyme: VK-P+	Hops: PK-V+		
			Nettles: PK-V+		

Brewer's yeast

Add turmeric to rice and vegetables

Alfalfa: PK-V+
Licorice: PV-K+
Lemongrass: PK-Vo
Motherwort: PK-V+
Dandelion: PK-V+
Shepherd's Purse: PK-V+
Black Currant: KP-V+
Turmeric: VK-Po
Cardamon: VK-P+ (in excess)

Dysmenorrhia Herbal Brew

See directions for preparing herbal brew on page 409

VATA		PITTA		KAPHA	
Cramp Bark	2 oz.	Yarrow	2 oz.	Raspberry Leaf	2 oz.
Shatavari	2 oz.	Shatavari	2 oz.	Ginger	1 oz.
Ginger	1 oz.	Motherwort	1 oz.	Vitex	1 oz.
Cinnamon	1 oz.	Fennel	1 oz.	Lemongrass	1 oz.
Licorice	1 oz	Vitex	1 oz.	Uva Ursi	1 oz.
Vitex	2 oz.	Nettles	1 oz.	Nettles	1 oz.

Drink 2-3 cups daily, beginning two weeks before menstruation.

Self-Care

Exercise — Regular sleep schedule

Compresses — Warm bath with essential oils of clary sage, lavender, and geranium.

Compress over the abdomen — Vaginal massage (by GYN, midwife, mate, or self)

Breathwork

EARACHE

Earaches are due to inflammation in the middle ear. This may be due to chronic or acute infections, eczema, wax, neuralgia or infected teeth. Other causes may be colds, tonsillitis, allergies, or measles. Vatas may experience dryness, scalyness, or severe pain and inflammation. Pittas may experience burning pain. Kaphas may experience congestion, pain, and drainage.

Feelings and Emotions: Not wanting to hear that which is being spoken about. For children, when there is too much fighting going on in the home, they may get an earache.

Cell Salts: Kalimur (Potassium Chloride)

Diet	Vitamin & Minerals (Daily)	Essential Oils (always dilute)	Herbs	Alternative Therapy	Avoid
Ayurvedic diet for body type	A: 100,000 IU	Camphor: KV-P+	Astralagus: VP-K+	Chiropractic	All dairy
	C: 2500 mg.	Lavender: PK-Vo	Mullein: PK-V+	Cranial sacral	Bread containing milk
	Thymus gland extract:	Cajeput: KV-P+	Echinacea: PK-V+	Reiki	
Elimination	50 drops per day	Niaouli: PK-V+	Hops: PK-V+	Therapeutic touch	Simple carbohydrates
diet for	Zinc: 100 mg.	Savory: KV-P+	Oregano: VKP+	Ear candling	Eggs
2 weeks	Bioflavonoids: 200 mg.	Clove: VK-P+	Boneset: PK-V+	Sound therapy	Wheat
	Evening Primrose: 200 mg.	Eucalyptus: VK-P+	Lobelia: K-PV+		Corn
Rotation diet	Flax Seed Oil: 200 mg.	Pine: KV-P+	Manjishta: PK-V+		Oranges
		Geranium: PK-V+	Dashmoola: VK-P+		Peanut butter
Lemon juice		Juniper: KV-P+	Castor Root: V-PK+		
		Immortele: PKV-	Vatsanabha: VPK+		
			Vitex: VPK-		
		Medicated Oil:	Bhringaraj: VPK=		
		Garlic with olive oil	Ginger: VK-P+		
		Mullein oil	Hing: VK-P+		

Earache Herbal Brew

See directions for preparing herbal brew on page 409

VATA & KAPHA

Lemon juice   1 oz.
Ginger, fresh   2-inch piece
Water   3 cups

In blender, mix ginger, water, and lemon juice; add honey or sucanat to taste. Blend well. Strain. Drink 3 times per day.

PITTA

Lemon juice   1 oz.
Fennel seed   1 Tbs.
Water   3 cups

In blender, mix fennel, water, and lemon juice; add maple syrup to taste. Blend well. Strain. Drink 3 times per day.

RECIPES

1. 40 drops pure lemon juice with 2 Tbs. of water. Put 3 drops in ear 3 times per day.

2. On a cotton ball put 2 drops of lavender, lemon or niaouli. Fold corners of ball and place cotton in outer ear.

3. From "Back to Eden", by Jethro Kloss: Bake a large onion until soft. Tie it over the ear.

4. A hot foot bath with 1-Tablespoon mustard seed vegetable oil and essential oil of your choice.

5. Mullein flower oil - 4 drops.

6. Use 1 pinch Hing (asafoetida) with one drop of essential oil and mix well. Place in the center of cotton ball and fold corners. Then place in ear and make sure the mixture on the cotton does not touch the ear.

Choose one of the above recipes. Then, using your thumbs, massage around the outside of the ear with a cooling essential oil of your choice. Massage with downward movements. Be sensitive.

Self-Care

Warm compresses around the ear.

ECZEMA (Atopic Dermatitis)

A disease of the skin which is not contagious but can be inflammatory. Causes of eczema can be due to disturbances of the digestive organs, blood conditions or external irritants such as heat, cold or irritants from plants. Eczema appears in three different varieties: Eczema rubrum, Eczema erythermatosum, or Eczema pustulosum. It is a skin condition with characteristic symptoms of itchiness, inflammation, thick or dry skin or skin lesions such as scratches, papules, patches of redness, weeping, scaling or blistering. Eczema is most commonly found on the face, wrists and insides of the elbows and knees.

Feelings and Emotions: Anger, guilt, blame

Cell Salts: Calc Sulph (calcium sulfate)

Diet	Vitamin & Minerals (Daily)	Essential Oils (always dilute)	Herbs	Alternative Therapy	Avoid
Ayurvedic diet for body type	B Complex: 200 mg.	Bergamot: VK-P+	Marshmallow: PV-K+	Therapeutic touch	Stress
	C: 3,000 mg.(ascorbate)	Chamomile: VPK	Bupleurum: PKV+	Reiki	Dairy
	D: 500 IU	Eucalyptus: VK-P+	Isatis: PKV+	Acupuncture	Wheat
Legumes	PABA: 200 mg.	Helichrysum: PKV+	Blackthorn: PKV+	Color therapy	Sugar
	Biotin: 300 mcg.	Juniper: KV-P+	Hawthorn Berry: V-KPo	Counseling	Caffeine
Wheatgrass	Choline: 200 mg.	Lavender: PK-Vo	Licorice Root: VP-K+		Fatigue
	Inositol: 100 mcg.	Melissa: PK-Vo	Burdock Root: KP-V+		Sour foods
Green vegetables	E: 500 IU	Patchouli: VPK	German Chamomile: VPKo		Pungent foods
	Niacin: 100 mg.	Rosewood: K-VP+	Neem: PK-V+		Salt
	Potassium: 500 mg.	Sage: VK-P+	Honeysuckle: PK-V+		Alcohol
Ghee	Flaxseed Oil: 1 teaspoon 3 x day (300 mg.)	Geranium: PKV+	Pau d'arco: PK-V+		
		Hyssop: PKV+	Red Clover: PK-V+		
		Rosemary: P-VP	Yellow Dock: PK-V+		

Evening Primrose Oil: 400 mg.
A: 50,000-75,000 IU for 3 months
Zinc: 50 mg.
Zinc Skin Ointment
Bioflavonoids: 200 mg.
Magnesium: 600 mg.
Sulfur Skin Ointment
Silica: 25 mg.

Myrrh: KV-P+
Rose: VPK=
Neem: PK-V+

Calendula: PK-V+
Aloe Vera: VPK=
Chickweed: PK-V+
Dandelion: KP-V+
Plantain: KP-V+
Yarrow: PK-V+
Turmeric: VK-Po
Barberry: PK-V+
Guggul: KV-P+
Milk Thistle: PV-K+
Shatavari: PV-K+

HERBS - Continued:
Aloe Vera Gel: VPK=
Saffron: VPK=
Goldenseal: PK-V+
Nettles: PK-V+
Gokshura: PK-Vo

See directions for preparing herbal brew on page 409

Eczema Herbal Brew

VATA		PITTA		KAPHA	
Chamomile	2 oz.	Pau d'arco	1 oz.	Red Clover	1 oz.
Licorice	1 oz.	Dandelion	2 oz.	Milk Thistle	1 oz.
Shatavari	2 oz.	Yarrow	2 oz.	Dandelion	2 oz.
Hawthorn	2 oz.	Plantain	1 oz.	Plantain	2 oz.
Marshmallow	1/2 oz.	Calendula	2 oz.	Burdock	2 oz.
Chickweed	1 oz.				

Drink throughout the day - as many as 6 cups.

RECIPE

Vidanga	1/2 tsp.
Honey	1 tsp.
Water	1/2 cup

Mix well.
Drink in the evening.

POULTICE

Mix Aloe Vera Gel or Ghee and Turmeric (equal amounts)
Make a paste
Apply to the area

IN THE MORNING

In blender mix Aloe Vera Gel and Turmeric (equal amounts)
Drink before breakfast

NEEM - LAVENDER SALVE   *See directions on page 409*

1 part beeswax
3 parts oil

Melt beeswax in a pan over low temperature. Remove from stove. Add vegetable oil or jojoba oil. Add essential oils (50 drops total). Put in refrigerator for 15 minutes to cool. Take out. Apply to areas needed.

Self-Care

Drink cilantro juice (fresh)   Turmeric creme
Colon cleanse   Neem-Lavender salve

EDEMA

Water retention caused by weakening of the kidneys. Most common during old age. A Kapha condition affecting all doshas. Vatas experience dry skin, and tissues become spongy; Pitta may experience swelling, inflammation, and the skin holding the imprint of the finger when pressed; Kapha's have moist skin and feels damp when pressed with fingers. Can be caused by poor diet, poor food combining, pregnancy, PMS, and food allergies. *Caution: Edema could be an indication of kidney or heart failure.*

Feelings and Emotions: Fear of letting go.

Cell Salt: Silica Natrium Phosphate

Diet	Vitamin & Minerals (Daily)	Essential Oils (always dilute)	Herbs	Alternative Therapy	Avoid
Kapha diet best for Pitta	A: 25,000 IU C: 2,500 mg. B-Complex: 200 mg.	Sandalwood: VP-Ko Lavender: PK-Vo Juniper: VK-P+	Ashwagandha: VP-K+ Sarsaparilla: VPK+ Marshmallow: VPK+	Sauna Massage (LymphDrainage)	Dry foods (Vata) Corn Salt
Rotation diet	B6: 100 mg.	Coriander: VPK Parsley: KVP+	Dandelion: PKV+ Nettles: PK-V+	Acupuncture Therapeutic touch	Sodas Foods high-sodium
Diet must be modified			Coriander: VKP- Chickweed: PK-V+ Uva Ursi: PKV+		White sugar Chips Pretzels
			Burdock: PKV+ Cleavers: PK-V+		Birth control pills
Cilantro			Goshkura: PKVo Lemongrass: VK-P+ Purnarnava: PKV+ Chandraprabha: VK-VP+		

Edema Herbal Brew

VATA		PITTA		KAPHA	
Sarsaparilla	1 oz.	Dandelion	1 oz.	Buchu Leaves	1 oz.
Coriander	1/2 oz.	Nettles	1/2 oz.	Juniper	1/2 oz.
Lemongrass	1/2 oz.	Fennel	1/2 oz.	Uva Ursi	1/2 oz.
Ashwagandha	1/2 oz.	Coriander	1/2 oz.	Nettles	1/2 oz.
		Burdock	1/2 oz.	Lemongrass	1/2 oz.

Fennel: VPK=
Chicory: PK-V+
Lavender: PK-Vo
Juniper: KV-P+
Kudzy: PVK+
Gotu Kola: PKV
Red Clover: PK-V+

See directions for preparing herbal brew on page 409

Self Care

Compress over kidneys	Exercise
Kidney Flush	Dry skin brushing

FEVER

A fever occurs when the body temperature becomes elevated due to a high Pitta state or due to an infection in the body. Fevers are good for the body during illness because they help burn out toxins in the body. Many natural physicians encourage a low fever (under 105° F) and do not recommend suppression of the fever.

Feelings and Emotions: Burning up inside.

Diet	Vitamin & Minerals (Daily)	Essential Oils (always dilute)	Herbs	Alternative Therapy	Avoid
Pitta Diet	C: 2,000 every 2 hours	Lavender: PK-V+	Yarrow: PK-V+		Iron
	A: 50,000 mg.	Rose: VPK=	Echinacea: PK-V+		Zinc
Many fluids		Chamomile: PK-Vo	Feverfew: PKV+		Aspirin
		Fennel: VPK=	Pokeroot: PK-V+		No minerals
Lots of		Coriander: PKV=	Hyssop: K-P+		
vegetable juices		Hyssop: KV-P+	Lobelia Extract: K-PV+		
		Basil: VK-P+	Lemongrass: PK-Vo		
Green juices		Sandalwood: PV-Ko	Coriander: VPK-		
		Geranium: PK-V+	Fennel: VPK=		
		Rose: VPK=	Tulsi: VK-P+		
		Cyperus: PKV-	Catnip: PK-Vo		
		Juniper: VK-P+	Blackthorn: PK-V+		
			Fenugreek: VK-P+		
			Rose petals: PKV=		
			Ginger: VK-P+		

Fever Herbal Brew

See directions for preparing herbal brew on page 409

VATA

Fenugreek	2 oz.
Basil	2 oz.
Ginger	2 oz.
Catnip	2 oz.

PITTA

Yarrow	2 oz.
Rose Petals	1 oz.
Fennel	1 oz.
Feverfew	1 oz.
Coriander	1 oz.
Erand	1 oz.

KAPHA

Ginger	2 oz.
Yarrow	2 oz.
Fenugreek	1 oz.
Basil	1 oz.
Pokeroot	1 oz.

TAKE

Echinacea & Goldenseal extract every 3 hours.

FOOT BATH

In a basin of very warm water, add 10 drops of essential oils

Sit in chair with feet in basin of water

Cover person with blankets

COLD SHEET TREATMENT

Prepare a hot bath.

Add essential oils: 10 drops yarrow, 10 drops cypress, and 10 drops juniper

Put a sheet in the freezer or in ice water.

Put the person in the bath with a cool compress on the head - add more hot bath water to tolerance.

Drink a cup of the herbal blend for specific body type. This will cause sweating.

When the sweat breaks, remove them from bath.

Wrap in cold sheet from freezer.

Around the cold sheet, wrap with wool blanket(s).

Crush 2 cloves garlic; mix with petroleum jelly; apply to bottoms of feet/ cover with wool socks.

Fever should spike in 10-15 minutes with profuse sweating; then fever drops to normal.

When you remove the sheet, it is often tinged brown with impurities from the skin.

Self-Care

Cold sheet treatment

Enemas

Cool sponge baths

FIBROCYSTIC BREAST

Fibrocystic breast consists of lumps of a soft, moveable nature found in the breast tissue. They can increase in size and cause pain during menstruation. The main cause is hormonal imbalance and it can be aggravated by poor diet and stress.

Feelings and Emotions: Old hurt and pain relating to male energy.

Diet	Vitamins & Minerals (Daily)	Essential Oils (always dilute)	Herbs	Alternative Therapy	Avoid
Ayurvedic diet for body type	A: 15,000 IU (until clear)	Dhavana: VPK-	Shatavari: PV-K+	Ayurvedic consultation	Alcohol
Whole grains	Beta-carotene: 20,000 IU	Clary sage: VKP-	Squaw vine: PKV+	Therapeutic Touch	Animal fat
Kelp	B-1: 150 mg.	Geranium: PK-V	Pokeroot: PK-V+	Colon cleansing	Rancid foods
Spirulina	B-6: 150 mg.	Sage: VK-P+	Mullein: PK-V+	Acupuncture	Meat
Bee pollen	C: 4,000 mg.	Cypress: VKP+	Red Clover: VK-P+		Coffee
Wheatgrass	E: 500 IU	Borage Oil: PK-V+	Dandelion: PK-V+		Black tea
Mushroom	Evening Primrose: 400 mg.	Castor Oil: V-KP+	Jatamasi: VK-P+		Soda
Kelp	Q10: 100 mg.		Black Pepper: VK-P+		
Seed nuts	Selenium: 200 mcg.		Cayenne: VK-P+		
	Germanium: 100 mcg.		Saffron: VKP=		
	Kelp: 6 tablets		Ginger: VK-P+		
			Noni Juice: VPK-		

Fibrocystic Breast Herbal Brew

See directions for preparing herbal brew on page 409

VATA		PITTA		KAPHA	
Shatavari	2 oz.	Shatavari	2 oz.	Shatavari	2 oz.
Jatamasi	1 oz.	Dandelion	1 oz.	Red Clover	1 oz.
Guggul	2 oz.	Red Clover	1 oz.	Poke Root	1 oz.
Black Pepper	1 oz.	Mullein	1 oz.	Guggul	1 oz.
		Squavine	1 oz.		

DRINK

Saffron with rice milk, soymilk or low fat milk - 3 times per day.

CLAY PACKS

Bentonite clay	1 tsp.
Lemon juice	one small lemon, or ½ large lemon

Make a paste. Apply to breast. Let dry. Wash with essential oils (of your choice) and water.

Self-Care

Warm compresses with castor oil

FIBROIDS

Fibroids are benign tumors that can occur throughout the body. They usually occur in the smooth muscle such as Uterine and Breast areas. Vata may experience pain and fear; Kapha's fibroids may swell and become damp; Pitta suffers from inflammation and excessive bleeding.

Feelings and Emotions: Wanting to give birth to something.

Cell Salt: Silica

Diet	Vitamin & Minerals (Daily)	Essential Oils (always dilute)	Herbs	Alternative Therapy	Avoid
Ayurvedic diet for body type	B-Complex: 200 mg. Niacin: 200 mg. Pantothenic Acid: 1000 mg. C: 2000 mg. F: 200 mg.	Lavender: PK-Vo Frankincense: KV-P+ Bergamot: VK-P+ Clary Sage: VPK- Dhavana: PVK- Tea Tree: VPK= Cyperus: PKV- Frankincense: VK-P+	Chaparral: PK-V+ Pau d' Arco: PK-V+ Yellow Dock Root: PK-V+ Wild Yam: VP-Ko Dandelion: PK-V+ Burdock: PK-V+ Yarrow: PK-V+ Ginger: VK-P+ Shatavari: PV-K+ Cotton Root Bark: V-KP+ Triphalla: VPKo Cyperus: PKV- Vitex: PKV-	Acupuncture Reiki Homeopathics Therapeutic touch	Hormone replacement drugs Dairy Eggs Red meat Fat Dong Quai
Dark green leafy vegetables Spirulina Whole grains Green drinks Fresh fruit					

Fibroids Herbal Brew

See directions for preparing herbal brew on page 409

VATA		PITTA		KAPHA	
Ginger	equal parts	Dandelion	equal parts	Pippali	equal parts
Wild Yam Root		Cyperus		Ginger	
Myrtle		Vitex		Barberry	

NIGHTLY
Trifala tablets	4
Saffron	3000 mg.

CASTOR OIL PACK
See directions in book on page 307.

CLAY PACKS
Bentonite clay	3 Tbs.
Lemon juice	1 lemon

Use over pelvic area. Mix into a paste. Apply to the lower abdominal area. Let dry. Wash off.

FLATULENCE

Flatulence is a collection of gas in the stomach or bowels. Gas may produce unpleasant rumblings in the bowels, farting, or burping. The cause is usually fermentation set up by yeast overgrowth, poor food combining, junk food diet, stress, or hurried eating. Vata people are very susceptible to gas. Vegetarians can become low in hydrochloric acid. Older people lose their digestive powers.

Feelings and Emotions: Gripping fear.   **Cell Salts:** Magnesium Phosphate

Diet	Vitamin & Minerals (Daily)	Essential Oils (always dilute)	Herbs	Alternative Therapy	Avoid
Ayurvedic diet for body type	B1: 100 mg.	Lavender: PK-Vo	Licorice: VP-K+	Homeopathics	Improper food combining
	B5: 2500 mg.	Bergamot: VK-P+	Rhubarb: PK-V+	Ayurvedic consultation	Unsoaked legumes
Acidophilus	B-Complex: 200 mg.	Chamomile: PK-Vo	Coriander: VKP-	Pancha Karma	Repressed emotions
	Multi-vitamin	Coriander: VPK-	Cumin: PK-V+		Too much vitamin C
	Multi-mineral	Eucalyptus: KV-P+	Garlic: KV-P+		Constipation
Primadophilus		Fennel: VPK=	Mustard: KV-P+		
		Ginger: VK-P+	Nutmeg: VK-P+		
Food combining		Juniper: VK-P+	Turmeric: KV-Po		
		Myrrh: VK-P+	Tarragon: KV-P+		
Cave man diet		Nutmeg: VK-P+	Fennel: VPK=		
		Peppermint: PK-Vo	Valerian: VK-P+		
More fibre		Rosemary: KV-P+	Asafoetida: VK-P+		
		Spearmint: KP-Vo	Pippali: VK-P+		
		Tarragon: KV-P+	Cardamon: VK-P+		
		Jatamasi: KV-P+	Clove: VK-P+		
		Fennel: VPK=	Cinnamon: VK-P+		

Flatulence Herbal Brew

Anise: VK-P+
Caraway: VK-P+
Catnip: PK-Vo
Ginger: VK-P+
Horseradish: VK-P+
Haritaki: VK-Po
Amalaki: VP-Ko
Bibhitaki: KP-Vo
Hingwastika: VK-P+

See directions for preparing herbal brew on page 409

VATA		PITTA		KAPHA	
Cardamon	equal amounts	Fennel	equal amounts	Cardamon	equal amounts
Ginger	equal amounts	Mint	equal amounts	Ginger	equal amounts
Anise	equal amounts	Coriander	equal amounts	Anise	equal amounts
Hing	1 pinch	Hing	1 pinch	Hing	1 pinch

Drink 1 cup before meals.

MASSAGE FORMULA FOR ABDOMEN

Fennel	10 drops	Anise	5 drops	Vegetable oil	4 oz.
Coriander	10 drops	Caraway	5 drops		

Self-Care

Take bitters before each meal
Pinch of baking soda in warm water
Castor oil
Take sea salt
Compress of ginger
Basti oil enema
Food combining
Compresses
Colon cleansing

GALL BLADDER

The gall bladder is a companion to the liver and found underneath it, storing the bile produced by the liver. This small sac releases the necessary bile for digestion of oils and fats. When the organ becomes weakened due to improper diet, it can produce gallstones, which are often crystallized forms of cholesterol combined with fat. Vata types experience gallstones with severe pain, nausea and dry stones; Pitta experiences yellow and green inflammation, and Kapha experiences weight gain with a lot of phlegm, especially around the abdominal area, with stones that are round and whitish in color. When someone says, "I stay away from fats and oils because they don't agree with me", there is often a gallstone problem.

Feelings and Emotions: Too controlling; not flowing with inner self. Indecisiveness. Not knowing when to be in control or when to let flow with life.

Cell Salts: Natrium Phosphate

Diet	Vitamin & Minerals	Essential Oils (Always dilute)	Herbs	Alternative Therapy	Avoid
Ayurvedic diet for body type	A: 25,000 IU (until clear) (beta-carotene best) B-Complex: 150 mg. 12: 1,500 mcg.	Lemon: PV-Ko Coriander: PVK- Turmeric: VK-P+ Peppermint: PK-Vo	Barberry Bark: PK-V+ Dandelion: PK-V+ Fennel: VPK= Coriander: VPK-	Pancha Karma Acupuncture Reiki Colonics	Sweets Fats Fried foods Hydrogenated oils
Liquid diet for 10 days	Choline: 500 mg. Inositol: 500 mg. C: 25,000 mg. D: 400 IU E: 700 IU	Ginger: VK-P+ Lime: PK-V+ Grapefruit: KV-P+	Peppermint: PK-Vo Gokshura: PK-Vo Katuka: PKV+ Corn Silk: PK-V+ Guduchi: PKV+ Ginger: VK-P+ Catnip: PK-Vo Gravel Root: PK-V+ Triphalla Guggulu: VK-P+	Chiropractic treatments Acupressure	Meat Sugars

Gall Bladder Herbal Brew

See directions for preparing herbal brew on page 409

VATA		PITTA		KAPHA	
Ginger	1 oz.	Dandelion	1 oz.	Guduchi	1 oz.
Fennel	1 oz.	Mint	1/2 oz.	Ginger	1 oz.
Coriander	1 oz.	Catnip	1 oz.	Mint	1/2 oz.
		Gravel Root	1 oz.	Corn Silk	1 oz.

GALLBLADDER CLEANSE

DAY 1: Cut out all meat-flesh or fowl.

DAY 2: Cut out all dairy products. Continue eating other foods.

DAY 3: Cut out all nuts and seeds.

DAY 4: Cut out all legumes, tofu and tofu products as well.

DAY 5: Cut out all grains.

DAY 6: Cut out all vegetables.

DAY 7: Cut out all fruits and drink nothing but apple juice; if allergic reaction to apple or oranges, use cranberry.

FOR 3 DAYS: Drink 8 ounces of juice every 2 hours with the 2 capsules of Barberry Bark. This will soften the stones. Drink lots of water in between. Take an enema or colima every night.

ON THE EVENING OF THE 3RD DAY:

Take 4 ounces of olive oil and 4 ounces of lemon juice. Go to bed.

Next morning you should pass an oily bowel movement with green stones.

Go back to eating starting with vegetables as of day #6 above, reintroducing foods of day 6 through day 1 consecutively. You are back to normal eating. Be kind to yourself.

Self-Care

Compresses with essential oils

Colon cleanse

Fasting

Castor oil pack

Basti oil enema

Gall Bladder cleanse

GLAUCOMA

A condition of the eye in which increased pressure results in an imbalance between production and outflow of fluid. In acute glaucoma, obstruction to outflow is the main factor responsible for the imbalance. Since collagen is the most generous protein in the body, in the eye it gives strength to the tissues. Faulty collagen metabolism is often associated with this condition. Symptoms include eye discomfort or pain, blurred vision, poor night vision, poor peripheral vision and/or halos around lights. Vatas may experience extreme pain and nausea; Pittas may experience redness and blurred vision; and Kaphas may experience vomiting with whitish mucous.

Feelings and Emotions: Not wanting to see clearly.

Diet	Vitamin & Minerals (Daily)	Essential Oils (always dilute)	Herbs	Alternative Therapy	Avoid
Ayurvedic diet for body type	C & Bioflavonoids: 10,000-15,000 mg.	Sandalwood: PV-Ko	Bhringaraj: VPK=	Marijuana extract: -need a doctor's	Belladonna
	E: 400 IU		Triphala: VP-Ko	prescription	Dairy
	Bioflavonoids: 1 gm.	**Hydrosol (essential oil water):**	Bibhitaki: KP-Vo		Red meat
	Corticosteroids	Lavender: PK-Vo	Chrysanthemum: PK-V+	Massage	Tobacco
Oranges	B-Complex: 150 mg.	Rose: VPK=	Eyebright: PK-V+	Netra Basti	Coffee
	A: 50,000 IU		Bilberry: VPK-	Acupuncture	Black tea
	Thiamine: 100 mg.				Stress
	Pantothenic Acid: 100 mg. 3 x day				
Grapefruit	Rutin: 50-mg. 3 x day				
	Trikatu: 2 tablets				
All citrus	3 x day before meals				
	Zinc (sulfate): 50 mg.				

Glaucoma Herbal Brew

See directions for preparing herbal brew on page 409

VATA

Chrysanthemum	1 oz.
Licorice	2 oz.
Lemon Peel	1 oz.

EYEWASH #1
Make an infusion:

Chrysanthemum	2 tsp.
Eyebright	2 tsp.

Strain, using a fine cotton cloth in strainer. Cool.
Fill an eyecup and wash eye 3-4 times per day.
Store leftover in refrigerator.

NETRA BASTI

Make ghee, heat to body temperature 98.6°-100° F.
Make thick bread dough (1/4 pound of flour and water).
Roll into a donut and place around the eye as a dam while lying on your back with one eye facing straight up.
Pour warm ghee into eye dam. With eyes open, look in all directions and relax for 5-10 minutes.
Drain by piercing dam with finger on outer side and draining ghee into small bowl or cup. Repeat on other eye.

PITTA & KAPHA

Eyebright	1 oz.
Chrysanthemum	2 oz.

EYEWASH #2
Make an infusion:

Triphalla Powder only 4 tsp.

Strain, using a fine cotton cloth in strainer. Cool.
Store leftover in refrigerator.
Fill an eyecup and wash eye 3-4 times per day.

Self-Care

Yoga (avoid inverted postures)
Topical application of Vitamin C
Eye Exercises

GOUT

This a type of arthritis caused by an increased concentration of uric acid in the body fluids. Inflammation is caused by uric acid crystals in the joints, kidneys, tissues and tendons. Gout is considered to be the "Rich Man's Disease". Nearly one-half of all first gout attacks occur in the first joint of the big toe. Pitta will experience burning inflammation and pain; Vata will find dryness of the toes and nails; while Kapha retains water throughout the foot and ankle.

Feelings and Emotions: Impatience, the desire to control events

Cell Salts: Sodium Sulfate

Diet	Vitamin & Minerals (Daily)	Essential Oils (always dilute)	Herbs	Alternative Therapy	Avoid
Ayurveda diet for body type	E: 800 IU Folic Acid: 100 mg. E: 200 mg.	Basil: VK-P+ Birch: PK-V+ Fennel: VPK=	Devil's Claw: PK-V+ Camphor: KV-P+ Mugwort: VK-P+	Colloidal nickel Energy work Therapeutic touch	Meat Wine Alcohol
Plenty of fluids	Potassium: 3000 mg. Phosphorus: 800 mg.	Hyssop: K-P+ Lemon: PV-Ko	Sarsaparilla: PV-Ko Amalaki: PV-Ko	Reflexology Homeopathics	Aspirin Excess of food
Cherries	Glutamic Acid: 200 mg. Magnesium: 1000 mg.	Nutmeg: VK-P+ Thyme: VK-P+	Gokshura: PK-Vo+ Guggul: VK-P+		Trauma Purines
Blueberries	C: 2500 mg. Niacin: 200 mg. Iron: 40 mg.	Cyperus: PKV- Juniper: VK-P+	Pippali: VK-P+ Skullcap: PK-Vo Valerian: VK-P+		Organ meats Yeast Poultry
Vegetarian diet	Pantothenic Acid: 8000 mg. Calcium: 1500 mg. 2-week vitamin therapy Germanium: 200 mg.		Blue Violet: VK-P+ Burdock: VKP+ Gentian Root: VKP+ Yarrow: VKP+		Lentils Anchovies Fats Overweight Protein

Ginger:
Refined carbohydrates
Protein supplements

Plantain: VKP+
Wood Betony: VKP+
Broom: VKP+
Buckthorn Bark: VKP+

See directions for preparing herbal brew on page 409

Gout Herbal Brew

VATA

Sarsaparilla	2 oz.
Amalaki	2 oz.
Ginger	2 oz.
Valerian	1 oz.

PITTA

Burdock	2 oz.
Gokshura	2 oz.
Yarrow	1 oz.
Skullcap	1 oz.
Plantain	1 oz.

KAPHA

Plantain	1 oz.
Ginger	2 oz.
Burdock	1 oz.
Guggul	1 oz.
Gokshura	2 oz.

Self-Care

Foot baths
Colon Cleanse

HEADACHE

This is a symptom rather than a disease. The possible causes of headaches include eyestrain, stress, tension, musculoskeletal problems, misaligned spine, sinus or ear infections, high blood pressure, allergies, caffeine withdrawal or coffee toxicity, P.M.S., chocolate, hormonal fluctuations, an imbalance in arteries in the head, TMJ problems, changes in barometric pressure, overdoses of vitamin A, low blood sugar, and hangovers. To treat headaches, you must become a detective. Vata headaches are severe and pounding and are often caused by constipation. Pitta headaches usually occur in the middle of the day and may be burning and throbbing relative to impure blood, anger, irritability, judgements, or too much heat in the body. Kaphas usually wake up with a headache; the pain is dull and could be related to sinus congestion.

Feelings and Emotions: Not being flexible. Stressed. What is it you don't want to do or look at?

Cell Salts: Kali-Phos; Mag-Phos; Natmuri; Silica

Diet	Vitamins & Minerals (Daily)	Essential Oils (always dilute)	Herbs	Alternative Therapy	Avoid
Ayurvedic diet for body type	Quercetin: 500 mg.	Eucalyptus: KV-P+	Feverfew: PK-V+	Acupuncture	Caffeine
	Magnesium: 500 mg.	Menthol: PK-V+	Yellow Jasmine: PK-V+	Massage	Cigarettes
	Evening Primrose: 1000 mg.	Camphor: VK-P+	Everlasting: VPK-	Colonics	Bad food
Rotation diet	A: 150 IU	Juniper: KV-P+ (in excess)	Valerian: VK-P+	Biofeedback	combinations
	B-Complex: 100 mg.	Bergamot: VK-P+	Sweet Woodruff: VPK+	Chiropractic	Wine
Plenty of water	B1: 100 mg.	Hyssop: K-P+Vo	Cayenne Pepper: KV-P+	treatments	Steroids
	B2: 10 mg. per meal	Lavender: PK-Vo	Eucalyptus: VK-P+	Dance	Dairy
Food diary	Pangamic Acid: 100 mg.	Tea Tree: VPK=	Goldenseal: PK-V+	therapy	Wheat
	Pantothenic Acid: 100 mg.	Cajeput: KV-P+	Willow Bark: PK-V+	Shiatsu	Beef

C: 1000 mg.
E: 1200 IU
Calcium: 1,500 mg.
Iron: 80 mg.
Potassium: 3,000 mg.
Natural Lithium: 300 mg.
Megadophilus:
  3 x day

Lemon: PV-Ko
Peppermint: PK-Vo
Geranium: PK-V+
Ginger: VK-P+
Chamomile: PK-V+

Peppermint: KP-Vo
Ginger: VK- P+

Trager work
Cranial sacral
Electrical
  stimulation

Blended Oils:
(do not dilute)
- *Headache Free: VPK-

Product of Earth Essentials - Florida

Headache Herbal Brew

See directions for preparing herbal brew on page 409

VATA		PITTA		KAPHA	
Ginger	2 oz.	Feverfew	2 oz.	Jasmine Flowers	2 oz.
Valerian	1 oz.	Sweet Woodruff	1 oz.	Mint	1 oz.
Eucalyptus	1 oz.	Willow Bark	1 oz.	Guduchi	1 oz.
Shatavari	1 oz.	Mint	1 oz.	Willow Bark	1 oz.
		Guduchi	1 oz.		

BATH

Rosemary   10 drops
Eucalyptus   10 drops
Lavender   10 drops

CINNAMON-GINGER PASTE

Cinnamon   1/2 tsp.
Ginger   1/2 tsp.
Water   2 Tbs.

Mix well. Apply to the head. Let dry for 5 minutes. Wash off. Add a cool cloth over the area.

HEADACHE-FREE

Essential oil blend (available through Earth Essentials Florida) can be directly applied to the area of pain. Massage. Keep away from the eyes. At night, massage the neck.

Self-Care

Meditation	Tai Chi	Food diary
Visualization	Yoga	Compresses at night with essential oils of your choice
Relaxation techniques	Dance	Diffusing essential oils at night
Hot baths	Basti oil enemas	Inhalation of relaxing oil blends

HEART ATTACK

When an adequate blood supply can no longer reach the heart, part of the heart muscle dies from lack of oxygen and other nutrients. This is classified as a heart attack or myocardial infarction. Individuals who have experienced heart attacks best describe the symptoms as an extreme tightening across the chest region or a feeling of heaviness in the chest/heart area. There may be radiating pain down left arm. Vata may experience tremors, extreme pain, contractions in the chest area, constipation, and dry cough; prone to myocarditis and pericarditis. Pitta may experience sweating, burning pain in chest, fever, and poor sleep patterns; prone to congestive heart failure. Kapha may experience a feeling of heaviness around the heart, difficulty with walking, congestion, phlegm, and tiredness; prone to cardiac arrest.

Feelings and Emotions: "Life pressing on my chest." Stressed, angry, always doing something. Attached. Holding on.

Cell Salts: Calcium Fluoride

Diet	Vitamin & Minerals (Daily)	Essential Oils (always dilute)	Herbs	Alternative Therapy	Avoid
Ayurvedic diet for body type	Linseed Oil - 200 mg.	Cypress: VPK+	Thyme: VK-P+	Bio-feedback	Stress
	E: 500 IU	Geranium: PK-V+	Hyssop: K-P+	Massage	Smoking
	D: 600 IU	Ginger: VK-P+	Cinnamon Bark:VK-P+	Acupuncture	Alcohol
	A:15,000 IU	Lavender: PK-Vo	Skullcap: PK-Vo	Color therapy	Cadmium
When high Vata,	B-Complex: 100 mg.	Rosemary: KV-P+	Arjuna: PK-V+	Chiropractic	Oral
do Kapha-Pitta	C: 25,000 mg.	Ylang-Ylang: PV-K+	Ashwagandha: VK-P+	treatments	contraceptives
diet with	F: 200 mg.	Melissa: KP-Vo	Guggul: KV-P+	Tarpana	Saturated fats
cooked foods		Orange: VK-P+	Vervain: PK-V+	Shirodhara	Gaining weight
		Peppermint: PK-Vo	Saffron: VPK=	Pancha Karma	Sugar
Drink colloidal		Rose: VPK=	Tansy: PK-Vo	Chelation therapy	Suppressing
water		Myrrh: KV-P+	Hawthorn Berries: V-KoP+		emotions
			Noni Juice: VPK-		

Greasy foods
Red meat
Table salt
Dairy

Sandalwood: PV-Ko
Angelica: VPK=
Borage: PKV+
Cardamon: VK-P+
(in excess)

Cardamon: VK-P+
Licorice: VP-K+
Comfrey: VP-K+
Solomon's Seal: PV-K+
Gotu Kola: VPK=
Motherwort: PK-V+
Blue Cohosh: KV-P+
Cayenne: KV-P+
Coriander: VPK-
Goldenseal: PK-V+
Sorrel: VKoP+
Valerian: VK-P+

See directions for preparing herbal brew on page 409

Heart Attack Herbal Brew

VATA TEA (*drink warm*)

Dashmoola	1 oz.
Ginger, fresh	1 oz.
Ashwagandha	2 oz.
Licorice	1 oz.
Guduchi	1 oz.
Sorrel	1 oz.
Hawthorn Berries	2 oz.

PITTA TEA (*drink at room temperature*)

Solomon Seal	2 oz.
Coriander	1 oz.
Gotu Kola	2 oz.
Licorice	1 oz.
Colloidal silver	30 drops

KAPHA TEA (*drink warm*)

Cardamon	2 oz.
Hawthorn Berries	2 oz.
Motherwort	1 oz.
Blue Cohosh	1 oz.
Chitrak	1 oz.

HERBAL FORMULA #1

Arjuna Powder	1/2 Tbs.
Dashmoola	1/2 tsp.
Triphalla Powder	1/2 tsp.
Guggul	1/4 tsp.

Mix all ingredients together with water as a tea; or put in a capsule. Take 3 times per day.

Vata & Kapha: Take with 6 Triphalla tablets at bedtime.

CHEST MASSAGE AT NIGHT

Sandalwood essential oil mixed into base oil,10 drops

Vata - use Sesame oil base

Pitta - use Sunflower oil base

Kapha - use castor oil base

Self-Care

Visualization

Relaxation techniques

Spend time in nature

Yoga

Meditation

Wearing gemstones:
ruby, garnet, gold, silver, pearl, moonstone, emerald, jade, yellow sapphire, yellow topaz

Experiencing love

Parasite cleanse

HERBAL FORMULA #2

Guduchi	1/2 tsp.
Arjuna	1/2 tsp.
Punarnava	1 tsp.
Shatavari	1 tsp.

Mix with 1 cup milk, rice milk, or soymilk.

HEMORRHOIDS (PILES)

Consists of a varicose and inflamed condition of the veins at the lower end of the bowel. Hemorrhoids can be divided into three types: external, internal and mixed. External piles, found outside the bowel, are covered by skin that is brown or purple in color. Internal piles are within the opening covered by a mucous membrane and are red or cherry colored. Mixed piles are situated on the margin and covered half by skin, half by mucous membrane. Pittas can experience much redness, inflammation, swelling, and bleeding with burning and diarrhea. Pain involves the bladder and all around the thigh area, with dry skin around the rectum and constipation. Kaphas may experience large, white swollen hemorrhoids, with mucus on the stool. Vatas experience dryness and cracking with sharp pain.

Feelings and Emotions: Anal-retentive. Holding on.
Cell Salts: Calcium Fluoride

Diet	Vitamin & Minerals (Daily)	Essential Oils (always dilute)	Herbs	Alternative Therapy	Avoid
Ayurvedic diet for body type	A: 25,000 IU B-Complex: 200 mg.	Cypress: VKP+ Cajeput: KV-P+	Bayberry: KV-P+ Aloe Vera Gel: VPK=	Acupuncture Reiki	Constipation Carbohydrates
	C: 2,000 mg.	Lavender: PK-Vo	Calamus: VK-P+	Therapeutic touch	Sedentary lifestyle
Plenty of fluids	E: 600 IU Bioflavinoids: 200 mg.	Myrrh: VK-P+ Tea Tree: VPK=	Black Pepper: KV-P+ Yellow Dock: PK-V+		Sitting in upright chair
	Calcium: 800 mg.	Chamomile: VPK-	Haritaki: VK-Po		
Low cellulose		Basil: VK-P+	Alum Root: PK-V+		
		Clary Sage: VPK-	Pomegranate: PK-Vo		
Salads		Frankincense: KV-P+	Red Raspberry: PK-V+		
		Helichrysum: PKV+	Marshmallow: PV-K+		
		Juniper: KV-P+	Mullein: PK-V+		

Green vegetables

Fresh fruits

Radish juice

Patchouli: VP-K+
Peppermint: PK-Vo
Yarrow: PK-V+
Tagetes: VK-P+

Ginseng: V-KPo
Astralagus: PVK+
Black Cohosh: PK-V+
Basil: VK-P+
Dry Ginger: KV-P+
Turmeric: KV-Po
Amalaki: PV-Ko
Trikatu: VK-Po
Triphala: PVK
Guggul: KV-P+

Hemorrhoids Herbal Blend

VATA	
Astralagus	2 oz.
Basil	1 oz.
Pippali	1 oz.
Ginger	1 oz.

PITTA	
Chamomile	2 oz.
Mullein	1 oz.
Yarrow	1 oz.

KAPHA	
Pomegranate	2 oz.
Basil	1 oz.
Pippali	1 oz.

See directions for preparing herbal brew on page 409

PITTA & KAPHA SUPPOSITORY RECIPE

1/2 oz. Witch Hazel Leaf or Bark
1/2 oz. Oak Bark (powdered)
1 oz. Cocoa Butter

VATA SUPPOSITORY RECIPE

Tumeric Powder	1/2 oz.
Aloe Vera gel	1/2 tsp.
Slippery Elm	1/2 tsp.

PITTA & KAPHA (cont'd)

Grind herbs

Melt cocoa butter in frying pan.

Add herbs

Remove from fire

Add essential oils: 5 drops of cypress

Form into bullet shaped suppositories 1/2" in diameter, 1" long

Lay on plate. Cover. Place in refrigerator to harden

VATA & KAPHA RECIPE

1 oz. vegetable oil

Add 5 drops Cypress essential oil (or any suggested essential oil)

Rub into anus and inject small amount with rectal syringe (or baby ear syringe)

Self-Care

Warm sitz bath

Witch hazel compresses

Wear pearls

Place 4-5 pears in water overnight and drink the water.

Ice packs

Crush black sesame seeds (3-4 gms.) in hot water and take a sitz bath.

When sitting for long periods, use a pillow

Vitamin E on rectum

VATA (cont'd)

n blender, mix 2 Tablespoons aloe vera gel with:

Ghee   2 tsp.

Castor oil   2 tsp.

Apply in rectal area

Refrigerate leftover

Use each night until well

HEPATITIS

A virus or bacteria that has several types: A, B, non-A, and non-B being the most common. Hepatitis A is transmitted mostly through fecal contamination. Hepatitis B is transmitted through infected blood or blood products and, occasionally, through saliva or sexual fluids. Hepatitis non-A and non-B is contacted most often through blood transfusions. Hepatitis can also be caused by Type D virus, cytomegaloveries and Epstein-Barr virus. Pitta usually displays the yellow eyes and fever, while the distinguishing characteristic in Vata is pain, loss of appetite, anger, and resentment.

Feelings and Emotions: Anger. Lashing out and dumping emotions onto others.

Cell Salts: Sodium Phosphates

Diet	Vitamin & Minerals (Daily)	Essential Oils (always dilute)	Herbs	Alternative Therapy	Avoid
Ayurvedic diet for body type	A: 1000 mg. C: 10-50 mg. B12: shots	Chamomile: PK-Vo Cinnamon: VK-P+ Cypress: VPK+	Aloe Vera: VPK= Barberry: PK-V+ Dandelion: PK-V+	Lymphatic drainage massage Homeopathics	Saturated fats Sugar Flour
Low in saturated fats	Folic Acid: 100 mg. Liver Extract: 500 mg. 3 x day	Eucalyptus: KV-P+ Melaleuca: VKP Peppermint: PK-Vo	Gentian: PK-V+ Rhubarb: PK-V+ Goldenseal: PK-V+	Acupuncture Chiropractic Ayurvedic	Fruit juice Honey Animal fat
Anti-Pitta diet	Choline: 1 gm. 3 x day Methionine: 1 gm. 3 x day Free Form Amino Acid:	Patchouli: VP-K+ Rosemary: KV-P+ Ginger: VK-P+	Amalaki: PV-Ko Bhringaraj: VKP= Manjishta: PK-V+	consultation	Meat Marijuana Cigarettes
Raw green vegetables & sprouts	2 gm. 3 x day Pangamic Acid: 100 mg. F: 200 mg.	Rose: VPK=	Ginger: VK-P+ Milk Thistle: PK-V+ Rose: VPK=		Amphetamines Hot, spicy, sour & salty foods

Green juices

Kicharee

Anger
Resentment
Depression
Fish

Licorice: VP-K+
Horsetail: PK-V+
Turmeric: KV-Po
Coriander: VPK-
Guduchi: PK-V+
Sudan Shan: PKV
Chiretta: VPK-
Katuka: VKP+

See directions for preparing herbal brew on page 409

Hepatitis Herbal Brew

VATA

Amla	1 oz.
Ginger	2 oz.
Licorice	1 oz.
Milk Thistle	2 oz.
Rose Petals	1 oz.

PITTA

Dandelion	1 oz.
Barberry	2 oz.
Katuka	2 oz.
Guduchi	1 oz.
Licorice	1 oz.

KAPHA

Guduchi	1 oz.
Ginger	2 oz.
Manjishta	2 oz.
Horsetail	1 oz.
Coriander	1 oz.

Add 10 drops goldenseal extract to 1 cup tea.

Liver Flush

VATA & KAPHA

Cayenne	1/2 tsp.
Ginger	1/2 tsp.
Aloe Vera	3 Tbs.
Lemon	1 juiced
Olive oil	2 Tbs.
Orange	1 fresh

Mix in blender. Drink first thing in the morning.

PITTA & KAPHA

Coriander	1/2 tsp.
Barberry	1/2 tsp.
Aloe Vera	3 Tbs.
Lemon	1 juiced
Olive oil	2 Tbs.
Apple	1 fresh

Mix in blender. Drink first thing in the morning.

Self-Care

Liver flush

Compresses

Dry skin brushing

Rebounder

HOT FLASHES

A condition that occurs with the onset of menopause and is accompanied by a decrease in estrogen levels. Hot flashes usually affect the head and upper body, but can cover the torso or entire body. The length and duration of hot flashes vary from a few seconds to more than ten minutes. After a hot flash, a woman can feel slightly damp or thoroughly drenched in perspiration; this occurs most commonly in Pitta types.

Feelings and Emotions: Stress. Lacking in trust.

Diet	Vitamin & Minerals (Daily)	Essential Oils (always dilute)	Herbs	Alternative Therapy	Avoid
Pitta diet	B-Complex: 200 mg.	Basil: VK-P+	Valerian: VK-P+	Biofeedback	Hot rooms
	C: 1300 mg.	Thyme: VK-P+	Wild Yam: VP-Ko	Homeopathics	Heat
	Magnesium: 2000 mg.	Lavender: PK-Vo	Red Clover: PK-V+	Dance therapy	Stress
Eat small meals	Potassium: 200 mg.	Calamus: VK-P+	Oatstraw: PV-K+	Massage	Tension
Salads	E: 1200 IU	Sage: VK-P+	Chickweed: PK-V+		Caffeine
Wild yams	Selenium: 200 mg.	Rose: VPK=	Elder: PK-Vo		Hot drinks
Cooling food	Bioflavenoids: 200 mg.	Myrrh: VK-P+	Violet: PK-V+		Tobacco
Soybeans	Black Current Oil: 100 mg.	Bergamot: VK-P+	Dandelion: KP-V+		Marijuana
Greens	Evening Primrose Oil:	Clary Sage: VKP-	Yellow Dock: PK-V+		Spicy foods
Protein	500 mg.	Fennel: VPK=	Black Cohosh: VK-P+		Acid foods
	D: 500 mg.	Peppermint: PK-Vo	Vitex: VKP-		Alcohol
	Iron: 30 mg.		Dong Quai: VK-Po		Fats
	B3: 100 mg.		Sage: VK-P+		
			Licorice: PV-Ko		

HERBS - Continued

Damiana: K-Vo-P+
Saffron: VPK=
Manjishta: PK-V+
Ginseng; V-KPo
Shatavari: PV-K+
+++Womans Treasure

Black Haw: VKP+
Alfalfa: PK-V+
Raspberry: PK-V+
Black Currant: PK-V+
Wormwood: PK-Vo
Fenugreek: VK-P+
Blessed Thistle: PK-V+
Elder Flower: PK-Vo
Chaparral: PK-V+

+++ *Product of Planetary Formulas*

Hot Flash Herbal Brew

VATA

Fenugreek	2 oz.
Shatavari	2 oz.
Valerian	1 oz.
Vitex	2 oz.
Licorice	1 oz.

PITTA

Red Clover	2 oz.
Vitex	2 oz.
Licorice	1 oz.
Red Raspberry	1 oz.
Alfalfa	1 oz.

KAPHA

Blessed Thistle	2 oz.
Elder Flowers	1 oz.
Sage	1 oz.
Red Clover	1 oz.
Damiana	1 oz.

See directions for preparing herbal brew on page 409

Self-Care

Cool footbaths
Exercise
Yoga: sun salutation
Mantra

Cool full body baths
Meditation
Essential oil patches
Breathing exercises

Wear silk
Positive mental attitude
Meditation

HYPOGLYCEMIA

Hypoglycemia represents a sudden drop in blood sugar. The brain is highly dependent on glucose as an energy source. A drop in blood sugar results in the release of hormones that work to increase those blood sugar levels, with adrenaline being one of those hormones. Vatas may experience tremors, anxiety, nausea, headaches, and dizziness. Pittas experience sweating, extreme hunger and an increase in heart rate; Kaphas experience clouded vision, confusion, and tiredness.

Feelings and Emotions: A powerless victim. Feeling "less than".

Diet	Vitamins & Minerals (Daily)	Essential Oils (always dilute)	Herbs	Alternative Therapy	Avoid
Ayurvedic diet for body type	B-Complex: 100 mg.	Ginger: VK-P+	St. John's Wort: PK-V+	Massage	Alcohol
	B-12: 1000 mcg.	Anise: VK-P+	Shatavari: PV-K+	Acupuncture	Skipping meals
	C: 3,000 mg.	Cardamon: VK-P+	Dong Quai: VK-Po	Reflexology	Candy bars
Low animal protein	Folic Acid: 800 mcg.	Basil: VK- P+	Barberry: PK-V+		Refined carbohydrates
	Magnesium: 340 mg. for 6 weeks	Rosemary: VK-P+	Aloe Vera: VPK=		Coffee
Shitaki mushrooms	Amino Acid Liquids: 1000 mg.	Oregano: VKP+	Trikatu: VK-P+		Marijuana
		Thyme: VK- P+	Triphala: VKPo		Chocolate
Blue-Green Algae	Alpa: 400 mg.	Geranium: PK-V+	Calumba: PK-V+		Milk
	Potassium: 200 mg.	Lemongrass: PK-Vo	Gentian: PK-V+		Goldenseal
	Digestive Aid: Best to take 2 before mealtime	Sandalwood: PV-Ko	Golden Thread: PK-V+		Black Tea
Frequent small meals	Comfrey/Pectin: before meals	Yarrow: PK-V+	Guduchi: PKV+		Soft Drinks
Bitter greens	2 tablets 2-x day		White Poplar: PK-V+		
			Peruvian Bark: PK-V+		
			Katuka: PVK		
			Neem: PK-V+		

Shilajit: K-VP+
Chiarata: PVK-
Yellow Dock: PK-V+
Hawthorn Berries: V-KoP+
Cardamon: VK-P+
Clove: VK-P+

Low carbohydrates	
Cinnamon	Chromium: 200 mg.
	Manganese: 200 mg.
	Aloe Vera Gel: 1 Tbs. 3 x per day with lemon & apple juice
Peanut butter	L-Tryptophan: 6 gms.
Spirulina	Bee Pollen: 1 tsp. per day

See directions for preparing herbal brew on page 409

Hypoglycemia Herbal Brew

VATA		PITTA		KAPHA	
Angelica	2 oz.	Nettles	2 oz.	Cardamom	2 oz.
Astralagus	2 oz.	Lemongrass	1 oz.	Ginger	1 oz.
Oat Straw	2 oz.	Licorice	1 oz.	Licorice	1 oz.
Ginger	1 oz.	Astralagus	2 oz.	Peppermint	2 oz.
Ashwagandha	2 oz.	Peppermint	2 oz.	Lemongrass	2 oz.
Licorice	1 oz.				

Pancreatic Soup

VATA		PITTA		KAPHA	
Ginger	2 inches	Green beans (cut in small pieces)		Spinach	1 bunch
Sweet Potatoes	1	Brussel sprouts	1/4 lb.	Ginger, fresh	2 inch
Carrots	4	Kale	1 bunch	Kale	1 bunch
Beet & Greens	1	Shitaki mushrooms	4 oz.	Brussel sprouts	1/4 lb.
Celery stalks	4	Sweet potato	1	Celery	4 stalks
Shitaki mushrooms	4 oz.	Mint	1/4 bunch	Parsley	1/2 bunch
Asparagus	1/2 lb.	Cilantro	1/2 bunch	Carrots	3
Turmeric	2 tsp.	Coriander	3 tsp.	Lemongrass	2 tsp.
Tomato	3	Water	1 quart	Onions	1
Onions	1			Garlic	2-3 cloves
Water	1 quart			Cumin	1/2 tsp.
				Water	1 quart

Chop all ingredients. Add potatoes, carrots and mushrooms (hardy vegetables) to the water. Bring to a boil. Sauté all herbs in ghee. Add sautéed herbs and greens to the pot of soup. Simmer for two hours.

DRINK

In a blender, mix 2 tsp. Aloe Vera Gel, the juice of 1 lemon. Add 4-oz. apple juice. Blend.

Self-Care

Massage feet with Immune Free* essential oils.   *Product of Earth Essential Florida

Tai Chi	Yoga	Walking
Sunbathing	MeditationI	Breathwork

INDIGESTION

Indigestion is when you experience burning and gas. This can be caused by too little hydrochloric acid as well as too much. It is more common for Pittas to experience hyperacidity with belching caused by sour food and too many sweets. Vatas can experience low hydrochloric acid and more gas fermentation due to weak digestion. Kaphas can experience excess mucous due to slow digestion. To determine if indigestion is excess acidity or lack of acidity, test your saliva with nitrosine paper. Average reading below 6.8 pH = hyperacidity. Average reading above 7.2 pH = lack of acidity.

Feelings and Emotions: Unable to bring thoughts and desires into reality

Cell Salts: Potassium Phosphate

Diet	Vitamin & Minerals (Daily)	Essential Oils (always dilute)	Herbs	Alternative Therapy	Avoid
Ayurvedic diet for body type	B-Complex: 100 mg. B1: 100 mg. B3: 100 mg.	Coriander: VPK- Bay: VKP+ Ginger: VK-P+	Asafoetida: VK-P+ Dill: PK-Vo Aloe Vera Gel: VPK=	Rotation diet Dairy diet Ayurvedic consultation	Coffee Tobacco Fats Beans Antacids
Small, frequent meals	B12: 400 mcg. Acidophilus: 2 tablets 30 minutes before meal	Cinnamon: VK-P+ Basil: VK-P+ Clove: KV-P+	Licorice: VP-K+ Black Pepper: VK-P+ Pippali: VK-P+		
Take time to chew	Lecithin: 800 mg. Digestive Enzymes:	Ajwan: VK-P+ Thyme: VK-P+	Mint: PK-Vo Coriander: VPK=		
Do not drink with meals	Papain - 2 before meals Amino Acids: 2 with meals	Mint: PK-Vo Angelica: VPK=,P+ Cardamon: VK-P+ Fennel: VPK=	Ajwan: VK-P+ Slippery Elm: VP-K+ Trikatu: VK-P+ Comfrey: PV-K+		
Bananas	Bromelain: 2 before meals	Peppermint: PK-Vo	Hingastash: VK-Po		

Cabbage juice   HCL: 2 tablets with
                 protein meal

Indigestion Herbal Brew

See directions for preparing herbal brew on page 409

VATA

Comfrey	1 oz.
Ginger	1/2 oz.
Cinnamon	1/2 oz.
Licorice	1/2 oz.

PITTA

Coriander	1 oz.
Fennel	1/2 oz.
Mint	1/2 oz.
Licorice	1/2 oz.

KAPHA

Clove	1 oz.
Ginger	1 oz.
Black Pepper	1/2 oz.
Coriander	1/2 oz.

Drink three cups per day before meals.

Drink First Thing in the Morning

VATA-KAPHA

Lemon	1 oz.
Ginger, fresh	2 inch piece
Water	3 cups

Blend all together. Strain. Drink.

PITTA & KAPHA

Lemon	1 oz.
Fennel or Coriander	1 tsp.

Blend all together. Strain. Drink.

VATA

Take hing (1/16 tsp. with ghee. Mix together. Follow with water - 3 times per day)

ESSENTIAL OIL FORMULA

Angelica	2 drops	Fennel	3 drops
Cardamon	2 drops	Peppermint	2 drops
Vegetable oil	2 oz.		

Mix together. Place 2 drops in 8-oz. water. Drink daily. Only use good quality essential oils when taking orally.

OLD TIME REMEDY

Baking soda	2 Tbs.
Water	8 oz. glass

DILL INFUSION

Dill	4 tsp.
Water	8 oz. glass

Boil water. Place herbs in container. Then add water to dill in container. Steep 15 minutes. Take 4 times per day.

Self-Care

Cook all beans with hing

Compress over the stomach area

Diet diary

INFECTION

Caused by a foreign organism entering the body, which the body is unable to destroy due to a weakened immune system. Infections can spread into other body parts as well as the blood, and become systemic. Pitta experiences swollen glands, boils, and redness; Vata may get a sore throat, dry cough, dizziness, and headaches; Kapha is plagued by respiratory and sinus problems.

Feelings and Emotions: I am weak. I am a victim.

Diet	Vitamin & Minerals	Essential Oils (always dilute)	Herbs Therapy	Alternative	Avoid
Immune support	A: 75,000 IU (until clear)	Thyme: VK-P+	Astralagus: VK-P+	Color therapy	Allergic foods
	Zinc: 50 mg.	Eucalyptus: KV-P+	Burdock: PK-V+	Colonics	Dairy
Yellow foods	C: 10,000 mg.	Oregano: VK-P+	Golden seal: PK-V+	Music therapy	Sugars
	Potassium: 1,000 mg.	Rosemary: KV-P+	Rosehips: V-PK+		Canned foods
Juice fasts	Bioflavinoids: 250 mg.	Saffron: VPK-	Manjishta: PK-V+		Meats
	Colloidal Silver: PK-V+	*Immune-Free: VP-K+	Katuka: PK-V+		
Vata immune			Echinacea: KP-V+		
soup			Bayberry: KV-P+		
			Isatis: VKP+		
Cleansing diet			Tumeric: KV-Po		
			Coriander: VKP=		
			Dandelion: KP-V+		
			Amla: PV-Ko		
			**ImmuniTea: VP-K+		
			Juniper Berries: KV-P+		
			(drink a lot of water)		

* *Product of Earth Essentials Florida*
** *Product of UniTea Herbs*

Infection Herbal Brew

See directions for preparing herbal brew on page 409

VATA		PITTA & KAPHA	
Amla	1 oz.	Barberry	1 oz.
Ginger	1 oz.	Fennel	2 oz.
Astralagus	2 oz.	Dandelion	2 oz.
Rosehips	2 oz.	Coriander	1 oz.
		Burdock	1 oz. (Kapha only)

Add goldenseal extract - 15 drops. Drink 6 cups per day, until symptoms are gone.

Self-Care

Warm & cold baths with essential oils

Colon cleanse

Steam

Rebounder

Dry skin brushing

INFLAMMATION

This is a heating condition in the body and is caused by injury, trauma, accident, toxic blood (Ama), stress, or infection. The internal organs can also become inflamed. This condition is more common for Pitta types.

Feelings and Emotions: Not feeling centered in life.

Cell Salts: Ferr Phos; Iron Phosphate

Diet	Vitamin & Minerals	Essential Oils (always dilute)	Herbs	Alternative Therapy	Avoid
Ayurveda Diet for body type	B Complex: 200 mg. B5: 2,500 mg. B12: 300 mg.	Lavender: PK-Vo Chamomile (blue): PV-K+ Cyperus: VPK-	Fenugreek: VK-P+ Goldenseal: PK-V+ Hops: PK-V+	Color healing Reiki	Hot, spicy food Alcohol
Raw foods for Pitta & Kapha	E: 150 IU Flaxseed: 500 mg.	Yarrow: PK-V+ Sandalwood: PV-Ko Juniper: KV-P+ (in excess)	Lobelia: K-PV+ Marshmallow: PV-K+ Mugwort: VK-P+	Chiropractic treatments Energy work	Sugar Junk food
Food combining		Geranium: PK-V+ Rose: VPK=	Sarsaparilla: PV-Ko Slippery Elm: VP-K+		
Lots of green juice		Trifolia: VK-P+	Solomon's Seal: PV-K+ Sorrel: V-PK+ Tansy: PK-Vo White Pond Lily: PV-K+ Cyperus: PK-Vo Witch Hazel: PK-V+		

Inflammation Herbal Brew

VATA

Slippery Elm	1 oz.
Sorrel	2 oz.
Fenugreek	2 oz.
Kava Kava	1 oz.

PITTA

Yarrow	2 oz.
Chamomile	2 oz.
Mint	2 oz.
Hops	1 oz.

KAPHA

Fenugreek	2 oz.
Witch Hazel	1 oz.
Chickweed	1 oz.

Smart Weed: PKV+
Hyssop: VK-P+
Chickweed: PK-V+
Gum Arabic: PV-K+
Chamomile: PK-Vo
Yarrow: PK-V+

See directions for preparing herbal brew on page 409

Self-Care

Cold compresses

Ice therapy

Charcoal poultice

INSOMNIA

Insomnia is an inability to sleep soundly and undisturbed. The most common causes of insomnia are anxiety and pain, but it may also be a symptom of a serious disease. A major factor in sleeplessness is linked to the inability to cope with stress.

Feelings and Emotions: Anxious, stressful. Too many fearful thoughts

Homeopathics: Kali Phos (potassium phosphate)

Diet	Vitamin & Minerals (Daily)	Essential Oils (always dilute)	Herbs	Alternative Therapy	Avoid
Ayurvedic diet for body type	B-Complex: 200 mg.	Lavender: PK-Vo	Hops: PK-V+	TherapeuticTouch	Late night TV
	B6:100 mg.	Chamomile: VPK-	Motherwort: PK-V+	Reiki	Caffeine
	B12: 100 mcg.	Camphor: VK-P+	Mullein: PK-V+	Counseling	Stimulants
Protein	Niacin: 100 mg.	Thyme: VK-P+	Vervain: PK-V+	Massage	Chocolate
Fish	Pantothenic Acid:	Marjoram: VK-P+	Skullcap: PK-Vo	Shirodhara	Soda
Baked potatoes	2,000 mg.	Neroli: VP-K+	Catnip: PK-Vo		Sugar
	C: 3,000 mg.	Rose: VPK=	Kava Kava: PVK		Stress
Sweetened milk	D:500 IU	Sandalwood: PV-Ko	Passion Flower: PK-V+		
	Calcium: 1000 mg. before bedtime	Ylang-Ylang: PV-K+	Valerian: VK-P+		
Bananas	Magnesium: 1000 mg. before bedtime	Orange:VK-P+	Chamomile: PK-Vo		
Herbal teas	Phosphorous: 2000 mg.	Coriander: VKP-	Jatamasi: KV-P+		
		Melissa: KP-Vo	Nutmeg: VK-P+		
Rice & hot sweetened milk	Potassium: 2500 mg.	Mandarin: PK-V+			
	Melatonin: 100 mg.	Rosemary: VK-P+			
	hGH Plus: 2 x per day	Basil: VK-P+			

Wheat	Co Q-10: 100 mg.
Oatmeal	DHEA: 50 mg.
Almonds	
Walnuts	
Oranges, Mandarins	
Raisins	
Foods containing	
Tryptophan	

Insomnia Herbal Brew

VATA

Valerian	1 oz.
Catnip	2 oz.
Nutmeg	2 oz.
Jatamasi	1 oz.

PITTA

Hops	1 oz.
Skullcap	1 oz.
Chamomile	2 oz.
Passion Flower	2 oz.
Gotu Kola	1 oz.

KAPHA

Skullcap	1 oz.
Valerian	1 oz.
Hops	2 oz.
Passion Flower	2 oz.

See directions for preparing herbal brew on page 409

Drink one cup after dinner. At bedtime, add milk.

INSOMNIA BLEND

Basil	1 drop
Lavender	1 drop
Chamomile	1 drop
Ylang Ylang	2 drops

Mix together. Place 2-3 drops on pillow at night.

Self-Care

Enemas

Warm baths

Soft music

Daily aerobic exercise

Massage head and shoulders

Aromatherapy: Diffuse essential oils near bed or put a few drops of essential oil on your pillow

Leisurely walk before bedtime

Hot bath before bed

Meditation

Yoga asana: "crocodile pose" (Makarasan)

Abyangha at night (self massage)

Swimming

Hot milk

Stress reduction techniques

Mantra repetitions

Self-Reiki

KIDNEY STONES

They are abnormal accumulations of mineral salts which form in the kidneys and are sometimes passed into the urinary tract. The formation of these stones may be due to overactivity of the parathyroid gland which causes elevated calcium levels in the blood. Stones are caused by poor diet, a weakening of the pancreas, and the reduction of enzymes. Pitta will manifest acute infections, with wet yellow stones; Vata experiences colon pain with brown to black stones; while Kapha may find puss in their urine, along with stones composed of calcium.

Diet	Vitamin & Minerals (Daily)	Essential Oils (always dilute)	Herbs	Alternative Therapy	Avoid
Ayurvedic diet for body type	A: 10,000 IU (until clear)	Juniper: KV-P+	Parsley: VK-P+	Massage	Dehydration
Apple juice	B2: 200 mg.	Cyperus: PKV-	Thyme: VKP+	Energy work	Infections
Cilantro	B5: 1000 mg.	Orange: VK-P+	Corn Silk: PK-V+	Acupuncture	Prolonged bed rest
Lemon juice	B6: 200 mg.	Lemongrass: PK-Vo	Dandelion: PK-V+		Vitamin B6 deficiency
Water	C: 2500 mg.	Myrtle: KP-V+	Juniper: VK-P+		Magnesium deficiency
Melon	E: 400 IU	Uva Ursi: PK-V+			Vitamin A deficiency
	F: 200 mg.	Marshmallow: PV-K+			Sugar
	Choline: 500 mg.	Horsetail: PK-V+			Food high in oxalic acid
	Potassium: 1000 mg.	Gokshura: PK-Vo			Coffee
	Magnesium: 500 mg.	Manjishta: PK-V+			Black tea
		Buchu Leaves: PK-V+			Red meat
		Plantain: PK-V+			Antacids
		Shilajit: VK-P+			Dairy
		Gravel Root: PK-V+			Alcohol
		Cleavers: PK-V+			Nightshade vegetables
		Pashanbheda: VPK			

Kidney Stone Herbal Brew

See directions for preparing herbal brew on page 409

VATA		PITTA		KAPHA	
Lemongrass	1 oz.	Horsetail	1 oz.	Cornsilk	2 oz.
Coriander	2 oz.	Cilantro	2 oz.	Buchu leaves	1 oz.
Goshkura	1 oz.	Plantain	1 oz.	Lemongrass	2 oz.
Marshmallow	2 oz.	Coriander	2 oz.	Horsetail	1 oz.

Take: 500 grams of Shilajit – 3 times per day with tea

Self-Care

Compresses
Kidney flush
Purgatives
Basti oil enemas

Kidney Stone Program

The following formulae will dissolve kidney stones, is soothing to inflammed tissues and will assist in smooth and painless release of stones.

Kidney Stone Formulae and Ingredients

KB-13 KIDNEY STONE HERBAL TEA BLEND

Hydrangea Root*	1 oz.
Gravel Root	2 oz.
Marshmallow Root	1 oz.

PARSLEY WATER

1 bunch fresh parsley
1 quart distilled water

KB-16 Kidney Herbal Tea Blend

Mix together 3 tsp. of each of the following:

Cornsilk
Horsetail
Uva Ursi
Parsley Root
Juniper Berries
Queen of the Meadow
Cascara Sagrada
Chickweed
Oregon Grape Root
Burdock Root
Chamomile
Cleavers

Cubeb Berries
Kidney Bean Pod
Watermelon Seed
Gravel Root
Golden Seal Root
Stone Root
Buchu
Marshmallow Root

OTHER INGREDIENTS:

2 quarts fresh squeezed apple juice (must be fresh)
2 eye droppers Golden Rod Tincture (optional)
2 Tablespoons Black Cherry Concentrate (optional)
1 Gallon Distilled Water

* *If allergic to Hydrangea Root, substitute Parsley Root*
** *If pain exists, add Lobelia and Ginger Root to regular formulae*

INSTRUCTIONS FOR PREPARATION

Mix together 4 oz. (1/2 cup) KB-13 Kidney Stone Herbal Tea Blend, and 4 oz. (1/2 cup) KB-16 Kidney Herbal Tea Blend. Soak for 4 hours (or overnight) in 1 gallon distilled water. Heat to boiling and then simmer for 15-20 minutes. Cool, strain and refrigerate "herbal mixture" for future use.

Parsley Water: Boil 1/2 bunch fresh parsley in 1 quart of distilled water for 3 minutes only. Cool, strain and refrigerate.

Stone Softening Method

Mix together the following Herbal Mixture:

2 quarts fresh squeezed apple juice
9 cups herbal mixture (KB-13 and KB-16) *(Preparation instructions on previous pages)*
1 cup parsley water

*Optional:
2 eyedroppers Golden Rod Tincture
2 Tablespoons Black Cherry Concentrate

INSTRUCTIONS FOR USE

DAY 1: Sip 2 oz. of the Herbal Mixture every hour (for 16 hours) up to one quart (32 oz.) - also drink 32 oz. extra distilled water any time during this period to flush the system.

DAY 2: Sip 1 oz. Herbal Mixture each hour up to 16 oz. Also 32 oz. distilled water and 32 oz. of fresh squeezed juices any time during this period.

DAY 3: Sip 1 oz. Herbal Mixture each hour up to 16 oz. Also 32 oz. distilled water and 32 oz. fresh squeezed juices.

DAY 4: Juice Fast: only consume 64 oz. distilled water and 64 oz. fresh squeezed juices. That's 4 oz. of each every hour for 16 hours.

SPECIAL INSTRUCTIONS

Absolutely no other liquids are allowed, especially alcoholic beverages, sodas or carbonated beverages, black tea, coffee, dairy products and no minerals. Diet during this time should be animal-free. Best is fresh juice fast for the 4 days. If this is not possible, do a raw food diet consisting of raw fruits and vegetables. Best are orange, distilled water with lemon or lime juice, cranberry, watermelon, or combination vegetables with carrot, parsley, garlic and ginger root.

LARYNGITIS

Inflammation of the mucous membrane of the larynx, and may be either acute or chronic. It can come by exposure to cold increasing Vata, or through a congestion extending from the nose above, or from the bronchial tubes causing great redness for Pittas. Kaphas may experience swelling, and Vatas may experience dryness. Vatas may experience dry throat, loss of voice, or hoarseness. Pitta may experience yellow mucous and inflammation with fever. Kaphas may experience swollen throat with much mucous.

Feelings and Emotions: Difficulty with speaking their truth.

Cell Salts: Kali Murr, Potassium Chloride

Diet	Vitamin & Minerals (Daily)	Essential Oils (always dilute)	Herbs	Alternative Therapy	Avoid
Ayurvedic diet for body type	A: 100,000 IU	Benzoin: VPK-	Amla: VP-K+	Breathing therapy	Dairy
	B-Complex: 200 mg.	Sandalwood: VPKo	Goldenseal: PK-V+	Sound therapy	Overexposure to cold
	C: 3000 - 5000 mg.	Cajeput: VK-P+	Echinacea: PK-V+	Lymphatic drainage	Protein foods
Elimination diet	Zinc: 50 mg.	Fennel: VPK=	Rosehips: V-PK+	Chakra annointment	
	Zinc lozenges every 2-3 hours	Anise: VK-P+	Lemon Peel: PV-Ko	Neck massage	
		Lemon: VP-Ko	Purnarnara: PK-V+		
		Thyme: VK-P+	Astragalus: PVK+		
		Oregano: VK-P+	Yarrow: KP-V+		
		Cinnamon: VK-P+	Angelica: VK-Po		
		Clove: VK-P+	Ginger: VK-P+		
		Coriander: VPK-	Boneset: PK-V+		
			Burdock: PK-V+		
			Mint: PK-Vo		

Laryngitis Herbal Brew

VATA		PITTA		KAPHA	
Rosehips	2 oz.	Yarrow	1 oz.	Sage	2 oz.
Lemon Peel or Orange Peel	1 oz.	Mint	1 oz.	Ginger	1 oz.
Astralagus	2 oz.	Burdock	2 oz.	Yarrow	1 oz.
Ginger	1 oz.	Jasmine	1 oz.	Elecampane	1 oz.
Cinnamon	1/2 oz.	Astralagus	1 oz.	Amalaki	2 oz.

See directions for preparing herbal brew on page 409

Add 10 drops of goldenseal tincture per cup for all body types.

Ephedra: K-VP+
Sage: VK-P+
Jasmine: PK-V+
Elecampane: VK-P+
Bibhitaki: KP-Vo
Turmeric: VK-Po
Licorice: VP-K+

GARGLE

4-5 times per day. Add to one cup of water:

Sandalwood   1 drop
Thyme   1 drop
Cajeput   1 drop

INHALATION *See directions for inhalation therapy on page 225*

Repeat every three hours with one of the following oils:

Sandalwood   3 drops
Thyme   3 drops
Cajeput   3 drops

THROAT SWAB

Dilute the oil with water: 50% water & 50% essential oil (use any of the above oils and/or Tea Tree).

Wet a Q tip with the solution.

Dab on tonsil or any area that is inflammed.

Self-Care

Steam bath

Inhalations

Fomentations

Vapor rub throat

LEUCORRHEA

A whitish, brown or yellow vaginal discharge with an abnormal odor and a stickiness. This condition creates irritation and discomfort. More common in Kapha women, yet all body types can be affected. Vata's get dryness with brown discharge and itchiness. Pitta's experience inflammation, external redness, burning, a cheese texture to the discharge, and a sour odor. Kapha's experience thick mucus, swelling and heaviness.

Feelings and Emotions: Feeling unsupported by male energies.

Diet	Vitamin & Minerals (Daily)	Essential Oils (always dilute)	Herbs	Alternative Therapy	Avoid
Ayurvedic diet for body type	A: 75,000 mg. (until clear)	Tea Tree: VPK=	Pau d'Arco: PK-V+	Vaginal massage	Refined sugar
	B-Complex: 4 tablets (yeast free)	Dhavana: VPK-	Goldenseal: KP-V+	Rebirthing	Fructose
Yeast free diet	Biotin: 100 mcg.	Trifolia: VK-P+	Raspberry Leaves: PK-V+	Tarpana	Fruit concentrates
	D: 100 IU		Myrrh: VK-P+		Mushrooms
	Calcium: 800 mg.		Echinacea: PK-V+		Yeasted breads
	Magnesium: 600 mg.		Wild Yam: PV-Ko		Frozen foods
	F: 200 mg.		Prickly Ash: KV-P+		Canned foods
	Evening Primrose: 200 mg.		Alum Root: PK-Vo		Pickles
	Capryllic Acid: 2 tablets		Turmeric: VK-Po		Smoked dried meat
	B6: 200 mg.		Aloe Vera: VPK=		Moldy foods
	Zinc: 40 mg.		Shatavari: PV-K+		
	Iron: 100 mg.		Katuka: KP-V+		
	Megadophilus: 3 x day		Oak Bark: VP-K+		
			Sarsaparilla: PV-Ko		

Leucorrhea Herbal Brew

See directions for preparing herbal brew on page 409

VATA
Wild Yam	1 oz.
Sarsaparilla	1 oz.
Shatavari	1/2 oz.
Prickly Ash	1 oz.

PITTA
Katuka	1 oz.
Raspberry Leaves	1 oz.
Shatavari	1/2 oz.
Wild Yam	1/2 oz.

KAPHA
Katuka	1 oz.
Raspberry Leaves	1 oz.
Sage	2 oz.
Alum Root	1/2 oz.

Drink until condition clears up. Take 10-15 drops of echinacea.

BOLUS OR PESSARY
An ancient herbal form of a vaginal suppository

Coconut oil	1/8 cup
Cocoa butter	1 oz.
Herb of your choice	3 oz.

(My preferences are goldenseal, pau d'Arco, shatavari, alum, myrrh and sage)

Sift all herbs well with a colander. Melt cocoa butter. Add vegetable oil.

Add herbs until mixture thickens. Remove from stove. Add essential oils.

Make into small cylinders, approximately 1/2 the size of your "pinky" in diameter

Place in refrigerator to harden for 1 hour. Remove from refrigerator. Store in container in cool place.

For use: insert into the vagina for 3 hours. Pitta's should wear a panty liner for protection. Remove. Douche to remove excess.

DOUCHE WITH STRONG DECOCTION

Yogurt	1/2 cup
Water	1/4 cup
Apple cider vinegar	1/4 cup
Tea tree essential oil	10 drops

When itching occurs, insert fresh aloe vera into the vagina.

DRYNESS

Essential oils	20 drops
Water	1 cup

Mix well. Soak a tampax. Squeeze excess water, then insert in vagina. Change when dry.

MONONUCLEOSIS

Characterized by chronic fatigue. Indicative of a chronically depressed immune system. It is an infectious disease believed to be caused by a virus. It affects the lymph nodes located in the neck, armpits and groin. Symptoms include sore throat, fever, chills, swollen glands, as well as fatigue.

Feelings and Emotions: Not wanting to deal with life; it's too much.

Diet	Vitamins & Minerals (Daily)	Essential Oils (always dilute)	Herbs	Alternative Therapy	Avoid
Ayurvedic diet for body type	A: 5,000 IU (until clear)	Eucalyptus: KV-P+	Saffron: VPK=	Counseling	Birth control pills
Protein	B1: 150 mg.	Lavender: PK-Vo	Echinacea: KP-V+	Massage	Stress
Fruit	B2: 100 mg.	Blue Chamomile: PV-Ko	Astralagus: VP-K+	Acupuncture	Cigarettes
Mineral water	B6: 200 mg.	Bergamot: VK-P+	Ashwagandha: KV-P+	Pancha karma	X-ray
Brewer's yeast	Biotin: 150 mcg.	Saffron: VPK=	Angelica: VK-Po	Lymphatic drainage	Fat
Eggs	Choline: 150 mg.	*Immune-Free: VPK	Red Root: PK-V+	Chiropractic treatments	Alcohol
Fish	Pantothenic Acid: 200 mg.		Lemon Peel: VP-Ko	Chakra balancing	
Shrimp	C (ascorbate): 6000 mg.		Ginger: VK-P+		
Brown Rice	Potassium: 800 mg.		Red Clover: PK-V+		
Basmati Rice	Cod Liver Oil Caps: 4 at night		Burdock: PK-V+		
Garlic, Onions	Raw Thymus Extract: 30 drops 3x/day		Lemongrass: PK-Vo		
Liver	Raw glandular complex: 40 drops or 2 tablets daily		**ImmuniTea: VP-K+		
Asparagus			Noni Juice: VPK-		

* *Product of Earth Essentials Florida*

** *Product of UniTea Herbs*

Mononucleosis Herbal Brew

See directions for preparing herbal brew on page 409

VATA		PITTA		KAPHA	
Astralagus	1 oz.	Red Root	1 oz.	Burdock	1 oz.
Angelica	1 oz.	Astralagus	2 oz.	Echinacea	1 oz.
Ginger	1 oz.	Coriander	2 oz.	Ginger	2 oz.
Lemon Peel	2 oz.	Echinacea	1 oz.	Lemongrass	1 oz.
Ashwagandha	2 oz.				

Self-Care

Hot baths

Rest

Yoga

Compresses

Inhalation of essential oils

Fasting

Abyangha - self massage (page 207)

Immune Broth (page 171)

MORNING SICKNESS

For some women, this becomes an irritating, uncomfortable experience. These symptoms, in most cases, go away within 3-4 months. This occurs due to the rapid hormonal changes. Very often this is caused by vitamin B deficiency or low enzyme function, particularly hydrochloric acid. Vata's women experience dizziness, flatulence, stomach problems, fatigue, and bloatedness. Pitta's experience irritability, diarrhea, becomes upset easily, heartburn, fevers, cravings of sour foods, and heat waves. Kapha's experience sleepiness, tiredness, sweet and starch cravings, water retention, rapid weight gain, nausea, vomiting, and depression.

Feelings and Emotions: Uneasiness and uncertainty about the birth process.

Diet	Vitamin & Minerals (Daily)	Essential Oils (always dilute)	Herbs	Alternative Therapy	Avoid
Ayurvedic diet for body type	B-Complex: 4 tablets daily (yeast free)	Ginger: VK-P+	Wild Yam: VP-Ko	Acupuncture	Cigarettes
Oatmeal	Digestive Aids	Fennel: VPK=	Fennel: VPK=	Ayurveda consultation	White sugar
	Multi-vitamin	Chamomile: VP-K+	Ginger: VK-P+	Music therapy	Coffee
Soup with digestive herbs		Lavender: PK-Ko	Dandelion: PK-V+	Energy work	Black Tea
		Lemon: PV-Ko	Vitex: VPK-	Homeopathics	Refined carbohydrates
Ginger snaps		Peppermint: PK-Vo	Peppermint: PK-Vo		Avoid yeasts
			Red Raspberry: PK-V+		
Peppermint snaps			Rose Petals: VPK-		
			Shatavari: PV-K+		
Whole grains			Slippery Elm: VP-K+		
			Cardamon: VK-P+		
			**MaterniTea: VPK-		
			Papaya Leaves: PK-V+		

** *Product of UniTea Herbs, Colorado*

Morning Sickness Herbal Brew

MaterniTea from UniTea Herbs for all doshas.

FOR ALL DOSHAS

| Ginger | equal amounts | Fennel | equal amounts |
| Mint | equal amounts | vegetable oil | 50% |

Massage on stomach a few times per day.

See directions for preparing herbal brew on page 409

Self Care

| Abyangha | Foot bath | Breathwork |
| Meditation | Mantra | Tai Chi |

MUMPS

Mumps is an infectious disease which is most common in children and is characterized by inflammatory swelling of the parotid and other salivary glands. Mumps, most often, affects the young and can be infectious one week or longer after the swelling of the glands has subsided. Once contracted, most people have lifetime immunity.

Cell Salts: Aconite, Belladonna

Diet	Vitamin & Minerals (Daily)	Essential Oils (always dilute)	Herbs	Alternative Therapy	Avoid
Ayurvedic diet for body type	A: 800 IU	Lavender: PK-Vo	Mullein: PK-V+	Reiki	Contact
	B-Complex: 300 mg.	Lemon: PV-Ko	Sage: VK-P+	Therapeutic Touch	Citrus
	Multi-Complex	Camphor: VK-P+	Bayberry: KV-P+	Color Therapy	Dairy
Acidophilus	RNA/DNA: 4 tablets/day	Geranium: PK-V+	Root Bark: VPK	Music Therapy	Sugar
Green juice	(children: 2 tablets)	Cypress: VK-P+	Echinacea: PK-V+		Poor food combining
Green vegetables	C: 3000 - Adults	Tea Tree: VPK=	Ginger Root: KV-P+		
	1500 - Children	Juniper: KV-P+	Lobelia: K-PV+		
Apples	1000 - under 12 years	Fennel: VPK=	Witch Hazel: PK-V+		
			White Oak Bark: PK-V+		
			Peppermint: PK-Vo PK-Vo		

See directions for preparing herbal brew on page 409

Mumps Herbal Brew

VATA	
Ginger	2 Tbs.
Root Bark	1 Tbs.
Chamomile	2 Tbs.
Add honey & lemon to taste	

PITTA & KAPHA	
Mullein	2 Tbs.
Witch Hazel	1 tsp.
Peppermint	1 tsp.
Chamomile	1 tsp.
Add equal amount of apple juice	

RECIPES

In blender mix:
Ginger, fresh - 2 inches
Fennel - 2 teaspoons
Lemon juice, fresh - 2 lemons
Blend well.
Add 1 dropperful of echinacea tincture.
Strain and drink 1 cup every two hours.

HIBISCUS-CHAMOMILE DRINK

Chamomile 1 oz.
Mullein 1 oz.
Hibiscus 1 oz.
Lobelia 1/2 oz.
Ginger 1/2 oz.
Mix with equal amounts of apple juice.
Add 1 dropperful of echinacea tincture.

COMPRESS

Make a paste with Slippery Elm powder and warm water.
Add 5 drops essential oil of your choice.
Apply on area.
Wrap with handkerchief around the jaw.
Keep on for 15 minutes.
Do once per day.

CLAY COMPRESS

Bentonite clay 1 teaspoon
Lemon juice, fresh 1/2 lemon
Mix well.
Apply. Let dry.
Wash with chamomile tea.

Self-Care

Poultice of flaxseed
Steam bath
Warm compresses

PARASITES

There are several different types of worms which can live in our intestines. Most commonly found are hookworms, tapeworms, roundworms, and pinworms. Because infestation of these parasites irritate the lining of the intestines, nutrient absorption from food is severely limited. Symptoms of parasites manifest itself in the form of weight loss, hunger pains, anemia, loss of appetite, and diarrhea.

Feelings and Emotions: Not caring for self.

Cell Salts: Natrium Phosphate, Sodium Phosphate

Diet	Vitamins & Minerals (Daily)	Essential Oils (always dilute)	Herbs	Alternative Therapy	Avoid
Ayurvedic diet for body type	A: 10,000 IU	Ginger: VK-P+	Mugwort: KV-P+	Colonics	Drinking ground water
Elimination diet	B1: 200 mg.	Lemon: VP-Ko	Black Walnut: V-PK+	Colloidal silver	Some raw ocean fish
	B2: 100 mg.	Tea Tree: VPK=	Bibhitaki: KP-Vo	Color therapy, esp. red	Sugar
Horseradish	B6: 100 mg.	Clove: VK-P+	Tansy: PK-Vo		Improper food combining
Mustard	B12: 30 mcg.	Fennel: VPK=	Neem: PK-V+		Insufficiently cooked meats, especially beef, pork, & fish
Onions	K: 200 mcg.	Neroli: VP-K+	Wormwood: PK-Vo		Walking barefoot
Acidophilus	F: 200 mg.	Tangerine: VP-Ko	Prickly Ash: KV-P+		Bad personal hygiene
Protein	D: 500 IU	Bergamot: VK-P+	Garlic: VK-P+		
Spices in cooking	Potassium: 800 mg.	Chamomile: VPK-	Basil: VK-P+		
	Calcium: 800 mg. 2000 mg.	Lavender: PK-Vo	Rhubarb: PK-V+		
	Magnesium: 600 mg.	Melissa: VP-Vo	Pysillium Husk: VP-K+		
		Angelica: VPK-	Hyssop: VK-P+		
		Camphor: VK-P+	Mountain Savory: VK-P+		

Small amount
of fruit

Sage: VK-P+
Trifolia: VK-P+
Hyssop: KV-P+

Oregano: VK-P+
Tarragon: VK-P+
Thyme: VK-P+
Nutmeg: VK-P+
Marjoram: VK-P+
Bayberry: VK-P+
Black Pepper: VK-P+
Bay Leaves: KV-P+
Cardamon: KV-P+
Cayenne: VK-P+
Horseradish: VK-P+
Mustard: VK-P+
Rosemary: VK-P+
Aloe Vera Gel: VPK=
Pomegranate: PK-Vo
Asafoetida: VK-P+

See directions for preparing herbal brew on page 409

Parasite Herbal Brew

VATA & KAPHA
Black walnut tincture:

Day 1 - Take 2 drops 4 times a day with milk or juice

1 wormwood capsule, 200-300 mg before supper

	3 capsules of cloves 3 times a day before meals
Day 2 -	Take 3 drops of black walnut tincture four times a day
	1 wormwood capsule before supper
	3 capsules of cloves before supper
Day 3 -	Take 3 drops of black walnut tincture
Days 4 through 10 -	Take 3 capsules of wormwood per day with 2 capsules cloves and 2 drops walnut tincture
After 10 Days -	Take 3 capsules of wormwood per week with 1 clove tablet and 1 drop walnut tincture

PITTA

Follow same procedure as above, except use barberry capsules instead of cloves.

Caution

Do not use during pregnancy.

Self-Care

Parasite cleanse

Zapper electrical device

Neem basti

Basti oil enema

PRE-MENSTRUAL SYNDROME (P.M.S.)

PMS consists of a reoccurrence of symptoms around the menstrual cycle. These symptoms include depression, feelings of being bloated, moodiness, anxiety, tension, tiredness, cramps, backache, forgetfulness, irritability, headaches, and weight gain. A poor diet contributes to these symptoms.

Feelings and Emotions: Dislike of feminine energy cycle.

Diet	Vitamins & Minerals (Daily)	Essential Oils (always dilute)	Herbs	Alternative Therapy	Avoid*
	Evening Primrose: 500 mg. 2 x day	Clary Sage: VPK- Rose: VPK=	Raspberry Leaf: PK-V+ Unicorn Root: VPK+	Acupuncture Chiropractic	Salt Caffeine
Ayurvedic diet for body type	Calcium/Magnesium: 1000 mg.	Cyperus: VPK- Valerian: VK-P+	Black Haw: PK-V+ Dong Quai: VK-Po	treatments Polarity	Chocolate Cola
Whole grains	A: 10,000 IU E mixed tocopherals:	Jasmine: KP-V+ Sandalwood: PV-Ko	Milk Thistle: PKV+ Licorice: PV-K+	Massage Shiatsu	Sugar Honey
Legumes	400 IU 2 x day	Gardenia: PK-V+ Cinnamon: VK-P+	Aloe Vera Gel: VPK- Turmeric: VK-Po		Maple syrup Dried fruit
		Black Pepper: K-PV+	Dill: PK-Vo		Fruit juices
Fruits	Zinc: 15 mg. Linseed oil: 2 Tbs.	Ginger: VK-P+	Fennel: VPK=		Dairy
Brewer's yeast	Bioflavonoids: 500 mg 2 x day	Calamus: VK-P+ Clove: VK-P+	Crampbark: KV-P+ Rosemary: VK-P+		Fats Cabbage
Acidophilus	B-Complex: 100 mg. C: 2,000 mg.	Myrrh: VK-P+ Ylang Ylang: PV-K+	Chamomile: PK-Vo Comfrey: VP-K+		Brussel sprouts Cauliflower
Protein	B5 - Pantothenic Acid: 2,500 mg.	*PMS Free: VKP Lavender: PK-Vo	False Unicorn: VK-P+ Saffron: VPK=		Tobacco Aspartame

Green leafy vegetables   Bromelin: 200 mg.

*Product of Earth Essentials
** Product of UniTea Herbs

Chamomile: PV-K+(excess)
Lemon Balm: KP-Vo

Coriander: PKV-
Gotu Kola: VPK-
Dandelion: PK-V+
Shatavari: PV-K+
Ashwagandha: VK-P+
Jatamasi: VK-P+
Asafoetida: VK-P+
**FeminiTea: VPK-

*Best to avoid 1-2 weeks before menstrual cycle.

Pre-Menstrual Syndrom (PMS) Herbal Brew

See directions for preparing herbal brew on page 409

VATA		PITTA		KAPHA	
Shatavari	2 oz.	Raspberry Leaves	2 oz.	Raspberry Leaves	2 oz.
Licorice	1 oz.	Mint	1 oz.	Rosemary	1 oz.
Ginger	1 oz.	Fennel	1 oz.	Ginger	2 oz.
Comfrey	1/2 oz.	Coriander	1 oz.	Shatavari	1 oz.
Rosemary	1/2 oz.	Chamomile	1 oz.	Coriander	2 oz
Vitex	1 oz.	Dandelion	2 oz.		
Ashwagandha	2 oz.	Shatavari	2 oz.		

Drink tea 2 weeks before menstruation 4 times per day. Also drink tea 1 day after menstruation ends.

Massage Formula

Chamomile	5 drops
Lemon Balm	5 drops
Clary Sage	5 drops
Ylang Ylang	2 drops
Vegetable oil	4 oz.

Self-Care

Exercise

Aromatherapy

Yoga

Women support groups

Wearing gemstones: pearl, moonstone, garnet, ruby

Apply warm sesame oil to head and lower abdomen

Kapha: Hot baths with essential oils that help eliminate water retention and are stimulating; Use: 10 drops Juniper, 10 drops Cypress, and 5 drops Orange.

Pitta: Refreshing cool baths which help relax and sweat: Use 5 drops Rose, 10 drops Clary Sage, and 10 drops Geranium.

Vata: Hot baths with essential oils to relax, calm the mind and assist with digestion. Use 10-15 drops Sandalwood, 5 drops Jatamasi, and 5 drops Ginger.

Wild Yam Cream (Progesterone cream)

SCIATICA

Sciatica may be either neuralgia or neuritis affecting the large sciatic nerve running down the back of the thigh. This sciatica nerve extends from the lower back down the leg to the heel of the foot. The chief symptom is pain and spasms along the line of the nerve at the back of the thigh usually caused by bulging lumbar discs rubbing against the sciatic nerve. Pain can also be felt on the side of the leg and the Achilles heel. Possible causes of sciatica are trauma or inflammation of the nerve itself, sprained joints in the lower back, rupture of a disc between the spinal bones, or a vertebra out of alignment causing neuritis.

Feelings and Emotions: Fear of going forward in life.

Cell Salts: Kali Sulph Potassium Sulfate

Diet	Vitamins & Minerals (Daily)	Essential Oils (Always dilute)	Herbs	Alternative Therapy	Avoid
Anti-Vata Diet (if appropriate)	B-Complex: 200 mg. A: 50,000 IU (until clear) E: 200 IU	Chamomile: VPK- Eucalyptus: VK-P+ Rosemary: VK-P+	Alfalfa: PK-V+ Castor Oil: VP-Ko Garlic: KV-P+	Acupuncture Chiropractic Massage	Tomatoes Rice Potatoes
Ayurvedic diet for body type	B5: 1500 mg. C: 3000mg. Calcium: 400mg. Magnesium: 400mg. Multi-Minerals	Valerian: VK-P+ Wintergreen: PK-Vo Lavender: PK-Vo Skullcap: PK-Vo Valerian: VK-P+	Ginger: VK-P+ Kava Kava: VKP Passion Flower: PK-V+	Shiatsu Physical Therapy Myotherapy	Eggplant Cauliflower Cold drafts

Note: Vata body types are susceptible to sciatica

Sciatica Herbal Brew

See directions for preparing herbal brew on page 409

VATA		PITTA		KAPHA	
Chamomile	2 oz.	Passion Flower	2 oz.	Alfalfa	2 oz.
Ginger	1 oz.	Kava Kava	2 oz.	Kava Kava	1 oz.
Scullcap	2 oz.	Peppermint	1 oz.	Ginger	2 oz.
Valerian	1 oz.	Scullcap	1 oz.	Scullcap	1 oz.

Self-Care

Warm compresses with lavender and valerian

Muscle strengthening (i.e. swimming, walking)

Inversion therapy

Rest

Yoga Mudras

Yoga Postures:

Backbends

Half wheel

Knee to chest

Plough

SHINGLES (Herpes Zoster)

This is an infection that irritates the nerve endings in the skin and is characterized by blister and crust formations. It is accompanied by severe pain which may last up to several weeks. The most common site for the infection is across the chest and abdomen. Herpes Zoster, or shingles, received its name from a Greek word signifying a surcingle, or girdle, because it spreads in a zone-like manner around half the body. This virus lies dormant until injury or stress weakens the body.

Feelings and Emotions: Wanting control, wanting things your own way.

Cell Salts: Silica Q Oxide

Diet	Vitamins & Minerals (Daily)	Essential Oils (Always dilute)	Herbs	Alternative Therapy	Avoid
Ayurvedic diet diets	B-Complex: 200 mg.	Bergamot: VK-P+	Aloe Vera: VPK=	Acupuncture	Arginine rich
for body type	2 x day	Camphor: VK-P+	Astralagus: VPK+	Chiropractic	Chocolate
Red grapes	B1: 200-300 mg.	Chamomile: VPK-	Chamomile: PK-Vo	Reiki	Coffee
	B12: 300 mcg.	Clove: VK-P+	Eucalyptus: VK-P+	Therapeutic Touch	Colas
Potatoes	B6: 200 mg.	Eucalyptus: VK-P+	Comfrey Root: VP-K+		Fatigue
	Beta-carotene:	Tea Tree: VPK=	Echinacea: PK-V+		Nuts
Brewer's yeast	100,000 IU	Geranium: PK-V+	Goldenseal: PK-V+		Rice
	(until clear)	Lavender: PK-Vo	Neem: PK-V+		Skin drying out
Fish	C: 2000 mg.	Clary Sage: VPK-	Shatavari: PV-K+		Stress
	Calcium: 500 mg.	Frankincense: VK-P+	Slippery Elm: PV-K+		Sun exposure
Liver	Chlorophyll: 3 Tbs.	Rose: VPK=	Uva-Ursi: PK-V+		Tea
	3 x day	Neem: PK-V+	Burdock: PK-V+		

Eggs

D: 600 IU
Iron: 100 mg.
L-Lysine: 750-1000 mg.
RNA/DNA: 7-10 capsules
Thymus extract:
    2-3 tabs 3 x day
E: 400 IU
Zinc: 50-60 mg.
Bioflavonoids: 1 gm.

Lemon: VP-Ko
Myrrh: VK-P+
Peppermint: PK-Vo
Thyme: VK-P+
Ylang Ylang: PV-K+

Noni Juice: VPK-

Shingles Herbal Brew

VATA		PITTA		KAPHA	
Shatavari	2 oz.	Shatavari	2 oz.	Shatavari	2 oz.
Slippery Elm	1 oz.	Burdock	1 oz.	Uva Ursi	1 oz.
Comfrey	1 oz.	Astralagus	1 oz.	Burdock	1 oz.
Chamomile	1 oz.	Red Clover	1 oz.	Red Clover	1 oz.

See directions for preparing herbal brew on page 409

Self-Care

Compress over the area twice per day with equal amounts of: Rose, Geranium, Lavender, Chamomile.

SHOCK

Due to trauma, accident, or receiving alarming news. More common in Vata as they are easily frightened and put into fear, fainting, and affecting the nervous system. Not able to cope. May experience convulsions.

Feelings and Emotions: Not feeling centered. Not able to handle the challenges of life.

Diet	Vitamin & Minerals (Daily)	Essential Oils (always dilute)	Herbs	Alternative Therapy	Avoid
Ayurvedic diet for body type	B-Complex: 300 mg. Multi-mineral B6: 200 mg.	Lemon: PV-Ko Lavender: PK-Vo Sandalwood: PV-Ko Basil: VK-P+	Calamus: VK-P+ Mistletoe: VK-P+ Horse Nettle: PK-V+ Astralagus: VPK+	Breathing therapy Counseling Therapeutic Touch Reiki	Sugar Animal proteins
Green vegetables	B15: 300 mg. C: 1,000 mg, D: 500 IU	*Mental Clarity: VP-K+ Myrrh: VK-P+	Ashwagandha: VK-P+ Shatavari: PV-K+	Chakra Anointment Bach Flower Rescue Remedy	
High minerals	E: 100 IU L-tyrosine: 100 mg.	Chamomile: VK-P+ Rosemary: VK-P+	Arjuna: PK-V+ Lady's Slipper: VK-Po	Shirodhara	
Berries	Digestive Enzyme: 3-x day before meals	Peppermint: PK-Vo Hyssop: VK-P+	Chamomile: PK-Po		
Bee Pollen	Pituitary Extract: 2 x day Bioflavinoids: 2000 mg.	Myrtle: PK-V+			

Shock Herbal Brew

See directions for preparing herbal brew on page 409

VATA

Lobelia	2 tsp.
Valerian	1 tsp.
Fennel	1 tsp.

PITTA

Chamomile	1 tsp.
Scullcap	1 tsp.
Mint	1 tsp.

KAPHA

Chamomile	1 tsp.
Fennel	1 Tbs.
Gotu Kola	1 tsp.

RECIPE FOR VATA

Ashwagandha	2 oz.
Astralagus	300 mg.
Shatavari	100 mg.

Mix with 1 glass warm milk or rice milk.
Drink twice per day.

PITTA & KAPHA

Arjuna	500 mg.

Mix with 1 glass warm milk or rice milk.
Drink twice per day.

Self-Care

Keep the person warm

Lay them down

Rescue Remedy

Anoint all chakras with essential oils

Wrap the body tight (mummy wrap) with a white sheet.

Breathwork

SINUS OR NASAL PROBLEMS

Congestion and inflammation of the nasal passages and upper respiratory system, clogging the inside passage of the nasal cavity and the cheek bones behind the bridge of the nose. This could be caused by injuries, allergies, environmental irritants, and food allergies. Vata experiences sinus pain and headaches, Pitta experiences inflammation, and Kapha loses their sense of smell and has thick mucous drainage. When the mucous becomes green or yellow it has turned into an infection. This can lead to sore throat, laryngitis, or lung infection.

Feelings and Emotions: Feeling stuck, held back, confused, blocked. Afraid to act. I don't want to see.

Diet	Vitamin & Minerals (Daily)	Essential Oils (always dilute)	Herbs	Alternative Therapy	Avoid
Ayurvedic diet for body type	A: 3,000-10,000 mg. Bioflavinoids: 300 mg. B-Complex: 200 mg./	Eucalyptus: VK-P+ Rosemary: VK-P+ Myrtle: PK-V+	Horehound: PK-V+ Echinacea: PK-V+ Fenugreek: VK-P+	Emetic Therapy Rebirthing Pancha Karma	Dairy Sugars Fried Foods
Mucousless diet	2 x day B6: 200 mg.	Lavender: PK-Vo Sandalwood: VP-Ko	Lobelia: K-PV+ Goldenseal: PK-V+	Ayurvedic consultation	Poor food combining
Cleansing foods	Pantothenic Acid: 200 mg.	Calamus: VK-P+ Sage: VK-P+	Garlic: KV-P+ Onions: KV-P+	Acupuncture	
Greens	3 x per day Germanium: 100 mg. C (ascorbate): 3,000+ mg.	Inula: KV-P+ Camphor: KV-P+ Angelica: VPK- P+ Basil: VK-P+	Marshmallow: VP-K+ Mullein: PK-V+ Rosehips: V-KPo+ (in excess) Basil: VK-P+ Angelica: VK-Po Chrysanthemum: PK-V+ Ginger: VK-P+ Astralagus: VP-K+		

Sinus & Nasal Herbal Brew

Sitoplad Churna: VKP
Pippali: KV-P+
Elecampagne: VK-P+
Trikatu: VK-P+

VATA

Ginger	1 oz.
Marshmallow	1 oz.
Rosehips	1 oz.
Astralagus	1/2 oz.

PITTA

Mullein	1 oz.
Marshmallow	1 oz.
Mint	1 oz.
Horehound	1 oz.

KAPHA

Calamus	1 oz.
Ginger	1/2 oz.
Mullein	1 oz.
Basil	1 oz.

See directions for preparing herbal brew on page 409

INHALATION FORMULA

Basil	2 drops
Eucalyptus	2 drops
Camphor	2 drops
Angelica	2 drops
Boiling water	4 cups

Mix essential oils in water. Tent head with towel and bend over water, inhaling vapors.

Self Care

Yoga
Inhalation of essential oils
Compresses
Upper cervical & facial massage
Vapor rub on sinus areas
Nasya Nosedrops

SORE THROAT

An infection of the throat when the adenoids become inflamed. Vata experiences dryness, Pitta experiences inflammation, and Kapha experiences swelling of the throat.

Feelings and Emotions: Holding back communication. Fear of speaking truthfully.

Diet	Vitamins & Minerals (Daily)	Essential Oils (always dilute)	Herbs	Alternative Therapy	Avoid
Ayurvedic diet for body type	C: 1000 mg. every 2 hours (until clear)	Sandalwood: VP-Ko	Echinacea: PK-V+	Therapeutic Touch	Sugar
Drink large amounts of water	A: 25,000 IU	Lemongrass: PK-Vo	Amalaki: PV-Ko	Reiki	Dairy
Fresh squeezed orange juice	Beta-Carotene: 1000 IU	Ginger: VK-P+	Sage: VK-P+	Lymphatic drainage	Fried foods
Hot water with lemons	Zinc: 50 mg.	Cardamom: VK-P+	Garlic: VK-P+		Alcohol
	Bioflavenoids: 1 gm. per day	Goldenseal: KP-V+	Sitopaladi: VP-K+		Poor food combining
	Thymus extract: 500 mg. 2 x day	Forsynthia: VPK+	Zedoaria: PK-V+		
		Talisadi: VPK-	Bibhitaki: PK-Vo		
		Cinnamon: VK-P+	Korean Ginseng: V-PKo		
		Black Pepper: VK-P+	Honeysuckle: VPK+		
		Chamomile: VPK-	Siberian Ginseng: V-PKo		
		Clary Sage: VPK-	Rosehips: V-PKo		
		Eucalyptus: VK-P+	Licorice: VP-K+		
		Lavender: PK-Vo	Haritaki: VK-Po		
		Tea Tree: VPK=			
		Lemon: VP-Ko			
		Cajeput: VK-P+			
		Bergamot: VK-P+			

Niaouli: PK-V+
Geranium: PK-V+
Thyme: VK-P+
Peppermint: PK-Vo
Pine: VK-P+

Sore Throat Herbal Brew

See directions for preparing herbal brew on page 409

VATA

Ginger	1 oz.
Cinnamon	1/2 oz.
Cardamon	1/2 oz.
Lemon Peel	1/2 oz.
Haritaki	1/2 oz.
Licorice	1 oz.
Amla	1/2 oz.
Anise	1 oz.

PITTA

Mullein	1 oz.
Honeysuckle	2 oz.
Chamomile	2 oz.
Licorice	2 oz.
Fennel	2 oz.
Lemongrass	1 oz.

KAPHA

Sage	1 oz.
Ginger	2 oz.
Bibhitaki	1 oz.
Basil	1 oz.
Lemongrass	2 oz.
Haritaki	1 oz.

PITTA GARGLE

Water	2 oz.
Sandalwood	2 drops
Cajeput or tea tree	2 drops

Gargle 4-6 times per day, or every two hours.

VATA GARGLE

Salt	1/2 tsp.
Warm water	4 oz.

Mix well. Gargle 4-6 times per day, or every 2 hours.

KAPHA THROAT SPRAY

Tea tree oil	1 drop
Cajeput	2 drops
Sandalwood	2 drops
Water	4 oz.

Put in spray bottle. Spray onto throat every hour.

STRESS

Stress is a built-in system designed to prompt the "fight or flight" response. During the course of a day, we experience many prolonged stresses, and we often tend to squelch the "fight or flight" response. After years of failing to respond, we inadvertently damage the body's immune system which, in turn, results in ill health. Side effects can manifest as ulcers, arthritis, cancer, high blood pressure, coronary heart disease, and a host of other conditions.

ALARM + RESISTANCE + EXHAUSTION = STRESS

Feelings and Emotions: Victim. Life is getting me. Caught in the illusion.

Diet	Vitamins & Minerals (Daily)	Essential Oils (always dilute)	Herbs	Alternative Therapy	Avoid
Ayurvedic diet for body type	B-Complex: 200 mg. B5 - Pantothenic Acid: 2,500 mg.	Lavender: PK-Vo Lemongrass: PK-Vo Basil: VK-P+	Echinacea: PK- V+ Goldenseal: PK-V+ Panax Ginseng: PKVo	Massage Biofeedback Acupuncture	Smoking Cadmium Salt
Whole grains	A - (Beta carotene): 25,000 IU Bioflavinoids: 1000 mg.	Pine: VK-P+ Savory: VK-P+	Licorice: VP-K+ Valerian: VK-P+	Polarity Reiki	Mental fatigue Physical fatigue
Legumes	C: 500 mg, every 2 hours for 1 week	Geranium: PK-V+ Cypress: VKP+	Skullcap: PK-Vo Lady's Slipper: VK-Po	Shirodhara	Sugar Gaining weight
Cauliflower	Iron: 50 mg. Zinc: 100 mg.	Hyssop: VK-P+ Juniper: VK-P+ (in excess)	Cayenne: VK-P+ Black Cohosh Root: PK-V+		Tea Coffee
Broccoli	Calcium: 800 mg. Magnesium: 800 mg.	Rose Otto: VPK=	Guduchi: PKV+		Dairy
Salmon	Potassium: 3-5 gms.	Chamomile: VPK-	Shatavari: PV-K+ Ashwagandha: VK- P+		Chocolate Anti-depres-sants

Liver
Sweet Potatoes

Tomatoes

Ghee

L-Carnitine: 200 mg.
L-Tyrosine: 100 mg.
Folic Acid: 200 mcg.
Phosphorus: 200 mg.
PABA: 200 mg.
Chromium: 200 mcg.
Copper: 100 mg.

Sandalwood: VP-Ko
Ylang Ylang; PV-K+
Orange Blossom: VK-P+
Vetiver: V-PK+
Kava Kava: VPK-

Chrysanthemum: PK-V+
Chamomile: PK-Vo
Passion Flower: PK-V+

Sleeping pills
Protein

See directions for preparing herbal brew on page 409

Stress Herbal Brew

VATA		PITTA		KAPHA	
Ashwagandha	2 oz.	Chamomile	2 oz.	Chrysanthemum	2 oz.
Licorice	1 oz.	Chrysanthemum	2 oz.	Guduchi	1 oz.
Lady's Slipper	1 oz.	Shatavari	1 oz.	Skullcap	1 oz.
Shatavari	2 oz.	Licorice	1 oz.	Chamomile	2 oz.
Chamomile	1 oz.	Passion Flower	1 oz.		

Self-Care

Meditation	Foot rubs	Whirlpool	Tai Chi
Steam	Exercise	Sports	Rest
Walking	Prayer, devotion	Yoga	Visualization
Laughter	Dancing	Aromatherapy bath with essential oils	
Chanting			

ULCERS

Ulcers are an inflammation of the mucous lining of the stomach or the duodenum. They are associated with pain and burning in that area of the body. In advanced stages, bleeding occurs and when perforated, they can be life threatening. Ulcers are caused by excess acid from the small intestine which accumulates in the stomach and burns through the lining. It can sometimes be triggered by nervous sensitivity.

Feelings and Emotions: Stress and irritability.

Cell Salts: Nat Sulph, Sodium Sulfate

Diet	Vitamins & Minerals (Daily)	Essential Oils (always dilute)	Herbs	Alternative Therapy	Avoid
Ayurvedic diet for body type	A: 25,000-50,000 IU	Coriander: VPK-	Amalaki: PV-Ko	Biofeedback	Stress
	B-Complex: 100 mg.	Mint: PK-Vo	Aloe Vera: VPK=	Reiki	Smoking
Bland diet	C: 2,000 mg.	Chamomile: VPK-	Shatavari: VP-K+	Therapeutic touch	Caffeine
	(in calcium ascorbate form)	Fennel: VPK=	Licorice: VP-K+	Polarity	Acid fruits
Milk	E: 600-1200 IU	Rose: VPK=	Marshmallow: VP-K+	Color therapy: blue, green, indigo	Spicy foods
	Calcium: 800 mg.	Lavender: PK-Vo	Comfrey: VP-K+	Music/Sound therapy	Sour foods
Acidophilus	Iron: 50 mg.		Barberry: PK-V+	Cranial Sacral	Alcohol
	U: 300 mg.		Gentian: PK-V+	Homeopathics	Spices, including salt
Fruits	Evening Primrose oil: 100 mg. 2-x day		Chiretta: PKV+		Pickles
			Katuka: PKV+		Vinegar
Vegetables			Sudarshan: PVK		Nightshade vegetables: tomato
			Mahasudarshan: PKV		peppers
Pureed protein			Coptis: PKV		
			Dry Ginger: KV-P+		
			Noni Juice: VPK-		
			Slippery Elm: VP-K+		

Eggs

Cabbage juice
3 x per day

Unsalted Millet

Potato Juice

potatoes
eggplant
Cold food
Raw food

Goldenseal: PK-V+
Trikatu: VK-P+
Triphala: VPK-
Guggul:KV-P+

Ulcers Herbal Brew

VATA

Slippery Elm	2 oz.
Coriander	1 oz.
Shatavari	2 oz.
Licorice	2 oz.

PITTA

Mint	2 oz.
Shatavari	1 oz.
Comfrey	1 oz.
Slippery Elm	1 oz.
Coriander	2 oz.

KAPHA

Marshmallow	1 oz.
Coriander	2 oz.
Fennel	2 oz.
Mint	2 oz.
Shatavari	1 oz.
Amalaki	1 oz.

See directions for preparing herbal brew on page 409

Self-Care

Cool Compresses on the stomach with cooling essential oils

Visualization

VAGINITIS

There are three different types of vaginitis: infectious, hormonal and irritant. Infectious vaginitis may be sexually transmitted or may be a disturbance to the ecology of a healthy vagina. Examples of infectious vaginitis is simplex, chlamydia, gonorrhea, trichomonas, or candida albicans. Hormonal vaginitis is usually a problem in post-menopausal women and those whose ovaries have been removed. Another indication of hormonal vaginitis is increased vaginal discharge. Irritant vaginitis is directly related to certain medications, an injury, or foreign bodies in the vagina which irritate the delicate membranes. Vata generally experiences itching, Pitta usually has hormonal involvement, and Kapha tends to have heavy mucous discharge.

Feelings and Emotions: Irritation by male energy

Diet	Vitamins & Minerals (Daily)	Essential Oils (always dilute)	Herbs	Alternative Therapy	Avoid
Ayurvedic diet for body type	A: 10,000 IU (until clear)	Anise: VK-P+	Alfalfa: PK-V+	Reiki	Alcohol
	Aloe Vera Gel: 1 Tbs. 2 x day	Bergamot: VK-P+	Red Clover: PK-V+	Therapeutic touch	Antibiotics
Acidophilus	B-Complex: 100 mg.	Dhavana: PKV-	Don Quai: VK-Po		Bad hygiene
1/2 tsp.	Beta-carotene: 2,000 IU	Fennel: VPK=	Echinacea: PK-V+		Coffee
2 x day	Bioflavonoids: 2,000 mg.	Lavender: PK-Vo	Garlic: VK-P+		Elevated vaginal pH
	C: 2,500 mg.	Myrrh: VK-P+	Ginseng: V-PKo		Fats
Raw garlic	Chlorophyll: 2-x day	Rose: VPK=	Goldenseal: PK-V+		Nylon tights
	Zinc: 15 mg.	Tea Tree: VPK=	Licorice: VP-K+		Oral contraceptives
Yogurt	E: 400 IU		Raspberry Leaves: PK-V+		Refined foods
	L-lysine: 2,000 mg.		Shatavari: PV-K+		Sexual activity
			Witch Hazel: PK-+		Steroids
			Yarrow: PK-V+		Sugar
			Yellow Dock: PK-V+		Excessive douching

Vaginitis Herbal Brew

See directions for preparing herbal brew on page 409

VATA		PITTA		KAPHA	
Shatavari	2 oz.	Red Clover	2 oz.	Alfalfa	1 oz.
Ginseng	1 oz.	Rose	2 oz.	Red Clover	2 oz.
Rose	2 oz.	Yarrow	1 oz.	Yarrow	2 oz.
Licorice	1 oz.	Licorice	1 oz.	Witch Hazel	1 oz.
				Raspberry Leaves	2 oz.

RECIPE

Bolus-Vagina suppositories (instructions on page 374)

VARICOSE VEINS

Varicose veins is a weakening in the wall of the veins, causing the lining to stretch and the pooling of blood in that area. Causes include poor circulation, lack of exercise, and long periods of either sitting or standing. This condition can be hereditary.

Feelings and Emotions: I am stuck. I am afraid to move.

Diet	Vitamins & Minerals (Daily)	Essential Oils (always dilute)	Herbs	Alternative Therapy	Avoid
Molasses	C: 5000 mg.	Geranium: KP-V+	Ginger: VK-P+	Steam	Long periods of standing or sitting
	Bioflavinoids: 200 mg.	Lavender: KP-Vo	Juniper: VK-P+	Body wraps	Crossed legs
Greens	B-Complex: 200 mg.	Cypress: VKP+	Triphalla: VKPo	Lymphatic drainage	Dairy
	D: 1500 mg.	Juniper: VK-P+ (in excess)	Cardamon: VK-P+	Massage	Red meats
Ayurvedic diet for body type	Magnesium: 100 mg	Ginger: VK-P+	Burdock: KP-V+		Congesting foods
	E: 600 IU	Cardamon: VK-P+	Aloe Vera Gel: VKP=		
	Zinc: 60 mg.	Orange: VK-P+	Cinnamon: VK-P+		
Peaches	K: 150 mg.	Lemon: VP-Ko	Rosehips: V-KP+		
		Parsley: KV-P+	Parsley: VK-P+		
Fresh spices		Lemongrass: PK-Vo	Grape leaves: PVK		
			Uva Ursi: PK-V+		
All berries			Stone Root: PK-V+		
			Buckhorn: PK-V+		
			Butcher Broom: VPK-		
			Noni Juice: VPK-		

Varicose Veins Herbal Brew

See directions for preparing herbal brew on page 409

VATA

Ginger	1 oz.
Cardamon	2 oz.
Lemon Peel	1 oz.
Cinnamon	1 oz.
Rosehips	2 oz.

PITTA

Burdock	1 oz.
Colistonia	2 oz.
Parsley	1 oz.
Butchers Broom	2 oz.
Witch Hazel	1 oz.

KAPHA

Burdock	1 oz.
Colistonia	2 oz.
Ginger	1 oz.
Uva Ursi	1 oz.
Juniper	2 oz.
Orange	1 oz.

MORNING

2 Tbs. of Aloe Vera Juice with lemon and lime juice.

NIGHT

Take 6 tablets of triphalla (500 mg).

Herbal Body Wrap

HERBAL SOLUTION:

Juniper berries	1 oz.
Uva Ursi	1 oz.
Buckhorn	2 oz.
Water	2 quarts
Parsley leaves	2 oz.
Butchers Broom	2 oz.
Colistonia	2 oz. (or any of the herbs listed above)

Add 40 drops each of the following essential oils: orange, juniper and cypress.

Bring water to boil. Add herbs. Immediately turn heat to low. Steep for two hours.

Add essential oils after herbs have steeped for two hours. Strain.Place this herbal liquid into a crock-pot.

Roll the surgical sleeves and let them soak for 8 hours in the crock-pot to keep them warm.

(Surgical sleeves can be purchased at medical supply store.)

Squeeze out bandages from the crock-pot. Wrap bandages around the body for one hour. Remove the wrap.

Next, massage body with the following essential oil mixture:

Cypress	10 drops	Juniper Berries	15 drops
Lavender	10 drops	Geranium	15 drops (or any of your favorite oils)
Vegetable oil	4 oz. (according to your body type)		

Massage towards the heart.

Save leftover mixture. Use daily.

CIRCULATION (do twice a week) – USE SAME MIXTURE AS FOR BODY WRAPS

To increase circulation:

Bentonite clay   3 Tbs.

Mix with herbal liquid to form a paste. Apply to leg. Let dry.

Squeeze out bandages from the crock-pot. Wrap leg from left to right while bandages are warm.

Elevate the legs until bandages become cool. Keep wrapped for at least one hour.

Massage Formula

Cypress	5 drops		Lemongrass	5 drops
Juniper	5 drops		Vegetable oil	2 oz.

Self-Care

Elevate legs	Wear loose clothing	Sitz baths
Walking on cool water	Clay packs	Steam
Body wraps	Lymphatic drainage	Basti oil enema

VOMITING

The expulsion of the stomach contents by way of the mouth, caused by irritation, food poisoning, the flu, viruses, or nerves.

Feelings and Emotions: I am nauseated by my life; I am sick of it.

Cell Salt: Natrium Sulfate

Diet	Vitamin & Minerals (Daily)	Essential Oils (always dilute)	Herbs	Alternative Therapy	Avoid
Cilantro juice (3x/day)	B-Complex: 150 mg. (yeast-free)	Anise: VK-P+	Poplar Bark: PK-V+	Ayurvedic consultation	Mucus forming foods
	C: 3,000 mg.	Fennel: VKP-	Spearmint: PK-Vo	Therapeutic touch	Poor food combining
Ayurveda diet for bodytype		Ginger: VK-P+	Peach Leaves: PK-V+		
		Mint: PK-Vo	Sweet Basil: VK-P+		
		Nutmeg: VK-P+	Fennel: VKP-		

Food combining

Cardamon: VK-P+   Cinnamon: VK-P+
                   Clove: VK-P+
                   Ginger: VK-P+
                   Nutmeg; VK-P+
                   Peppermint: PK-Vo
                   Raspberry Leaves: PK-V+

See directions for preparing herbal brew on page 409

Vomiting Herbal Brew

VATA

Ginger	1 oz.
Nutmeg	1/2 oz.
Cardamon	1 oz.
Fennel	1 oz.

PITTA

Mint	1 oz.
Coriander	1/2 oz.
Peach Leaves	1/2 oz.
Raspberry leaves	1 oz.

KAPHA

Raspberry leaves	1 oz.
Ginger	1 oz.
Spearmint	1/2 oz.
Cardamon	1/2 oz.

Self-Care

Meditation
Relaxation techniques
Breathwork
Compress over stomach
Nosedrops
Aromatherapy inhalation after vomiting and in-between
Induce vomiting

TO MAKE AN HERBAL BREW

1. Mix all herbs together in a bowl. Pray or chant as you sit, to add potency and increase the healing effect.

2. Bring water to a boil and add one teaspoon of herb mix per cup of water. Cover. Remove from heat and allow to steep (sit) ½ hour or more (overnight.)

3. Strain into a jar and refrigerate for future use. Makes up to one gallon at a time. Pitta may drink the blend cool, and Vata should warm the blend before consuming.

4. Herbs are best cut and sifted or whole.

HOW TO MAKE AN HERBAL SALVE

The basic recipe for making a salve is:

Beeswax   1 part
Medicated vegetable oil   4-6 parts

Medicated vegetable oil is made much like medicated ghee:

Soak herbs in vegetable oil for 30-60 days

Then strain to remove the herbs

OR

Adding essential oils to any vegetable oil will immediately make your vegetable oil medicated.

GENERAL DIRECTIONS

Use a small stainless steel (or ceramic) pan to slowly melt the beeswax.

Add the vegetable oil. Stir to blend well.

To check consistency, take a cold spoon from the freezer (which you placed there earlier), and dip it into your mixture. The salve should immediately harden on the spoon. If you find it is too hard, add more oil. If it is too soft, add more beeswax. When it is the exact consistency you want, remove the pan from the stove.

If using essential oils, you can then add 20-40 drops per ounce of salve.

For a preservative, use wheat germ oil, benzoin, or squeeze a capsule or two of Vitamin E into your mixture.

Stir well. Pour into a wide mouth container (baby food jar, recycled cosmetics container.)

FORGIVENESS

We can be on the best diet, take the best vitamins, herbs, oils, or use alternative therapies, yet, without forgiveness the highest state of health is not actualized.

Forgiveness is a letting go, a transformation of the way we see the world. Our pain comes from our holding on. Forgiveness and letting go releases us. We can choose to see situations for the value of the experience and for the gifts that they offer. See problems as challenges. Forgiveness is "For The Forgiver". We then no longer carry the anger or sorrow. Each experience has a gift within it regardless of how hard it may be to see it. In becoming "clear" with what the message is, and by taking responsibility (the ability to respond), freedom from past fears can be attained.

Ayurveda offers a wonderful ceremony called "Tarpana" (relationship healing) which is a forgiveness ritual. It is a process of applying forgiveness to everyone in your life, even your ancestors, for whatever may have occurred. It is an opportunity to bring us into our true essence which is Divine Love. When we truly forgive, we no longer have a "charge" or a holding on the experience. We no longer need to tell any "stories". The answer is simple - Loving, Serving, and Remembering who you truly are (see page 200).

This book is written to support to the creation a healthy, holy, and happy family environment so that each person can find blissfulness and wellbeing. The alternative recipes, diets, herb formulas, and wholistic approaches are a collection of many years of practice. It reflects a combination of East-West practices; a spiritually guided adventure. As healing occurs through each person, it simultaneously contributes to a healing of families, communities, societies, and ultimately, the world. It all begins with oneself. Let us each embrace and practice our own healing, peace, joy, prosperity, and longevity.

CHAPTER 14

DISCOVERING YOUR AYURVEDIC TYPE

INTRODUCTION

Examination is a way of knowing and understanding yourself. A good place to start is evaluating the Prakriti (basic nature, Humor or Doshic type) to see "who" you are in Ayurvedic terms. Then, when diagnosing the Vikriti (imbalance, disease or symptom) you will have a reference point from which to judge. Example: If a Vata body type complains of dry skin, you would not be too concerned. Simply add more oil to the diet and oil the skin. But if a Pitta or Kapha type complains of dry skin, you are going to be looking seriously for problems.

QUESTIONNAIRE

This questionnaire is important because it covers multiple areas of health quickly. We have divided the questions into Prakriti (things which do not change), Vikriti (things which do change), the mind, and the emotions.

Prakriti (Part I) does not change because it is who you are. Unless you get a strange bone disease, Vatas always have small bones, Pittas medium bones, and Kaphas large bones.

Vikriti (Part II) will change often, especially if you make lifestyle or diet changes. It can be instructive to Part II after a period of treatments.

The Mind and the Emotions change as a person spiritually evolves.

Totaling parts II, III and IV will give you a total *now* picture of the individual body, mind and emotions.

AYURVEDIC CONSTITUTIONAL QUESTIONNAIRE

On each line check the statement which best describes you. Occasionally no statement, or more than one will best describe you.

PART I
THINGS WHICH DO NOT CHANGE & CHILDHOOD

Interpreting Part I - Characteristics that do not change. The choices that you pick here reveal your original metabolic type. This is the body type that you were born into that you were meant to experience the world in. Of course, lifestyle, diet, climate, etc. can and will shift you from this (see Part II characteristics which change), but the result will be compromised immunity and health. The distribution of your answers may reveal you to be predominately one type or a mixed type, and this basic configuration VPK is where your health lies. Remember your numbers here and compare them to your Part II configuration.

VATA	PITTA	KAPHA
❑1. Frame: small & thin, tall or thin, underdeveloped	❑1. Frame: medium build, moderate physique, balanced & proportional	❑1. Frame: thick, tall or short, well developed
❑2. Head: small, thin, unsteady	❑2. Head: medium	❑2. Head: large
❑3. Forehead: small	❑3. Forehead: medium, receding hairline	❑3. Forehead: large

❏4. Eyes: gray sclera, brown or black, unsteady, jumpy, small

❏5. Eyebrows & Lashes: thin, small

❏6. Nose: crooked, thin, small

❏7. Lips: thin, small, irregular

❏8. Teeth: irregular, crooked, large

❏9. Hair: thin, coarse, curly, black or brown

❏10. Chin & Jaw: receding, small, pointing

❏11. Neck: unsteady, small, thin

❏12. Shoulders: narrow, thin

❏13. Chest: narrow, twisted, pigeon or concave

❏14. Hips: narrow

❏15. Hands & Feet: small & thin or long & thin

❏16. Joints: irregular, protruding

❏17. Nails: cracked, brittle, hang nails

❏18. Body Hair: dark, coarse, scanty or ever-abundant

❏4. Eyes: red sclera, green, amber, gray, blue, sharp, penetrating, medium

❏5. Eyebrows & Lashes: medium

❏6. Nose: medium, reddish

❏7. Lips: medium, red, pink

❏8. Teeth: even, medium

❏9. Hair: thin, soft, fine, straight, red or light brown

❏10. Chin & Jaw: medium

❏11. Neck: medium

❏12. Shoulders: medium, balanced

❏13. Chest: medium, balanced

❏14. Hips: medium

❏15. Hands & Feet: medium

❏16. Joints: medium, regular

❏17. Nails: red nail beds, nails bend

❏18. Body Hair: fine, light texture

❏4. Eyes: clear, white sclera, blue-black, liquid, large

❏5. Eyebrows & Lashes: thick, bushy

❏6. Nose: large, wide, thick

❏7. Lips: large, full

❏8. Teeth: gleaming

❏9. Hair: thick, wavy, soft, dark brown

❏10. Chin & Jaw: thick, large

❏11. Neck: thick, large sturdy

❏12. Shoulders: thick, broad, firm

❏13. Chest: large, broad

❏14. Hips: large

❏15. Hands & Feet: large fingers, square/thick toes

❏16. Joints: large, fleshy

❏17. Nails: thick nails, don't break

❏18. Body Hair: moderate, wavy

VATA	PITTA	KAPHA
❑19. Skin: dark complexion relative to your family, tans easily	❑19. Skin: fair skin, sunburns easily, freckles, moles	❑19. Skin: tans evenly, pale, white
❑20. Skin Thickness: thin, less than 1/4" on forearm	❑20. Skin Thickness: medium, 1/4-1/2" on forearm	❑20. Skin thickness: thick, 1/2"+ on forearm
❑21. Childhood: thin as a child, difficulty gaining weight	❑21. Childhood: medium build, periods of gaining & losing weight	❑21. Childhood: large build, gained weight easily
_____	_____	_____
Total Vata	Total Pitta	Total Kapha

PART II
THINGS WHICH CHANGE QUESTIONNAIRE

Symptoms within the last year

Part II - Characteristics That Change. This shows where your balance is now. Total your VPK here and compare them to your original VPK to see how you've shifted. Many of these characteristics are symptoms of imbalance and you may wish to be free of them. Example, if you were born primarily Vata but in part II demonstrate a shift into Kapha symptoms like weight gain, fluid retention, craving sweets, this shows a Kapha imbalance that needs correcting.

VATA	PITTA	KAPHA
❑1. Difficulty gaining weight.	❑1. Can gain or lose weight if puts mind to it.	❑1. Gains weight easily, hard time losing unless exercise.
❑2. Gains around belly.	❑2. Gains evenly, especially chest.	❑2. More weight in hips and bust.
❑3. Cold hands and feet.	❑3. Skin warm to the touch.	❑3. Skin cool but not cold.
❑4. Dry skin, chaps easily, prone to corns and calluses.	❑4. Oily skin, prone to pimples and rashes.	❑4. Thick skin, well lubricated.

❑5. Suffers cracked, chapped lips often.

❑5. Lips tendency toward cold sores, fever blisters.

❑5. Full, moist lips.

❑6. Dry hair, luster-less, split ends

❑6. Oily or early gray hair, early thinning or baldness possible.

❑6. Thick, slightly wavy hair, a little oily, lustrous.

❑7. Dislikes dryness and cold and wind (craves warmth).

❑7. Dislikes heat and sun, craves cool.

❑7. Dislikes humidity, craves dryness.

❑8. Tongue dry with thin, grayish coating.

❑8. Tongue coating yellowish, orange or reddish.

❑8. Tongue swollen with thick, curdy, white coating.

❑9. Eyes often dry and scratchy.

❑9. Sclera has reddish or yellow tinge (sclera= whites of eye). Sties.

❑9. Tendency toward eye puffiness.

❑10. Bowel movement can be irregular, hard, dry or constipated

❑10. Bowels loose - more than twice a day/diarrhea.

❑10. Large full move-ment, once a day/ mucous, itching.

❑11. If ill: Nervous disorders, sharp pain likely.

❑11. If ill: Fevers, rashes or inflammation likely.

❑11. If ill: Swelling, fluid, retention, mucous, congestion.

❑12. Sexual interest variable, fantasy life active.

❑12. Over-sexed, arouses easily.

❑12. Steady sex, slow to arouse.

❑13. Menses irregular, scanty flow, severe painful cramps.

❑13. May bleed heavily and long-loose stool accompanies period.

❑13. Prone to water weight during menses, slight cramps if any.

❑14. Either indulge in rich food or on strict diet.

❑14. Loves proteins, caffeine and hot, spicy and salty foods.

❑14. Loves sweets, dairy, bread and pastry.

❑15. Receding gums.

❑15. Inflamed bleeding gums.

❑15. Thick gums.

❑16. Joints - painful, unsteady, cracking or stiff

❑16. Joints - hot, swollen, burning.

❑16. Joints - loose, aching, watery, swollen

❑17. Thirst: irregular

❑17. Thirst: strong, excessive

❑17. Thirst: slight

❑18. Appetite: variable	❑18. Appetite: strong, excessive	❑18. Appetite: steady, slow
❑19. Sweat: lack of. Odor: astringent	❑19. Sweat: profuse. Odor: sour, sharp	❑19. Sweat: moderate. Odor: sweet, pleasant
❑20. Urine: scanty, cloudy, colorless	❑20. Urine: profuse, yellow	❑20. Urine: moderate
❑21. Endurance: poor	❑21. Endurance: medium	❑21. Endurance: strong
❑22. Resistance: poor, tendency to acute allergies	❑22. Resistance: medium, prone to infections	❑22. Resistance: strong, tendency to chronic
❑23. Tongue: grey, coated, cracked	❑23. Tongue: red, yellow, coated	❑23. Tongue: white coated, scalloped edges

Total Vata	Total Pitta	Total Kapha

PART III
THE MIND QUESTIONNAIRE

Part III - The Mind. The mind of each metabolic type demonstrates favorable and unfavorable characteristics. Vatas are creative thinkers but change their mind often. Pittas have good memory and organization skills but can tend toward snap decisions and running over people in their drive to get things done. Kaphas work well with routine and follow directions thoughtfully but are slow to make decisions and can lack creativity. Knowing yourself and understanding how you think can save you much discomfort. For example, if your questionnaire reveals that you have predominately Vata mind characteristics, you will be much happier in a job using your creativity rather than in management or repetitive routines.

VATA	PITTA	KAPHA
❑1. Concentration is short, short-term memory good, but forgets quickly.	❑1. Good short and long-term memory, logical, rational, thoughts.	❑1. Takes time to learn things, once learned, never forgets.

❑2. Dislikes routine - and hard to structure	❑2. Enjoys planning & organizing, especially if you created it	❑2. Works well with routine
❑3. Difficulty deciding, changes mind easily	❑3. Rapid decision making, sees things clearly	❑3. Takes time making decisions, sticks with it
❑4. Restless, active, likes movement	❑4. Aggressive, likes competitive activities	❑4. Calm, likes to relax, leisure activities
❑5. Creative thinker	❑5. Organized thinker	❑5. Prefers to follow a plan or idea
❑6. Do many projects all at once	❑6. Constantly organizing, likes to proceed orderly	❑6. Resists change, new projects - likes simplicity
❑7. Know a lot of people, few close friends	❑7. Very selective, but creates warm friendships, makes enemies easily	❑7. Loyal with many friends
❑8. Spends impulsively, money is to be used	❑8. Plans spending. Money is for achieving purpose	❑8. Spends reluctantly, likes to save
❑9. Speech: rapid, variable, changes subjects	❑9. Speech: sharp, orderly, serious, fluid	❑9. Speech: slow, thoughtful, melodious

Total Vata	Total Pitta	Total Kapha

PART IV
THE EMOTIONS QUESTIONNAIRE

Part IV - Emotions. The emotional characteristics of each type have positive and negative aspects. Vata people become easily anxious or fearful yet can forget quickly and don't often hold a grudge. Pittas anger comes quickly, but they have the ability to transform it to competitiveness or in overcoming a challenge. Kaphas sensitivity means a slight is not easily forgiven, but that sensitivity makes them loyal and romantic.

Look at your choices in this section and note where you are emotionally: are you manifesting positive or negative aspects, are your emotions in line with your initial type (Part I), current balance (Part III), or have you developed characteristics outside of your dosha (summary of questionnaire).

VATA	PITTA	KAPHA
❑1. Experiences fear	❑1. Experiences hate	❑1. Experiences apathy
❑2. Practices secretiveness	❑2. Can be vindictive	❑2. Can be uncaring
❑3. Can be self-destructive	❑3. Can be destructive	❑3. Feels victimized
❑4. Anxious	❑4. Irritable	❑4. Attached
❑5. Sneaky	❑5. Manipulative	❑5. Greedy, loves possessions
❑6. Nervous	❑6. Angry	❑6. Desirous
❑7. Dynamic	❑7. Perceptive	❑7. Harmonious
❑8. Communicative	❑8. Caring	❑8. Devoted, loyal
❑9. Flexible, takes change well	❑9. Tolerant, accepts things when no other choice	❑9. Patient, accepts all
❑10. Feelings and emotions change easily	❑10. Aggressive about opinions and feelings, gives opinions even if they are not asked for	❑10. Avoids giving opinions in difficult situations
❑11. Dreams about flying, running restless nightmares	❑11. Dreams in color, fast, passion, conflicts	❑11. Romantic, short dreams, often involve water

_____	_____	_____
Total Vata	Total Pitta	Total Kapha

SUMMARY OF QUESTIONNAIRES

Part I - shows where we started constitutionally and where we may need to return to "feel ourselves."

Part II - shows our immediate state of balance and makes us aware of symptoms that we may wish to see changed. This section will be your guide in choosing a lifestyle regime and diet to reduce your most aggravated dosha.

Part III - shows our mind strengths and weaknesses. Understanding our mental nature can help us choose work that suits our innate abilities and avoid those activities that do not suit us.

Part IV - if our negative or destructive emotions match our "dosha imbalance" (Part IV), they will be taken care of by the appropriate diet and lifestyle regime. If they fall out of pattern, they are associated with a different dosha (VPK). Specific essential oils to reduce those emotions can be used.

Totals for Parts II, III, IV

Total VATA _____   Total PITTA _____   Total KAPHA _____

This three-part total shows where you are operating physically, mentally and emotionally at this moment. After initiating therapies, diet, and lifestyle changes to balance your doshas, you can retake these parts and see a shift. Part I will always remain the same and so is not included in the total, nor is it retaken.

DIET FOR REDUCING VATA IMBALANCE

Grains		Vegetables	
YES	AVOID/ REDUCE	YES	AVOID/ REDUCE
Basmati rice	Barley	Well cooked with butter, lemon	Bean sprouts
Brown rice	Rye		Peas
Oats	Corn	Beets	Brussel sprouts
Wheat	Granola	Cucumber	Cauliflower
Couscous	Millet	Carrots	Lettuce
Spelt	No dry cereals	Yams	Fresh corn
Amaranth	Corn chips unless eaten with cheese	Jerusalem artichokes	Raw vegetables
Buckwheat		Mushrooms	(these vegetables may be eaten in small quantities – always cooked)

Vegetables (cont'd)

YES

All tubers
Okra
Pickled veggies
Celery
Potato
All squash
Kale
Turnip
Spachetti &
winter squash
Asparagus
Yucca

Animal Foods

YES	AVOID/ REDUCE
Pork	Rabbit
Seafood	Beef
Turkey	
Chicken	
Duck	

Spices

YES	AVOID/ REDUCE
Anise	Chili
Bay	Tarragon
Juniperberry	Cayenne
Asafoetida	Caraway
Basil	Peppermint
Caraway	
Cardamon	

Spices (cont'd)

Cinnamon
Black pepper (small amounts)
Clove
Coriander
Sage
Cumin
Fennel
Garlic
Ginger
Onion
Thyme
Turmeric
Fenugreek
Nutmeg
Allspice
Horseradish

Fruits

YES	AVOID/ REDUCE
Avocado	Apple
Banana	Cranberry
Cantaloupe	Dried fruits
Cherries	Melon
Coconut	Pear
Fresh figs	Pomegranate
Peaches	Jujube
Grapefruit	
Kiwi	
Dates	
Lime	
Lemon	
Mandarine	

Fruit (cont'd)

Mango
Papaya
Grapes
Persimmons
Sweet berries
Sweet fruits
Sweet oranges
Sweet pineapple
Sweet plums

Dairy

YES

All dairy products unless there is an allergy. Especially fermented like yogurt, buttermilk, keifer, cream cheese

Beans

All beans should be avoided except for pulses (dahl), green beans and tofu. Make into a paste or dahl: chick peas (hummus), mung beans, pink lentils

Oils

YES	AVOID/ REDUCE
All oils, although the best are: sesame oil, ghee & mayonnaise	Canola Corn oil Mustard oil

Nuts & Seeds

YES	AVOID/ REDUCE
All nuts – best soaked. Peanuts in butter	Peanuts – dry roasted Pumpkin

Sweeteners

YES	AVOID/ REDUCE
Sugar cane products Molasses Stevia Rice syrup Sucanat Cooked honey	Raw honey Carob

Beverages

YES	AVOID/ REDUCE
Hot herbal teas 1 small glass wine – (no sulfates) with meals. Warm rice milk No carbonated drinks	Cold drinks Coffee Black tea All other alcohols

Note: Avoid/Reduce means: When balanced, decrease consumption & eat occassionally. When imbalanced, avoid completely. If unclear as to your body type, consult an Ayurvedic practitioner

DIET FOR REDUCING PITTA IMBALANCE

Grains

YES – WELL COOKED	AVOID/ REDUCE
Barley with spices	Brown rice
Buckwheat	Corn (yellow)
Quinoa	Yeasted breads
Oats	
Kumut	
Soda breads & pancakes	
Wheat	
Rye	
Millet	
White basmati rice	
Corn (blue is best)	

Vegetables

YES	AVOID/ REDUCE
Asparagus	Beets
Broccoli	Carrots
Alfalfa sprouts	Chard
Brussel sprouts	Chilis
Artichokes	Eggplant
Cabbage	Garlic
Green bell peppers	Onions
Cauliflower	Hot peppers
Celery	Mustard greens
Eggplant	Tomatoes
Cucumber	Parsley
Green beans	Pickles
Lettuce	Purple peppers
	Radish
	Spinach

Vegetables (cont'd)

Mushrooms
Okra
Peas
Potatoes
Pumpkin
Turnips
Sweet potatoes
Steamed sweet onions
Turnips
Zucchini
Lots of greens

Animal Foods

YES	AVOID/ REDUCE
Chicken (white meat)	Beef
Egg white	Egg yolk
Pork	Lamb
Turkey	Duck
Pheasant	
Freshwater fish	

Spices

YES	AVOID/ REDUCE
Cilantro	Clove
Milk curries	Fenugreek
Cinnamon	Ginger
Turmeric	Pepper
Coriander	Mustard seed
Mint	Nutmeg
Cumin	Horseradish
Fennel	Oregano

Spices (cont'd)

Lotus seeds
Dill
Lemongrass
Lemon skin
Braggs Aminos

Rosemary
Sage
Salt
Asofoetida
Hing
All other spices;
hot spices

Beverages

YES	AVOID/ REDUCE
Cold drinks	Alcohol
Soy milk	Coffee
	Tea
	Hot drinks

Fruit

YES	AVOID/ REDUCE
Coconut	Grapefruit
Cherries	Lemon juice
Grapes	Limes
Melon	Olives
Pear	Papaya
Pomegranate	Peaches
Sweet fruit	Persimmon
Sweet oranges	Sour oranges
Sweet pineapples	Sour pineapple
Sweet plums	Mango

Dairy

YES	AVOID/ REDUCE
Butter	Cheese (highly fermented)
Cottage cheese	

Dairy (cont'd)

Cream cheese
Ghee (best)
Milk
Rice dream
Soybean
ice cream

Cultured
buttermilk
Kefie
Salty cheeses
Sour cream
Yogurt

Beans

YES

Most beans OK, especially Mung, tofu, aduki, black, chickpeas, lima, soybeans, fava

Oils

AVOID/REDUCE

Sesame
Corn
Others

Nuts

YES	AVOID/ REDUCE
Lotus seed	Peanuts
Sunflower	Almonds
Cashews (best to skip in the summer)	Pine nuts
	Pumpkin
	Sesame seeds

Sweeteners

YES	AVOID/ REDUCE
Maple syrup	Honey
Rice syrup	Molasses
Stevia	White sugar
Barley syrup	Chocolate

Best to Avoid/Reduce

Fermented products
Vinegars
Red meat
Salt
Tobacco

Note: Avoid/Reduce means: When balanced, decrease consumption & eat occasionally. When imbalanced, avoid completely. If unclear as to your body type, consult an Ayurvedic practitioner

DIET FOR REDUCING KAPHA IMBALANCE

Grains

YES – WELL COOKED (with spices)	AVOID/ REDUCE
Basmati rice	Millet
Buckwheat	Brown rice
Corn	Wheat
Rye	White rice
Dry cereals	Oats
Roasted grains	
Quinoa	
Couscous	
Barley	

Vegetables
(75% of diet)

YES	AVOID/ REDUCE
Artichokes	Cucumber
Beets	Okra
Fresh corn	Sweet potatoes
Turnips	Tomatoes
Asparagus	Zucchini
Bok choy	Sweet & juicy veggies
Bitter melon	
Bell peppers	

Vegetables (cont'd)

Carrots
Broccoli
Cabbage
Spinach
Swiss chard
Celery
Eggplant
Green salads
Leafy greens
Lettuce
Mushrooms
Chili peppers
Mustard greens
Onions
Sprouts
Potatoes
Squash
Hot peppers
Radish

Animal Foods

YES	AVOID/ REDUCE
Freshwater fish	Beef
Rabbit	Chicken
Turkey (dark meat)	Duck

Animal Foods (cont'd)

Venison

Beef
Chicken
Duck

Beverages

YES

Almond milk
Ginger tea
Coffee (1 cup per day)
Cranberry juice
Tea
Carbonated drinks
1 small glass wine with meals

AVOID/ REDUCE

Ice cold drinks

Avoid

All Vinegars

Fruits

**YES –
(especially dry)**

Apple
Cranberry
Dried fruits
Lemons
Grapefruit
Pears
Persimmons
Pomegranate
Raisins
Papaya
Blueberries

AVOID/ REDUCE

Bananas
Coconut
Dates
Figs
Prunes
Grapes
Kiwi
Melons
Orange
Pineapple
Sweet fruits

Fruits (cont'd)

Strawberries
Apricots
(moderation)

Dairy

YES

Small amounts unsalted ghee, soft cheese, cottage cheese

AVOID/ REDUCE

Fermented, aged dairy

Beans

YES

All beans, especially aduki, fava, kidney, lentils, lima

AVOID/ REDUCE

Tofu in extreme Kapha
Chickpeas
Hummus

Oils

**YES –
(Small Amounts)**

Best cold pressed
Canola
Flax
Corn
Mustard
Almond
Sunflower
Soy
Mayonnaise
Peanuts

AVOID/ REDUCE

All others

Sweeteners

YES	AVOID/ REDUCE
Small amounts of raw uncooked honey	All other sweeteners

Nuts & Seeds

YES	AVOID/ REDUCE
Best if sprouted	All others
Flax	Peanuts

Nuts & Seeds (cont'd)

Pumpkin

Sunflower

Spices

YES

All spices, especially ginger

Avoid/Reduce

Pickles

Salt vinegar

Note: Avoid/Reduce means: When balanced, decrease consumption & eat occassionally. When imbalanced, avoid completely. If unclear as to your body type, consult an Ayurvedic practitioner

DIET FOR REDUCING VATA-KAPHA OR KAPHA-VATA IMBALANCE

When Vata is obstructed, it is best to follow a Kapha diet

Grains

YES – (cooked well)	AVOID/ REDUCE
Basmati rice	Barley
Oats	Buckwheat
Wheat	Corn
Couscous	Granola
Spelt	Millet
Amaranth	Rye
	No dry cereals
	Corn chips unless eaten with cheese

Vegetables – (well cooked)

YES	AVOID/ REDUCE
With butter, lemon	Bean sprouts
Beets	Brussel sprouts
Cilantro	Raw vegetables
Carrots	Cauliflower
Yams	Lettuce
Cucumber	Fresh corn
Celery	(the above vegetables may be eaten in small quantities – always cooked)
Jerusaleum artichokes	
Mushrooms	
Okra	
Green beans	

Vegetables (cont'd)

Broccoli
Pickled veggies
Spinach
Potato
Acorn & all
squash
Cooked kale
Turnips
Asparagus
Cooked greens
Cooked eggplant

Animal Foods

YES	AVOID/ REDUCE
Pork	Rabbit
Seafood	Beef
Turkey	
Chicken	
Duck	

Spices

YES	AVOID/ REDUCE
Anise	Chile
Bay	Cayenne
Asofoetida (hing)	Peppermint
Basil	
Caraway	
Cardamon	
Cinnamon	
Juniper	
Black pepper (small amounts)	
Clove	

Spices (cont'd)

Coriander
Sage
Cumin
Fennel
Garlic
Ginger
Onion
Caraway
Tarragon
Turmeric
Thyme
Fenugreek
Nutmeg
Allspice
Horseradish

Fruits

YES	AVOID/ REDUCE
Avocado	Apple
Banana	Cranberry
Payaya	Dried fruits
Cantelope	Pear
Cherries	Pomegranate
Grapes	Jujube
Coconut	Melons
Fresh figs	
Peaches	
Grapefruit	
Kiwi	
Dates	
Lemons	
Lime	
Mandarine	
Mango	

Fruits (cont'd)

Persimmons
Sweet berries
Sweet plums
Sweet fruit
Sweet oranges
Sweet pineapple
Add spices to fruits

Dairy

YES

All dairy products unless there is an allergy. Especially fermented like yogurt, buttermilk, keifer, cream cheese, soy, rice, almond cheeses

Beans

All beans should be avoided except for pulses (dahl), ghee, beans & tofu.

Make into a paste or dahl: Chick peas (hummus), Mung beans, Pink lentils

Oils

YES	AVOID/ REDUCE
All oils, although the best are:	Canola
	Corn oil

Oils (cont'd)

sesame, ghee, mayonnaise	Mustard oil

Nuts & Seeds

YES	AVOID/ REDUCE
All nuts – best soaked	Peanuts – dry roasted
	Pumpkin

Sweeteners

YES	AVOID/ REDUCE
Cooked honey	Raw honey
Molasses	Carob
Stevia	
Rice syrup	
Sucanat	

Beverages

YES	AVOID/ REDUCE
Hot herbal teas	Cold drinks
1 small glass wine (with no sulfates) with meals.	Coffee
	Black tea
Warm rice milk	All other alcohols
	No carbonated drinks

Note: Avoid/Reduce means: When balanced, decrease consumption & eat occasionally. When imbalanced, avoid completely. If unclear as to your body type, consult an Ayurvedic practitioner

DIET FOR REDUCING PITTA-VATA OR VATA-PITTA IMBALANCE

When there is extreme imbalance or allergies, diet may have to be modified

Grains

YES (well cooked)	AVOID/ REDUCE
Basmati rice	Barley
Spelt	Brown rice
Oats	Wheat
Amaranth	Buckwheat
Couscous	Corn
Rye	Granola
Quinoa	Millet
	No dry cereals
	Corn chips unless eaten with cheese

Vegetables

YES (Well cooked with butter & lemon)	AVOID/ REDUCE
Carrots	Bean sprouts
Yams	Peas
Cucumber	Brussel sprouts
Okra	Cabbage
Jerusalem artichokes	Cauliflower
Mushrooms	Lettuce
Broccoli	Green beans
Celery	Fresh corn
Sweet potato	Eggplant
	Raw vegetables (these vegetables may be eaten in small quantities, always cooked)

Vegetables (cont'd)

Acorn squash & all squash
Kale
Turnips
Spaghetti & winter squash
Asparagus
Steamed onion
All greens
Dandelion
Fennel

Animal Foods

YES	AVOID/ REDUCE
Seafood	Rabbit
Turkey	Beef
Chicken	
Duck	

Spices

YES	AVOID/ REDUCE
Anise	Chili
Bay	Juniper berries
Asofoetida	Sage
Basil	Cayenne
Cilantro	Caraway
Cardamon	Clove
Cinnamon	Garlic

Spices (cont'd)

Black pepper
(small amounts)
Coriander
Sage
Cumin
Fennel
Fresh garlic
Onion
Sea salt
Tarragon
Thyme
Fenugreek
Nutmeg
Allspice
Turmeric
Peppermint
Milk curries
Braggs Aminos

Fruits

YES	AVOID/ REDUCE
Avocado	Apple
Banana	Cranberry
Cantaloupe	Dried fruits
Melon	Pomegranate
Cherries	jujube
Coconut	
Fresh figs	
Peaches	
Grapefruit	
Kiwi	
Dates	
Lime	
Lemon	

Fruits (cont'd)

Mandarine
Mango
Papaya
Grapes
Persimmon
Sweet berries
Sweet fruit
Sweet oranges
Sweet pineapple
Sweet plums
Cooked apples
Cooked pears

Dairy

YES

All dairy products unless there is an allergy.

Beans

All beans should be avoided except for pulses (dahl), beans with ghee & beans with tofu

Make into a paste or dahl: Chick peas (hummus), Mung beans, Pink lentils

Nuts & Seeds
(all nuts best soaked)

YES	AVOID/ REDUCE
Sunflower, sprouted	Peanuts – dry roasted
Peanuts in butter	Pumpkin

Sweeteners

YES	AVOID/ REDUCE
Sucanat	Raw honey
Fructose	Carob
Stevia	
Rice syrup	
Cooked honey	

Beverages

YES	AVOID/ REDUCE
Herbal teas	Cold drinks
1 small glass wine (no sulfates) with meals.	Coffee
	Black tea
	All other alcohols
Warm rice milk	No carbonated drinks

*Note: **Avoid/Reduce means:** When balanced, decrease consumption & eat occassionally. When imbalanced, avoid completely. If unclear as to your body type, consult an Ayurvedic practitioner*

DIET FOR REDUCING PITTA-KAPHA OR KAPHA-PITTA IMBALANCE

Grains

YES (well cooked)	AVOID/ REDUCE
	Millet
Barley	Brown rice
Basmati rice	Wheat
Buckwheat	White rice
Corn	
Rye	
Dry cereals	
Roasted grains	
Quinoa	
Couscous	

Vegetables
(75% of diet)

YES	AVOID/ REDUCE
Artichokes	Cucumber
Asparagus	Okra

Vegetables (cont'd)

Bell peppers
Beets
Turnips
Bitter melon
Bok choy
Fennel
Broccoli
All greens
Spinach
Swiss chard
Cabbage
Cauliflower
Celery
Eggplant
Green pepper
Lettuce
Green salads
Leafy greens

Sweet Potatoes
Tomatoes
Zucchini
Sweet & juicy vegetables
Radish
Carrots
Hot peppers
Chili peppers

Vegetables (cont'd)

Mushrooms
Mustard greens
Dandelion
Onions
Sprouts
Potatoes
Squash

Animal Foods

YES	AVOID/ REDUCE
Freshwater fish	Beef
Turkey (dark meat)	Seafood
Venison	Chicken
	Duck
	Lamb
	Port
	Fatty foods
	Fried, greasy meats

Spices

YES	AVOID/ REDUCE
Coriander	Pickles
Mint	Salt
Cardamon	Vinegar
Cilantro	
Ginger	
Fennel	
Turmeric	
Anise	
Cinnamon	
Milk curries	

Fruits

YES (especially dry)	AVOID/ REDUCE
Apple	Banana
Dried fruits	Coconut
Lemon	Dates
Grapefruit	Figs
Pear	Prunes
Persimmon	Grapes
Pomegranate	Kiwi
Raisins	Melons
Papaya	Oranges
Strawberry	Pineapple
Apricot (moderation)	Sweet fruits
Blueberries	

Dairy

YES	AVOID/ REDUCE
Goatmilk (small amount, unsalted)	Fermented, aged dairy
Ghee	
Soft cheese	
Cottage cheese	

Beans

YES	AVOID/ REDUCE
All beans, especially aduki, fava, kidney, lentils, lima	Tofu in extreme Kapha
	Chickpeas
	Hummus

Oils

YES (small amounts)	AVOID/REDUCE
Best cold pressed:	All others
Canola	
Flax	
Corn	
Mustard	
Almond	
Sunflower	
Soy	
Mayonnaise	
Peanut	

Sweeteners

YES	AVOID/REDUCE
Small amount only – raw uncooked honey	All other sweeteners

Nuts & Seeds

YES	AVOID/REDUCE
Best if sprouted:	All others
Flax seed	Peanuts
Pumpkin seed	
Sunflower	

Beverages

YES	AVOID/REDUCE
Almond milk	Ice cold drinks
Ginger tea	
Coffee (1 cup per day)	
Lemonade	
Tea	
Carbonated drinks	
Wine – 1 small glass with meals	

*Note: **Avoid/Reduce** means: When balanced, decrease consumption & eat occassionally. When imbalanced, avoid completely. If unclear as to your body type, consult an Ayurvedic practitioner*

AYURVEDIC DAILY CHECKLIST

Name: _____

Date:_____   Arising Time: _____

(If you awake feeling imbalanced - review your previous day's Checklist)

Food Intake

A.M.: _____
_____

Mid A.M.:_____
_____

Mid Day: _____
_____

Mid Afternoon: _____
_____

P.M.: _____
_____

P.M. Snack: _____
Supplements: _____
_____

Herbs: _____
_____

Other

Environment/Mood: _____
_____

Stress Level:_____
_____

P.M. Activities: _____
_____

Time to Bed: _____

Resources

Aromatherapy Video and Home Study Program

Michael Scholes (founder of Aroma Vera)
3384 South Robertson Pl.
Los Angeles, CA 90034
Ph: 800-677-2368

Jeanne Rose Aromatherapy and Herbal Healing Intensives
Attn: Jeanne Rose
219 Carl Street
San Francisco, CA 94117

London School of Aromatherapy
P.O. Box 780
London NW5 1DY
England

Pacific Institute of Aromatherapy
Attn: Kurt Schnaubelt
P.O. Box 8723
San Rafael, CA 94903
Ph: 515-479-9121

Quintessence Aromatherapy
Attn: Ann Berwick
P.O. Box 4996
Boulder, CO 80306
Ph: 303-258-3791

Ayurveda Centers and Programs

Australian Institute of Ayurvedic Medicine
19 Bowey Avenue
Enfield S.A. 5085
Australia
Ph: 08-349-7303

Australian School of Ayurveda
Dr. Krishna Kumar, MD, FIIM

27 Blight Street
Ridleyton, South Australia 5008
Ph. (08) 346-0631

Ayur-Veda AB
Box 78, 285 22 Markaryd
Esplanaden 2
Sweden
0433-104 90 (Phone)
0433-104 92 (Fax)
E-Mail: info@ayur-veda.se

Ayurveda for Radiant Health & Beauty
16 Espira Court
Santa Fe, NM 87505
Ph: 505-466-7662

Ayurvedic Healing Arts Center
16508 Pine Knoll Road
Grass Valley, CA 95945
Ph: 916-274-9000

Ayurvedic Healings
Dr.'s Light & Bryan Miller
P. O. Box 35214
Sarasota, FL 34242
Ph: 941-346-3581

Ayurvedic Holistic Center
82A Bayville Ave.
Bayville, NY 11709

The Ayurvedic Institute and Wellness Center
11311 Menaul, NE
Albuquerque, NM 87112
Ph: 505-291-9698
Fax: 505-294-7572

Ayurvedic Living Workshops
P.O. Box 188
Exeter, Devon EX4 5AB
England

California College of Ayurveda

1117A East Main Street
Grass Valley, CA 95945
Ph: 530-274-9100
Web: ayurvedacollege.com
E-Mail: info@ayurvedacollege.com
Clinical training in Ayurveda

Center for Mind, Body Medicine
P.O. Box 1048
La Jolla, CA 92038
Ph: 619-794-2425

The Chopra Center for Well Being
7590 Fay Avenue
Suite 403
LaJolla, CA 92037
Ph: 619-551-7788
Fax: 619-551-7811

John Douillard
Life Spa, Rejuvenation through Ayur-Veda
3065 Center Green Dr.
Boulder CO 80301
Ph: 303-442-1164, Fax: 303-442-1240

East West College of Herbalism Ayurvedic Program
Represents courses of Dr. David Frawley and Dr. Michael Tierra in UK
Hartswood, Marsh Green, Hartsfield
E. Sussex TN7 4ET
United Kingdom
Ph: 01342-822312
Fax: 01342-826346
E-Mail: ewcolherb@aol.com

EverGreen Herb Garden and Learning Center, Candis Cantin Packard
PO Box 1445, Placerville CA 95667

Ph. and Fax: 530-626-9288
E-Mail:
evrgreen@innercite.com

Himalayan Institute
RR1, Box 400
Honesdale, PA 18431
800-822-4547
E-Mail: earthess@aol.com
Web: ayurvedichealing.com

Inside Ayurveda
Bi-monthly, independent
publication for ayurvedic
professionals.
Niika Quistgard
PO Box 3021
Quincy CA 995971-3021
Ph: 530-283-3717
E-Mail: oflife@inreach.com

Institute for Wholistic
Education
33719 116th Street
Box AWF
Twin lakes, WI 53181
Ph: 262-877-9396
Beginner and Advanced
Correspondence Courses
in Ayurveda

Integrated Health Systems
3855 Via Nova Marie,
#302D
Carmel, CA 93923
Ph: 408-476-5130

International Academy
of Ayurved
NandNandan, Atreya
Rugnalaya
M.Y. Lele Chowk
Erandawana, Pune: 411
004, India
Ph/Fax: 91-212-378532/
524427
E-Mail: avilele@hotmail.com

International Ayurvedic
Institute
111 Elm Street
Suite 103-105

Worcester, MA 01609
Ph: 508-755-3744
Fax: 508-770-0618
E-Mail:
ayurveda@hotmail.com

International Federation
of Ayurveda
Dr. Krishna Kumar
27 Blight Street
Ridleyton S.A. 5008
Australia
Ph: 08-346-0631

Kaya Kalpa International
Dr. Raam Panday
111 Woodster Rd.
Satto, NY 10012

Life Impressions Institute
Attn: Donald VanHowten,
Director
613 Kathryn Street
Santa Fe, NM 87501
Ph: 505-988-2627

Light Institute of Ayurveda
Drs. Bryan & Light Miller
P.O. Box 35284
Sarasota, FL 34242
E-Mail: earthess@aol.com
Web: ayurvedichealings.com

Lotus Ayurvedic Center
4145 Clares St. Suite D
Capitola, CA 95010
Ph: 408-479-1667

Maharishi Ayurved
at the Raj
1734 Jasmine Avenue
Fairfield, IA 52556
Ph: 800-248-9050
Fax: 515-472-2496

Maharishi Health Center
Hale Clinic
7 Park Crescent
London, W14 3H3
England

Natural Therapeutics Center
'Surya Daya'

Gisingham, Nr. Iye
Suffolk, England

New England Institute of
Ayurvedic Medicine
111 N. Elm Street
Suites 103-105
Worcester, MA 01609
Ph: 508-755-3744
Fax: 508-770-0618
E-Mail:
ayurveda@hotmail.com

Rocky Mountain Ayurvedic
Health Retreat
P.O. Box 5192
Pagosa Springs, CO 81147
Ph: 800-247-9654;
970-264-9224

Atreya Smith
Represents Dr. David
Frawley's course in Europe,
particularly France, Germany
and Switzerland.
13Q, Rue de Rivoli,
Paris, France
Tel: 33-0-1-40-28-42-20,
Fax 33-0-1-42-19-02-91
E-Mail:
Atreya@compuserve.com

Victoria Stern, N.D.
P.O. Box 1814
Laguna Beach, CA 92652
Ph: 714-494-8858

Vinayak Ayurveda Center
2509 Virginia NE, Ste D
Albuquerque, NM 87110
Ph: 505-296-6522
Fax: 505-298-2932
Web: ayur.com

Wise Earth School
of Ayurveda
Attn: Bri. Maya Tiwari
RR1 Box 484
Candler, NC 28715
Ph: 704-258-9999
Teachers and Practitioners
Training Programs Only

Ayurvedic Cosmetic Companies

Auroma Int'l
P.O. Box 1008
Dept. AWF
Silver Lake, WI 53170
Ph: 262-889-8569
Fax: 262-889 8591
importer and master
distributor of Auroshikha
Incense, Chandrika
Ayurvedic Soap and Herbal
Vedic Ayurvedic products

Bindi Facial Skin Care
A Division of Pratima Inc.
109-17 72nd Road
Lower Level
Forest Hills, New York
11375
Ph: 718-268-7348

Devi Inc. (for Shivani
product line)
Attn: Anjali Mahaldar
P.O. Box 377
Lancaster, MA 01523
Ph: 800-237-8221
Fax: 508-368-0455

Gajee Herbals
The Khenpo Company
Attn: Gayatri Puri, Owner
17595 Harvard St., C531
Irvine, CA 92714
Ph: 714-250-6027

Internatural
33719 116th St.
Box AWF
Twin Lakes, WI 53181
USA
800-643 4221 (toll free
order line)
262-889 8581 (office
phone)
262-889 8591 (fax)
E-Mail:
internatural@lotuspress.com
Web: internatural.com
Retail mail order and
internet reseller of essential

oils, herbs, spices,
supplements, herbal
remedies, incense, books and
other supplies

Lotus Brands, Inc.
P.O. Box 325
Dept. AWF
Twin Lakes, WI 53181
Ph: 262-889-8561
Fax: 262-889-8591
E-Mail:
lotusbrands@lotuspress.com
manufacturer and distributor
of natural personal care and
herbal products, massage oils,
essential oils, incense and
aromatherapy items

Lotus Light Enterprises
P O Box 1008
Dept. AWF
Silver Lake, WI 53170 USA
800-548 3824 (toll free
order line)
262-889 8501 (office
phone)
262-889 8591 (fax)
E-Mail:
lotuslight@lotuspress.com
wholesale distributor of
essential oils, herbs, spices,
supplements, herbal
remedies, incense, books and
other supplies. Must supply
resale certificate number or
practitioner license to obtain
catalog of more than 10,000
items.

Siddhi Ayurvedic
Beauty Products
C/O Vinayak
Ayurveda Center
2509 Virginia NE, Suite D
Albuquerque, NM 87110
Ph: 505-296-6522
Fax: 505-298-2932

Swami Sada Shiva Tirtha
Ayurvedic Holistic Center
82A Bayville Avenue

Bayville, NY 11709
Ph/Fax: 516-628-8200

TEJ Beauty
Enterprises, Inc.
(an Ayurvedic
Beauty Salon)
162 West 56th St. Rm 201
New York, NY 10019
(owner: Pratima Raichur,
founder of Bindi)
Ph: 212-581-8136

Ayurvedic Herbal Suppliers

Auroma Int'l
P.O. Box 1008
Dept. AWF
Silver Lake, WI 53170
Ph: 262-889-8569
fax: 262-889 8591
importer and master
distributor of Auroshikha
Incense, Chandrika
Ayurvedic Soap and Herbal
Vedic Ayurvedic products

Ayur Herbal Corporation
P.O. Box 6390
Santa Fe, NM 87502
Ph: 262-889-8569

Ayurveda Center
of Santa Fe
1807 Second St., Suite 20
Santa Fe, NM 87505
Ph: 505-983-8898

Ayush Herbs, Inc.
10025 N.E. 4th Street
Bellevue, WA 98004
Ph: 800-925-1371

Banyan Trading Company
Traditional Ayurvedic Herbs
- Wholesale
P.O. Box 13002
Albuquerque, NM 87192
Ph: 505-244-1880
800-953-6424
Fax: 505-244-1878

Bazaar of India
Imports, Inc.
1810 University Avenue
Berkeley, CA 94703
Ph: 800-261-7662; 510-
548-4110

Dhanvantri Aushadhalaya
Herbs of Wisdom and Love,
Ayurvedic Herbs and
Classical Formulas.
PO Box 1654, San Anselmo
CA 94979
Ph: 415-289-7976, Email:
ayurveda@dhanvantri.com

Dr. Singha's Mustard Bath
and More
Attn: Anna Searles
Natural Therapeutic Centre
2500 Side Cove
Austin, TX 78704
Ph: 800-856-2862

Bio Veda
215 North Route 303
Congers, NY 10920-1726
Ph: 800-292-6002

Earth Essentials Florida
Dr.'s Bryan and Light Miller
4067 Shell Road
Sarasota, FL 34242
941-316-0920

Frontier Herbs
P.O. Box 229
Norway, IA 52318
Ph: 800-669-3275

HerbalVedic Products
P.O. Box 6390
Santa Fe, NM 87502

Internatural
33719 116th St.
Box AWF
Twin Lakes, WI 53181 USA
800-643-4221 (toll free
order line)
262-889-8581 (office
phone)
262-889-8591 (fax)

email:
internatural@lotuspress.com
Web: internatural.com
Retail mail order and internet
reseller of essential oils, herbs,
spices, supplements, herbal
remedies, incense, books and
other supplies

Kanak
P.O. Box 13653
Albuquerque, NM
87192-3653
Ph: 505-275-2469

Lotus Brands, Inc.
P.O. Box 325
Dept. AWF
Twin Lakes, WI 53181
Ph: 262-889-8561
Fax: 262-889-8591

Lotus Herbs
1505 42nd Ave. Suite 19
Capitola, CA 95010
Ph: 408-479-1667

Lotus Light Enterprises
P O Box 1008
Dept. AWF
Silver Lake, WI 53170 USA
800-548-3824 (toll free
order line)
262-889-8501 (office
phone)
262-889-8591 (fax)
email:
lotuslight@lotuspress.com
wholesale distributor of
essential oils, herbs, spices,
supplements, herbal
remedies, incense, books and
other supplies. Must supply
resale certificate number or
practitioner license to obtain
catalog of more than 10,000
items.

Maharishi Ayurveda Products
International, Inc.
417 Bolton Road
P.O. Box 541
Lancaster, MA 01523

Info: 800-843-8332
Ext. 903
Order: 800-255-8332
Ext. 903

Planetary Formulations
P. O. Box 533
Soquel, CA 95073
Formulas by Dr. Michael
Tierra

Quantum Publication, Inc.
P.O. Box 1088
Sudbury, MA 01776
Ph: 800-858-1808

Seeds of Change
P. O. Box 15700
Santa Fe, NM 87506-5700
Catalog of rare Western and
Indian seeds.

Vinayak Panchakarma
Chikitsalaya
Y.M.C.A Complex, Situbuldi
Nagpur (Maharastra State)
India 440 012
Ph: 011-91-712-538983
Fax: 011-91-712-552409
Retail/Wholesale

Yoga of Life Center
2726 Tramway N.E.
Albuquerque, NM 87122
Ph: 505-275-6141

Ayurvedic Practitioners (by state and country)

ARIZONA

Jeffrey Armstrong
4820 N. 35th St.
Phoenix, AZ 85018
602-468-9448
Ayurvedic Astrologer, Author,
Lecturer, Teacher

Darcy Frankell
9750 North 966 St, Ste 125
Scottsdale, AZ 85258
614-979-9799
Ayurvedic Consultant

CALIFORNIA

Changing Worlds
Gail Ann Shwartz
329 Strawberry Village
Mill Valley, CA 94941
415-383-3223
415-383-9933
Ayurvedic Consultant

Donna Panagajus
329 Strawberry Village
Mill Valley, CA 94941
415-388-0260
Ayurvedic Consultant

COLORADO

Brigitte Mars
1919-D 19th Street
Boulder, Colorado 80302
303-442-4967
Herbalist, Lecturer,
Ayurvedic Consultant

CONNECTICUT

William Rasmussen
Box 616
Sugar Hill
New Hampshire, CT 03585
Ayurvedic Consultant

FLORIDA

Ayurvedic Healings
Drs. Bryan & Light Miller
P. O. Box 35214
Sarasota, FL 34242
941-346-3220
Ayurvedic herbs, personalized
perfumes, starter kits, books

Marie Abeles
P.O. Box 691
Osprey, FL 34229
941-724-3054
Ayurvedic Practitioner

Bodyworks
Carla Polins
3801 Beed Ridge
Sarasota, FL 34233
941-923-7546
Ayurvedic Consultant,
Massage, Weight Loss,
Aromatherapy

Jackie Buchanan
P.O. Box 372
Collinsville, IL 62234
618-344-8896
Ayurvedic Practitioner

Cary Caster
3065 St. James Drive
Boca Raton, FL 33434
561-852-0296 (fax)
Ayurvedic practitioner,
Aromatherapy

Dian DeMaio
17352 Terry Ave
Port Charlotte, FL 33948
941-627-2100 (B)
Ayurvedic Consultant,
Licensed Nutritionist

Richard and Diana Dafner
P.O. Box 35195
Sarasota, FL 34242
941-346-1024
E-Mail Rdaffner@juno.com
Tantra, Tai Chi, Workshops

Suzanne Dameron
P.O. Box 3722
941-955-2583
Ayurvedic Practitioner

Brian Fields
3426 Clark Drive
Sarasota, FL 34234
941-355-4663

Margie Green
P.O. Box 19601
Sarasota, FL 34276
941-926-8006
Ayurvedic Consultant,
Lymphatic Drainage

Healing Heaven - Namaste
Katya Kudrow
818 Plymouth St
Sarasota, FL 34242
941-346-1972
Ayurvedic Consultant,
Indian Massage, Pancha
Karma, Lomi Lomi Massage,

Indian Dance, Yoga,
Meditation,
Aromatherapy Bar

Sandra Hoy
11185 Rockwell Avenue
Englewood, FL 34224
941-474-1760
Ayurvedic Practitioner

Kevin O'Bryan
2574 Hawthorne
Sarasota, FL 34239
941-955-7435
Ayurvedic Consultant,
Lecturer, Wholistic
Personal Trainer

Paula Olton
71 Emerald Woods Drive
NOF6
Naples, FL 34108
941-513-2313
Ayurvedic Consultant

Options for Growth, Inc.
Gloria DeVoss, LCSW
4523 Park Lane Terrace N.
Bradenton, FL 34209
941-798-6949
941-794-2115 (Fax)
E-Mail GDeV99@aol.com
Ayurvedic Consultant, NLP,
Aromatherapy, Massage,
Hypnosis, Workshops, Classes

Tahnia Palczynski
28701 SW 182nd Avenue
Homestead, FL 33030
309-247-9442
Ayurvedic Consultant

John Riccio, D.D.
4917 Remington Dr.
Sarasota, FL 34234
941-358-7902
941-351-5642 (fax)
Ayurvedic Consultant

Matthias Saretzky
P.O. Box 3122
Sarasota, FL 34230
Ph/Fax: 941-355-6036

Ayurvedic Consultant, Yoga, Chanting, Meditation

SwanSong
4740 Oak Hill Drive
Sarasota, FL 34232
Compassionate complementary therapies for the end of life

GEORGIA

Jyoti Leaf
7 Waite Drive
Savannah, GA 31406
912-354-9274
Ayurvedic Consultant, Aromatherapy, Lymphatic Drainage, Yoga

NEW MEXICO

David Bigdon, D.C.
Professional Plaza,
Cruz Alta Rd, Ste A
P.O. Box 1446
Taos, NM 87571
505-758-2038
505-751-7896 (Pager)
Ayurvedic Consultant, Gentle Chiropractic Techniques
Neuromuscular Therapist

Lehsa Orcutt, LMT
Professional Plaza,
Cruz Alta Rd, Ste A
P.O.Box 1446
Taos, NM 87571
505-758-2038
505-751-5263 (Pager)
800-369-4618
E-Mail dblo@newmex.com
Neuromuscular Therapist,
Ayurveda Indian Massage

NEW YORK

Allyson Best
184 Porterfield Place
Freeport, NY 11520
516-868-6531
Ayurvedic Consultant,
Ayurvedic Massage

Scott Gerson, M.D.
13 West 9th St
New York, NY 10011
212-505-8971
Ayurvedic Medical Physician

David Hendry
116 Jefferson St
East Islip, NY 11730
516-224-7869
Ayurvedic Consultant,
Pancha Karma, Massage

Jeanne McDougall
16 Greenwood St.
Rochester, NY 14608-2236
716-454-1036
Ayurvedic Consultant

TEXAS

Anita Fuller
2213 Bluff Circle
Salado, TX 76571-9344
254-947-4523
Ayurvedic Consultant,
Ayurvedic Massage

VIRGINIA

Vedic Health
Joyce O'Mally
149 Old Field Rd.
Williamsburg, VA 23188
540-786-7960
Ayurvedic Consultant

David Mathis, MD, FAAFP
213 Loudoun St, SW
Leesburg, VA 20175-2794
703-777-4203
703-777-0045 (Fax)
NVaNamaste@AOL.COM
Family Medicine, Ayurveda,
Mind-Body Medicine

WEST VIRGINIA

Joyce Marie McCoy
P.O. Box 1118
Harpers Ferry, WV 23451
304-535-2512
Ayurvedic Consultant,
Ayurvedic Massage

AUSTRALIA

Dr. Krishna Kumar, MD,
FIIM
Australian School of
Ayurveda
27 Blight Street
Ridleyton, South Australia
5008
Tel. 08 346-0631
Ayurvedic Medical Physician

CANADA

Liora Bruck
7445 fWest 14th - Apt 501
Vancouver, BC
Canada V6H 1R5
Ayurvedic Consultant,
Ayurvedic Cooking

Debra Drummond
2056 West 15th Avenue
VanCouver, B.C., Canada
V6J 2L5
604-739-3926
Ayurvedic Consultant,
Ayurveda Massage,
Lymphatic Massage,
Aromatherapy

Marilyn Carriere
55 Longshire Circle
Nepcan, Ontario K2J 4K7
613-825-3124
Ayurvedic Consultant

Saida Desilets
3002 West 3rd Ave
Vancouver, BC
V6K 1N1 Canada
Phone: 604-731-4835
Aromatherapist,
Aromabodywork,
Reiki, Tui Na Chinese
Massage, Goddess Workshops

Mina Kormam
438 Muller Drive
Thomhill, Ontario
Canada
905-763-1786
Ayurvedic Consultant,
Lecturer

Soulcare Consulting
Kelly Banah
7716 Patterson Avenue
Burnaby, B.C.
V5J 3P5 Canada
604-430-3662
Ayurvedic Consultant

Pamela J. Uyeyama
North Vancouver, B.C.
604-985-4206
604-977-5206 (pager)
Bodywork, Lymphatic
Drainage, Spa Treatments,
Healing Touch, Energy Work

Moona Wilds
516 Ballantree Place
West Vancouver, B.C.,
Canada V7S 1W5
Ayurvedic Practitioner,
Aromatherapy

Christina Young
2465 West 8th Ave
Vancouver, BC
Canada V6K 2B2
Ayurvedic Consultant,
Ayurvedic Indian Massage,
Cross Fibre Massage

GERMANY

Matthias Saretzky
Binnerstr, 23
92637 Weiden
Germany
Ph/Fax: 0961-419499
Ayurvedic Consultant, Yoga,
Chanting, Meditation

MEXICO

Gregory Soucy & Selene Ruiz
521 Aldama
Puerto Vallarta, Jalisco 48300
011 52-322 23344
E-Mail:
ayurvedasoucy@hotmail.com
tridosha@com.
Ayurvedic Consultants,
Indian Massage,
Pancha Karma

SPAIN

Paul Votava
Aptdo 135
11520 Rota Cadiz
Spain
E-Mail: pvotava@teleline.es

SWEDEN

Eva Georgsson
Smultronstigen 1 C
27138 Ystad
Sweden
01146-411-14668

Vijay Ralhoe
Rutensvag - 18
13436 Gustansberg
Sweden
Ayurvedic Consultant,
Ayurvedic Cooking

Ebba Palmcratz
Slipgatan
11739 Stockholm, Sweden
Ayurvedic Consultant

UNITED KINGDOM

Dr. Nicholas G. Kostopoulos
MC, MF
354 Finchley Road
London NW3 7AJ
Ayurvedic Medical Physician

WEST INDIES

Allyson Best
22 Purple Heart
Homeland Gardens
Cunupia
Trinidad, West Indies
868-671-3505
Ayurvedic Practitioner

Transformational Seminars

ClearMind
Duane O'Kane
22778 72nd Avenue
Langley, B.C., V2Y 2K3
Canada
800-210-0372
604-513-2219

Michael Rice
c/o Heartland
Rt. 3, Box 3280
Theodosia, MO 65761
417-273-4838

Sandy Levey-Lunden
Skraddarod 24
272 97 Garsnas, Sweden
Phone: 011 46-414-24320
Fax: 011 46-414-24395
E-Mail:
On.Purpose@Swipnet.se
Contacts: P.O. Box 2071
Mill Valley, CA 94942
408-2966962, and:
c/o Light & Bryan Miller
P.O. Box 35284
Sarasota, FL 34242
941-346-3518

Bodywork Training

The Center For Release and
Integration
450 Hillside Drive
Mill Valley, CA 94941

Dr. Jay Scherer's Academy of
Natural Healing
1443 St. Francis Drive
Santa Fe, NM 87505

The Rolf Institute
205 Canyon Blvd.
Boulder, CO 80302

The Upledger Institute
]1211 Prosperity Farms Rd.
Pal Beach Gardens, FL
33410

The Feldenkrais Guild
524 Ellsworth St. SW,
P.O. Box 489

Correspondence Courses

Light Institute of
Ayurvedic Teaching
Drs. Bryan & Light Miller
P.O. Box 35284
Sarasota, FL 34242

Ph: 941-346-3518
Fax: 941-346-0800
E-Mail: earthess@aol.com
www.ayurvedichealing.com
Ayurvedic Pratitioner
Training, Correspondence
Course, Books

American Institute of
Vedic Studies
Dr. David Frawley, Director
P.O. Box 8357
Santa Fe, NM 87504-8357
Ph: 505-983-9385
Fax: 505-982-5807
E-Mail: vedicinst@aol.com
Web: consciousnet.com/vedic
correspondence courses in
Ayurveda and Vedic
Astrology

Lessons and Lectures
in Ayurveda by
Dr. Robert Svoboda
P.O. Box 23445
Albuquerque, NM
87192-1445
Ph: 505-291-9698

Institute for Wholistic
Education
33719 116th St. Box AWF
Twin lakes, WI 53181
Ph: 262-877-9396

To train in Ayurvedic Facial Massage and Beauty practices

Melanie Sachs
"Invoking Beauty with
Ayurveda" Seminars
P.O. Box 13753-3753
San Luis Obispo, CA 93406

Beauty and Quality Ayurvedic Supplements

Auroma Int'l
P.O. Box 1008
Dept. AWF
Silver Lake, WI 53170
Ph: 262-889-8569

fax: 262- 889 8591
importer and master
distributor of Auroshikha
Incense, Chandrika
Ayurvedic Soap and Herbal
Vedic Ayurvedic products

Ayur Herbal Corporation
P.O. Box 6390 YA
Santa Fe, NM 87502
Ph: 262-889-8569
fax: 262-889 8591
Manufacturer of Herbal
Vedic Ayurvedic products

Internatural
33719 116th St.
Box AWF
Twin Lakes, WI 53181
USA
800-643-4221 (toll free
order line)
262-889-8581 (office
phone)
262-889 8591 (fax)
E-Mail:
internatural@lotuspress.com
Web: internatural.com
Retail mail order and internet
reseller of essential oils, herbs,
spices, supplements, herbal
remedies, incense, books and
other supplies

Lotus Brands, Inc.
P.O. Box 325
Dept. AWF
Twin Lakes, WI 53181
Ph: 262-889-8561
Fax: 262-889-8591
E-Mail:
lotusbrands@lotuspress.com
manufacturer and distributor
of natural personal care and
herbal products, massage oils,
essential oils, incense and
aromatherapy items

Lotus Light Enterprises
P O Box 1008
Dept. AWF
Silver Lake, WI 53170 USA

800-548-3824 (toll free
order line)
262-889-8501 (office
phone)
262-889-8591 (fax)
E-Mail:
lotuslight@lotuspress.com
wholesale distributor of
essential oils, herbs, spices,
supplements, herbal
remedies, incense, books and
other supplies. Must supply
resale certificate number or
practitioner license to obtain
catalog of more than 10,000
items.

Maharishi Ayur-Veda
Products International, Inc.
417 Bolton Road
P.O. Box 54
Lancaster, MA 01523
Ph: 800-ALL-VEDA
Fax: 508-368-7475

New Moon Extracts
P.O. Box 1947
Brattleborough, Vermont
05302-1947
Ph: 800-543-7279

Spectrum Natural
Omega 3 Oil
The Oil Company
133 Copeland Street
Petaluma, CA 94952

Universal Light, Inc.
P O Box 261
Dept. AWF
Wilmot, WI 53192
Ph: 262-889 8571
Fax: 262-889 8591
Importer and Master
Distributor for Vicco Herbal
Toothpaste

Color, Sound, and Gems

PAZ
P.O. Box 4859
Albuquerque, NM 87196

For open-backed gemstone settings

Color Therapy Eyewear
C/O Terri Perrigone-Messer
P.O. Box 3114
Diamond Springs, CA 95619

Lumatron (light device)
C/O Ernie Baker
515 Pierce Street #3
San Francisco, CA 94117
Ph: 415-626-0083

Genesis (sound device)
Medical Massage Therapy
Attn: Tina Shinn
1857 Northwest Blvd.
Annex
Columbus, Ohio 43212
Ph: 614-488-5244

Essential Oil Supplies

Aromatherapy Supply
Unit W3
The Knoll Business Center
Old Shoreham Road
Hove, Sussex BN3 7GS
England

Aroma Vera
3384 South Robertson Pl.
Los Angeles, CA 90034
Ph: 800-669-9514

Auroma Int'l
P.O. Box 1008
Dept. AWF
Silver Lake, WI 53170
Ph: 262-889-8569
fax: 262- 889 8591
importer and master distributor of Auroshikha Incense, Chandrika Ayurvedic Soap and Herbal Vedic Ayurvedic products

Earth Essentials Florida, Inc.
P.O. Box 35214
Sarasota, FL 34242
800-370-3220
Fax: 941-346-0800

E-Mail: earthess@aol.com
Rare Essential Oils

Fenmail Tisserand Oils
P.O. Box 48
Spalding, LINCS PE11 ADS
England

Internatural
33719 116th St.
Box AWF
Twin Lakes, WI 53181 USA
800-643 4221 (toll free order line)
262-889 8581 (office phone)
262-889 8591 (fax)
E-Mail:
internatural@lotuspress.com
Web: internatural.com
Retail mail order and internet reseller of essential oils, herbs, spices, supplements, herbal remedies, incense, books and other supplies

Lotus Brands, Inc.
P.O. Box 325
Dept. AWF
Twin Lakes, WI 53181
Ph: 262-889-8561
Fax: 262-889-8591
E-Mail:
lotusbrands@lotuspress.com
manufacturer and distributor of natural personal care and herbal products, massage oils, essential oils, incense and aromatherapy items

Lotus Light Enterprises
P O Box 1008
Dept. AWF
Silver Lake, WI 53170 USA
800-548 3824 (toll free order line)
262-889 8501 (office phone)
262-889 8591 (fax)
E-Mail:
lotuslight@lotuspress.com
wholesale distributor of essential oils, herbs, spices,

supplements, herbal remedies, incense, books and other supplies. Must supply resale certificate number or practitioner license to obtain catalog of more than 10,000 items.

Private Universe
P.O. Box 3122
Winter Park, FL 32790
Ph: 407-644-7203

Oshadi Ayus -
Quality Life Products
15, Monarch Bay Plaza Suite 346
Monarch Beach, CA 92629
Ph: 800-947-1008
Fax; 714-240-1104

Primavera
D 8961 Sulzberg
Germany
08376-808-0

Original Swiss Aromatics
P.O. Box 606
San Rafael, CA 94915
Ph: 415-459-3998

Smitasha
26961 Ayamonte Dr.
Mission Viejo, CA 92692
949-982-8777
714-785-6891

Exercise Programs and Information

Callanetic Headquarters
1700 Broadway
Suite 2000
Denver, CO 80290
Ph: 303-831-4455

Diamond Way Health
Associates
214 Girard Blvd. NE
Albuquerque, NM 87106
Ph: 505-265-4826
(for Sotai, Tibetan Rejuvenation Exercises)

Partners Yoga
4876 Darvin Court
Boulder, CO 80301
303-415-0199

Vega Study Center
1511 Robinson Street
Oroville, CA 95965
Ph: 916-533-7702
(for Sotai instructions -
books)

Satori Resources
732 Hamlin Way
San Leandro, CA 94578
(for Tai Chi Chih)

Kushi Institute
P.O. Box 7
Becket, MA 01223
Ph: 413-623-5741
(for Do-in)

Natural Ingredients

Aloe Farms
Box 125
Los Fresnos, TX 78566
Ph: 800-262-6771
(for aloe vera juice, gel,
powder and capsules)

Arya Laya Skin Care Center
Rolling Hills Estates, CA
90274
(for carrot oil)

Aubrey Organics
4419 North Manhattan
Avenue
Tampa, FL 33614
(for rosa mosquita oil and a
large variety of natural
cosmetics and shampoos)

Body Shop
45 Horsehill Road
Cedar Knolls, NJ 07927-
2014
Ph: 800-541-2535
(aloe vera, nut and seed oils,
cosmetics, make-up, brushes,
loofahs, and much more)

Culpepper Ltd.
21 Bruton Street

London W1X 7DA
England
(variety of natural seed, nut,
and kernal oils, essential oils,
herbs, books, and cosmetics)

Desert Whale Jojoba Co.
P.O. Box 41594
Tucson, AZ 85717
Ph: 602-882-4195
(for jojoba products and
many other natural oils,
including rice bran, pecan,
macadamia nut and apricot
kernal)

Everybody Ltd.
1738 Pearl Street
Boulder, CO 80302
Ph: 800-748-5675
(large variety of oils, oil
blends, and cosmetics)

Flora Inc.
P.O. Box 950
805 East Badger Road
Lynden, WA 98264
Ph: 800-446-2110
(for flax seed oil, herbal
supplements for skin, hair,
nails and cosmetics)

Green Earth Farm
P.O. Box 672
65 1/2 North 8th Street
Saguache, CO 81149
(for calendula oil, creme, and
herbal bath)

The Heritage Store, Inc.
P.O. Box 444
Virginia Beach, VA 23458
Ph: 804-428-0100
(castor oil, organic ghee,
cocoa butter, massage oils,
flowerwaters, essential oils,
cosmetics, and natural home
remedies)

Internatural
33719 116th St.
Box AWF
Twin Lakes, WI 53181 USA

800-643 4221 (toll free
order line)
262-889 8581 (office
phone)
262-889 8591 (fax)
E-Mail:
internatural@lotuspress.com
Web: internatural.com
Retail mail order and internet
reseller of essential oils, herbs,
spices, supplements, herbal
remedies, incense, books and
other supplies

Janca's Jojoba Oil and
Seed Company
456 E. Juanita #7
Mesa, AZ 85204
Ph: 602-497-9494
(jojoba oil, butter, wax, and
seeds. Also a large variety of
naturally pressed unusual
oils, such as camellia, kukui
nut, and grapeseed. Also
have clay, aloe products,
essential oils, and their own
line of cosmetics)

Lotus Brands, Inc.
P.O. Box 325
Dept. AWF
Twin Lakes, WI 53181
Ph: 262-889-8561
Fax: 262-889-8591
E-Mail:
lotusbrands@lotuspress.com
manufacturer and distributor
of natural personal care and
herbal products, massage oils,
essential oils, incense and
aromatherapy items

Lotus Light Enterprises
P O Box 1008
Dept. AWF
Silver Lake, WI 53170 USA
800-548 3824 (toll free
order line)
262-889 8501 (office ph.)
262-889 8591 (fax)
E-Mail:
lotuslight@lotuspress.com

wholesale distributor of essential oils, herbs, spices, supplements, herbal remedies, incense, books and other supplies. Must supply resale certificate number or practitioner license to obtain catalog of more than 10,000 items.

Weleda, Inc.
841 South Main Street
Spring Valley, NY 10977
(for calendula oil and a large variety of natural cosmetics)

Non-Denominational Meditation Training

Shambhala Training International
Executive Offices
1084 Tower Road
Halifax, Nova Scotia
Canada B3H 265

Organic Milk/ Certified Raw Milk Suppliers

Alta Delta Certified
Raw Milk
P.O. Box 388
City of Industry, CA 91747
Ph: 818-964-6401
(non pasteurized, non-homogenized milk)

Natural Horizons, Inc.
7490 Clubhouse Road
Boulder, CO 80301
Ph: 303-530-2711
(organic/pasteurized, non-homogenized milk; whole, low-fat, skim buttermilk and cream)

Organic Valley Family of Farms
C/O Cropp Cooperative
La Farge, WI
Ph: 608-625-2602
(organic butter, non-homogenized low-fat milk)

Pancha Karma Kitchen Equipment

Earth Fare
Attn: Roger Derrough
66 Westgate parkway
Asheville, NC 28806
Ph: 704-253-7656
Carries hand grinders and suribachi clay pots and bowls.

Garber Hardware
49 Eighth Avenue
New York, NY 10014
Carries hand grinders, but no mail order.

Sesam Muhle Natural Products
RR1
Durham, Ontario
Canada, NOG 1RO
Ph: 519-369-6326
Carries a line of hand grinders and flakers for grains and legumes, made in Germany.

Taj Mahal Imports
1594 Woodcliff Drive, N.E.
Atlanta, GA 30329
Ph: 404-321-5940
Carries a full line of Indian kitchen equipment.

Pancha Karma Supplies

Vicki Stern
P.O. Box 1814
Laguna Beach, CA 92651
Ph: 714-494-8858
(for steam boxes)

To Receive Pancha Karma

Ayurvedic Healings
Dr. Bryan & Light Miller
P.O. Box 35284
Sarasota, FL 34242
Ph: 941-3518

Fax: 941-346-0800
E-Mail: earthess@aol.com
www.ayurvechealing.com
Panch Karma, Kaya Kalpa, Jarpana, Shirodhara

Diamond Way Health Associates
214 Girard Blvd., NE
Albuquerque, NM 87106
Ph: 505-265-4826

Dr. Lobsang Rapgay
2931 Tilden Ave.
Los Angeles, CA 90064
Ph: 310-477-3877

Spa Medicine

Ancient Way Ayurvedic Health Spa
Attn: Dr. Dennis Thompson
11510 N. Foothills HWY (Hwy 36)
Longmont, CO 80503
Ph: 303-823-0522; 800-601-9707
E-Mail: drtdrt@concentric.net

Transformational Seminars

ClearMind Institute
Duane O'Kane
22778 72nd Avenue
Langley, B.C., V2Y 2K3
Canada
800-210-0372
604-513-2219

Michael Rice
c/o Heartland
Rt. 3, Box 3280
Theodosia, MO 65761
Ph: 417-273-4838

Sandy Levey-Lunden
Skraddarod 24
272 97 Garsnas, Sweden
Phone: 011 46-414-24320
Fax: 011 46-414-24395
E-Mail: On.Purpose@Swipnet.se

Vedic Astrology

American Council of Vedic
Astrology (ACVA)
PO Box 2149
Sedona, AZ 86339
Ph: 800-900-6595; 520-
282-6595
Fax: 520-282-6097
Web: vedicastrology.org
E-Mail: acva@sedona.net
Conferences, tutorial and
training programs

American Institute of Vedic
Studies
Dr. David Frawley, Director
P.O. Box 8357
Santa Fe, NM 87504-8357
Ph: 505-983-9385
Fax: 505-982-5807
E-Mail: vedicinst@aol.com
Web: consciousnet.com/vedic
correspondence courses in
Ayurveda and Vedic
Astrology

Jeffrey Armstrong
4820 N. 35th St.
Phoenix, AZ 85018
602-468-9448
Ayurvedic Astrologer, Author,
Lecturer, Teacher

Videos

Feldenkrais Resources
Ph: 800-765-1907

Wishing Well Video
P.O. Box 1008
Dept. AWF
Silver Lake, WI 53170
Ph: 262-889-8501
(wholesale & retail)

Tantra Tai Chi: Exercise for
Couples to Enhance
Intimacy & Sexual Awareness
Diana & Richard Daffner
P.O. Box 35195
Siesta Key, FL 34242

E-Mail:
info@TanraTaiChi.com
www.TanraTaiChi.com

Additional Resources Mentioned in this Book:

Mary Murphy
"Noni" product
207 K Paseo Del Pueblo Sur
Taos, NM 87571
505-753-0083

James Minckler's Book,
*Energy Balancing for Natural
Health*
406-549-4373

The National Association of
Child Bearing Centers
3123 Gottschall Rd.
Perkiomenville, PA 18074
215-234-8068

UniTea Herbs
Brigette Mars
1919 D
Boulder, CO 80302
303-442-4967

*The resources and suppliers
listed in this guide are not
necessarily endorsed by the
author.*

Bibliography

The Yoga of Herbs, An Ayurvedic Guide to Herbal Medicine, by Dr. David Frawley and Dr. Vasant Lad. Lotus Press, Twin Lakes, WI, 1986.

Ayurvedic Medicine, by Birgit Heyn. Thorsons Publishing Group: Wellingborough, Northamptonshire, England, 1987.

Quantum Healing, by Deepak Chopra. Harmony Books, New York, NY.

Back to Eden, by Jethro Kloss. Back to Eden Press.

Nutritional Almanac, by John D. Kirschmann. McGraw Hill Book Co.

Kaya Kalpa, by Dr. Chandrasekhar Thakkur. Ancient Wisdom Publication, 1960.

Definitive Guide to Cancer, by W. John Diamond, M.D., W. Lee Cowden, M.D. with Burton Goldberg. Future Medicine Publishing, Inc., 1977.

BIOGRAPHY

As a child, Dr. Light Miller, or Jyoti (her Indian name), traveled all over the world learning and assimilating the natural ways of living in many cultures. Her East Indian background gives her a strong connection to her roots in Ayurveda, which she learned from her Grandmother, who practiced with Ayurvedic herbs. Her mother introduced her to the uses of essential oils and herbal products for skin care. Her familiarity with tropical flowers and herbs comes from time spent in the Caribbean.

In 1968, Light graduated from the University of California, Berkeley, and shortly thereafter graduated from the Los Angeles School of Massage, where she felt her calling as a healer. This experience awakened her natural interest in meditation, yoga and Eastern philosophy. She has 30 years experience as a health practitioner, and has trained over 1000 in the field of massage.

Currently, Light provides individual Ayurvedic counseling, Pancha Karma treatments, and trains Ayurvedic practitioners through her Ayurvedic Correspondence Course. She has also written a book, Ayurveda & Aromatherapy with her husband, Dr. Bryan Miller. Light also gives special Kaya Kalpa treatments and is the first woman in the world to practice this art. She was trained by Dr. Raam Panday of New York, and her 115-year-young master, Dr. Panchu Wai Chotay, of Santa Cruz, India.

For information regarding treatment programs, seminars or the Correspondence Course, you may contact the author by calling or writing:

AYURVEDIC HEALING
P.O. Box 35284
Sarasota, FL 34242
Phone: 941-346-3518
Fax: 941- 346-0800
e-mail: earthess@aol.com
website: www.ayurvedichealings.com

INDEX